Volume 9 in the Series

Major Problems in Neurology

JOHN N. WALTON, T.D., M.D., D.Sc., F.R.C.P.

Consulting Editor

OTHER MONOGRAPHS IN THE SERIES

PUBLISHED

Barnett, Foster and Hudgson: **Syringomyelia,** *1973*
Dubowitz and Brooke: **Muscle Biopsy: A Modern Approach,** *1973*
Pallis and Lewis: **The Neurology of Gastrointestinal Disease,** *1974*
Hutchinson and Acheson: **Strokes,** *1975*
Gubbay: **The Clumsy Child,** *1975*
Hankinson and Banna: **Pituitary and Parapituitary Tumours,** *1976*
Donaldson: **Neurology of Pregnancy,** *1978*
Behan and Currie: **Neuroimmunology**

FORTHCOMING

Cartlidge and Shaw: **Head Injury**
Lisak and Barchi: **Myasthenia Gravis**

Myotonic Dystrophy

PETER S. HARPER, M.A., D.M., F.R.C.P.

Reader and Consultant in Medical Genetics,
Welsh National School of Medicine and
University Hospital of Wales,
Cardiff, United Kingdom

1979

W. B. Saunders Company Philadelphia • London • Toronto

major problems
in neurology

W. B. Saunders Company: West Washington Square
                           Philadelphia, PA   19105

                           1 St. Anne's Road
                           Eastbourne, East Sussex BN21 3UN, England

                           1 Goldthorne Avenue
                           Toronto, Ontario M8Z 5T9, Canada

Myotonic Dystrophy   ISBN   0-7216-4527-5

Last digit is the print number: 9   8   7   6   5   4   3   2   1

To the memory of my father, Dr. Richard Harper

Foreword

Myotonic dystrophy, also known as dystrophia myotonica, less often as myotonia atrophica, is a unique disorder since, although rightly classified as one of the forms of human muscular dystrophy, it is a disease in which many tissues and organs of the body other than voluntary muscle are also affected. This topical, detailed and comprehensive monograph by Dr. Harper in my opinion will become recognised as quite the best work yet published on this tragic progressive disorder. Yet it is more than a treatise dealing with a single disease, for within it the reader will find detailed descriptions of other muscle disorders from which the condition must be distinguished, as well as a great deal of material on methods in common use in clinical genetics, whose importance is exemplified by their application to this condition.

Beginning with a lucid historical introductory chapter, Dr. Harper goes on to describe the clinical features and differential diagnosis of myotonic dystrophy, illustrating his arguments with superb clinical photographs of patients and of clinical phenomena as well as with diagrams, pedigrees and Tables through which he analyses previous reports from the abundant world literature as well as the fruits of his own extensive clinical experience. He then considers successively the evidence relating to smooth muscle involvement and deals in depth with cardiorespiratory, endocrine, neurological and ophthalmological manifestations and complications. His own special interest and expertise in clinical genetics stands out in the excellent chapters on inheritance, preclinical detection and genetic counselling, and especially in the very full chapter on the infantile variety of this condition, in which he draws special attention to the unexplained predominance of this variety of myotonic dystrophy in children born to affected mothers. He completes his outstanding monograph with chapters on pathology and electrophysiology and with a concluding essay on what is at present known of the fundamental biochemical basis of the disease.

I am convinced I shall be the first of many to confess that I have learned a great deal from reading this superbly organised volume, which deals with a fascinating disease whose mysteries are gradually being elucidated. Well-written and organised, beautifully illustrated, scholarly and complete, I believe that it represents a major achievement that will be read with pleasure and profit by neurologists, paediatricians, geneticists and many other physicians.

JOHN N. WALTON

Newcastle upon Tyne
July, 1978

Preface

The origins of this book lie nearly ten years in the past, when I began to work on myotonic dystrophy as a research fellow at the Johns Hopkins School of Medicine, Baltimore, with Dr. Victor McKusick. The immediate objective of that work was to detect genetic linkage, but it soon became clear that myotonic dystrophy was not a disorder that could be studied piecemeal, and that a genetic analysis was impossible without at the same time undertaking careful clinical investigations. On numerous occasions family members supposed to be normal proved to be affected, and like previous investigators I rapidly found a high index of suspicion developing for early features of the disease.

By the end of my initial study I found that valuable data had been collected on such aspects as preclinical detection and endocrine abnormalities, quite apart from the basic genetic data that were the original aim. As is so often the case, more questions had been raised than answered, especially regarding the puzzling features of myotonic dystrophy in infancy, at that time hardly recognised. On return to Britain, I was thus faced with some intriguing problems to solve, but with my patients scattered across America! My initial reaction was that further work would be impossible, but I soon realised that myotonic dystrophy, even the childhood form, was no rarity, and that time, not lack of patients, was the limiting factor.

The stimulus to write this book was the realisation that most patients with myotonic dystrophy are seen and treated not by specialists in muscle disease but by a wide variety of clinicians who may have had little experience with the disease previously. I myself have keenly felt the lack of an up-to-date book giving a balanced picture of this many-faceted disorder, and for this reason I have attempted to cover the clinical aspects as well as the genetic, and to relate these to some of the more recent experimental work which is bringing us nearer to an understanding of the primary underlying abnormality. Inevitably, approaching

ix

the subject from so many different angles will have led to omissions and perhaps to errors; I hope readers will inform me of these.

I owe a debt to many people for their help in the writing of this book and the research which underlies it. Wherever possible specific contributions, especially illustrations, are mentioned in the text, but I should like here to record my thanks to the following:

Firstly, the patients and their families, who were almost always helpful and appreciative that someone was taking an interest in them, even though they realised that I could often give little practical help. Likewise, many clinicians have been generous both of their time and in sharing their experience and allowing access to unpublished data. Among my clinical colleagues in Cardiff, special encouragement has been received from Robert Mahler, Peter Gray, John Graham and Charles Wells, while in America Drs. Victor McKusick and Paul Dyken were largely responsible for my entering the field in the first place. The genetic aspects have been the subject of some spirited and enjoyable discussions (not always ending in agreement!) with Sarah Bundey, Cedric Carter, Sir Cyril Clarke and Alan Emery, while Nick Thomas has kept me from going too far astray in the biochemical field.

Valuable criticism on specific chapters has come from Shirley Bryant, Victor Dubowitz, Alan Emery, David Gardner-Medwin, John Graham, Barrie Jay, Caroline Sewry and Nick Thomas, while the quality of the illustrations is largely due to the skill of Ralph Marshall and his Department of Medical Illustration in Cardiff. The patient and enthusiastic secretarial help of Edna Long, Laureen Mace and Caroline James has been invaluable. Working with the editorial staff of W. B. Saunders has been a pleasure, and a special debt is due to Professor John Walton, whose wise advice and encouragement was especially appreciated at times when the subject seemed too big for a single worker.

The Muscular Dystrophy Associations of America and the Muscular Dystrophy Group of Great Britain have both supported my work over the past ten years, and it is quite certain that without them and their supporters the book would not have been written, nor would the general interest in myotonic or other dystrophies be as widespread as it is.

Finally to my wife Elaine and my children I am especially grateful for support and patience during the long gestation of this book. Time spent writing has meant less time spent with them, but has not prevented the writing of the book from being an enjoyable and worthwhile experience.

PETER S. HARPER

Cardiff, September, 1978

Contents

CHAPTER ONE

Introduction

Myotonic dystrophy, the subject of this book, is a disorder that is highly distinctive in many of its features, yet difficult to define or classify satisfactorily. A clear definition is essential before clinical, genetic and pathological details are described, for without this one cannot accept or challenge the existence of this disease as a specific entity, nor can it be accurately related to other conditions that appear to be closely allied.

The essence of a definition is provided by the name used throughout this book — "myotonic dystrophy". Like the other commonly used titles, "dystrophia myotonica" and "myotonia atrophica", the combination of the phenomenon of myotonia with progressive muscle disease is the essential hallmark of the disorder. It relates it on the one hand to other conditions characterised by myotonia — impaired muscular relaxation resulting from a specific form of repetitive discharge arising within the muscle fibre itself; on the other hand it indicates its affinity to the group of muscular dystrophies in which genetically determined progressive primary muscle disease is the common feature. The term "myotonic muscular dystrophy" has been preferred by some as relating the disorder more closely to the other muscular dystrophies, but the simpler term "myotonic dystrophy" has the advantage that it does not restrict the concept to a single system and provides a framework for consideration of the third cardinal feature of the disease: the existence of a variety of specific non-muscular abnormalities that on occasion may be more prominent than the abnormalities of muscle. A working definition of myotonic dystrophy may be given as follows:

"A genetically determined disorder in which a characteristic pattern of dystrophic muscle disease is accompanied by myotonia and by specific abnormalities of a variety of other systems".

The difficulty of confining the features of myotonic dystrophy within this or any other definition will rapidly become clear as the detailed characteristics of the disease are discussed.

In the century that has passed since myotonia was first recognised, the myotonic disorders, and in particular myotonic dystrophy, have been the subject of a large amount of work, much more perhaps than might be expected from the frequency with which they occur. Why this is so should become clearer in subsequent chapters, but one thing is certain: myotonic dystrophy is a disorder that has posed problems to and attracted the attention of workers from all branches of clinical medicine and the basic medical sciences. It has not remained the preserve of neurologists; ophthalmologists, general physicians, paediatricians and geneticists have all made essential contributions to our knowledge of it, and it is noteworthy that in many instances the nature of the disease has made the investigator step beyond the bounds of his own speciality. It is perhaps this many-sided nature of the disease that has attracted and challenged many workers, including the author; as a clinical problem myotonic dystrophy may present in a bewildering variety of ways and in unexpected situations, and as an investigative problem it offers the opportunity to attempt to unify these various manifestations by the discovery of a common underlying factor. There is also the very real hope that an understanding of myotonic dystrophy will lead to corresponding advances in our knowledge of other muscular dystrophies and of some of the other dominantly inherited and poorly understood neurological diseases.

Despite past work and present interest, myotonic dystrophy remains very much an enigma. Although we now know a great deal about the physiological basis of myotonia and the pathological basis of the muscle changes, we are still unable to relate these changes adequately to the variety of other clinical manifestations of the disease, and are only just beginning to glimpse the likely area in which the primary biochemical defect lies. Our methods of prevention are unsatisfactory and the active treatment that we can offer patients is almost non-existent. There is clearly a long way to go before the disease is understood, let alone controlled.

This book aims to bring together our current knowledge about myotonic dystrophy so that those encountering the disease in clinical practice or working on it experimentally are able to assess all facets of the problem, not just the particular aspect with which they are involved. It is 15 years since the last monograph on the disease by Caughey and Myrianthopoulos (1963) and 30 years since the only other comprehensive account, that of Thomasen (1948). A glance at the areas not known to these authors shows how the subject has advanced, and that another synthesis is required. On the clinical side the congenital form of the disease was still unrecognised, and retinal involvement had escaped the attention of generations of ophthalmologists. The genetics of myotonic dystrophy have been advanced by location of the gene and by the application of this in prediction of genetic risks, and the recognition of a maternal influence in the congenital disease has posed problems that extend well beyond myotonic dystrophy itself. The experimental study of the disease, hardly begun at the time that Caughey and Myrianthopoulos were writing, has expanded dramatically. Not only do we now have a clear, though still incomplete picture of the physiological basis of myotonia, but biochemical and ultrastructural studies are also beginning to converge on the basic molecular defect that, it is generally agreed, must underlie both the myotonia and the dystrophic aspects.

The study of myotonic dystrophy can be seen as falling into three main periods. In the initial phase the disorder was discovered, delineated and its cardinal features established; this occupied the last quarter of the 19th century and the first quarter of the current one. During the second period, covering the next 30 years, the clinical aspects were expanded, the detailed involvement of the various systems was accurately studied, along with the pathological basis, and considerable interest also developed regarding the inheritance of the disease. During the past 20 years, work on the disease has steadily moved from a descriptive to an investigative phase, with the application of an ever-increasing variety of experimental techniques. The main part of this book examines the various aspects of myotonic dystrophy in the light of our current knowledge, but to set this in perspective the remainder of this chapter will trace the development of our knowledge during the initial phase when the main features were being recognised.

Anyone who attempts to trace the early story of myotonic dystrophy is immediately struck by the dominance in the field of the German Schools of Neurology, for not only are most of the relevant papers found in the German neurological literature, but it is clear that a number of active and flourishing centres existed which were in close contact with each other and which combined a meticulous and detailed recording of clinical data with a vigorous experimental approach in both pathology and early electrophysiology. Some of the key developments will be discussed here. Full reviews of the early literature from Germany, and to a lesser extent from other countries, are given in the work of Rohrer (1916), Curschmann (1936) and Thomasen (1948).

The history of myotonia in fact begins not with myotonic dystrophy but with myotonia congenita, and Dr. Julius Thomsen's account of this disease in himself and his family (1876) is the foundation for the subject. Earlier descriptions supposed to represent myotonia, such as that of Bell (1836), appear on closer inspection to be of uncertain nature. Thomsen's own life is well described by Thomasen (1948), who himself interviewed and examined a number of his descendants. Originally a Danish citizen, he lived in Schleswig-Holstein, which was transferred to Germany after a plebiscite, and it was the refusal of the Prussian military authorities to recognise his son's symptoms as genuine that prompted Dr. Thomsen to publish his account of the disorder affecting himself and four generations of his family.

Thomsen clearly described the three cardinal features of the disease that soon became known as myotonia congenita or "Thomsen's disease": the myotonia itself, its hereditary nature, and the essentially static and benign nature of the condition. Thomsen had information on 20 members of his family who were affected, and herein lay the remarkable value of his observations: coming from a single family they all clearly had the same disorder, and the advantage of numbers provided a balanced picture of the clinical features and natural history of the disease, something rarely seen in initial descriptions of a new disorder. Thomsen was also fortunate in living in the orbit of German medicine, for his paper was not neglected (in contrast to Mendel's original work on inheritance!) but was recognised by Wilhelm Erb, Professor of Medicine at Heidelberg, perhaps the most influential neurologist in Germany at that time, as an important contribution.

Erb's own monograph, "Die Thomsensche Krankheit" (1886), put myotonia congenita on a sound clinical and scientific footing, with study of the electrical reactions of the muscle and of the histology. However, by collecting together other cases from various families, Erb unwittingly had encountered the problem of "genetic heterogeneity" that ever since has been both a problem and a stimulus in the study of inherited disease. Among Erb's cases of "Thomsen's disease" were some with muscle wasting that almost certainly represented what was later to be recognised as myotonic dystrophy.

During the next 15 years a series of reports appeared of "atypical Thomsen's disease" or "myotonia congenita with muscle atrophy", and it is clear that this subject must have been much debated in Germany, for Curschmann (1906) in a case report of one such patient states that this individual had already been presented and written up by no fewer than five previous authors, including Hoffmann and Steinert.

One of the earliest and best documented reports, often claimed as the first undoubted case of myotonic dystrophy, came not from Germany but New York. Dana (1888) described a 35 year old man in whom myotonic symptoms began at the age of 20. Subsequently, there was mental deterioration and loss of potency, and ptosis was noted on examination. Interestingly a retinopathy was noted but no cataract. A unilateral talipes had required correction in adolescence. Against a diagnosis of myotonic dystrophy were the lack of facial weakness in the patient and the generalised nature of the myotonia, and overall it is difficult to accept the case conclusively as one of myotonic dystrophy. Dana took a muscle biopsy from the patient's supinator muscle, which showed increased internal nuclei, clearly seen in the drawings illustrating his paper. Modern investigators should note that to provide a normal control Dana "harpooned a piece of this same muscle from my own arm".

Much more convincing are the cases described by Hoffmann (1896, 1900). His initial report, part of a series of neurological case reports from the Heidelberg clinic, described a 35 year old man with myotonia who showed muscle wasting, particularly of the facial, sternomastoid and forearm muscles. Four years later, in a "Festschrift" volume in honour of Wilhelm Erb, he described a brother and sister similarly affected. The brother had suffered progressive weakness of grip since the age of 20, and when seen at age 35 showed marked atrophy and weakness of the forearm muscles, as well as of the face and sternomastoids. Myotonia was present in the thenar muscles. The 32 year old sister showed a similar pattern of weakness and myotonia, but was symptom-free.

A further undoubted case of myotonic dystrophy was provided by Rossolimo (1902), published in both the French and German literature, and it was this author who used the "myotonia atrophica" by which it was commonly known in the early years (and is still preferred by some today). Rossolimo's patient was a 37 year old man with progressive weakness since 20 years of age and more recent myotonic symptoms. He was noted to have had a mask-like face with weakness of facial muscles and wasting of both the upper and lower limbs. Rossolimo examined a muscle biopsy and his accurate drawings give a clear indication of the characteristic increase in internal nuclei, arranged in longitudinal chains.

Other early case reports include those of Nonne (1905), Pässler (1906) and Fürnrohr (1907), but the two reports that mark the clear delineation of myotonic dystrophy as a disorder in its own right are those of Steinert and Batten and Gibb, both published in 1909.

Steinert's study was a direct development of the previous work of the German Schools of Neurology, and its detailed treatment of the subject fully justifies the eponymous use of the term "Steinert's disease" in subsequent literature from continental Europe, even though "myotonic dystrophy" or "dystrophia myotonica" subsequently became preferred and Steinert's name never quite achieved the general acceptance that Thomsen's has done for myotonia congenita.

Steinert described nine cases in all: three were presented to a meeting of the Leipzig Medical Society in 1904, and the other six, two of whom were brothers, were reported in detail in his major paper. He noted the characteristic distribution of muscle weakness and wasting in his patients, with facial weakness and ptosis, selective atrophy of the sternomastoids among the neck muscles, and with the forearms more affected than the small hand muscles. He commented on the weak speech and laryngeal involvement in one patient. He also noted absence of reflexes and some distal sensory loss in some of his cases, features that have been the subject of subsequent debate (see Chapter 7). Of particular importance was Steinert's observation of testicular atrophy in four of his patients, the first documentation of an abnormality outside the nervous system.

Steinert not only made a thorough clinical observation of his patients but studied an autopsied case in detail, although his pathological findings proved somewhat misleading since he concentrated on the spinal cord, which showed marked degeneration of the dorsal columns, probably due to coincidental tabes. However, he showed extensive fibrosis and degenerative changes in a variety of skeletal muscles, and was able to demonstrate atrophy of muscle spindles and to note that the intramuscular nerves appeared normal. Steinert contributed a further brief note on the disease in 1910, and from the title of his original paper it is clear that it was planned as the first of a series of major studies in muscle disease. Sadly, these never took place, for he died young soon afterwards, and a note of his death appears in Curschmann's paper of 1912. However, the number of active workers in the field in Germany at the time meant that others soon took up the subject where he left off.

Although Steinert clearly recognised myotonic dystrophy as a distinct disorder, he remained convinced that the atrophy was a phenomenon secondary to the myotonia, debating the various possible alternatives in his paper. Batten and Gibb (1909), in the other publication that firmly established the disease, were much more convinced that they were dealing with a primary degenerative disease, quite separate from myotonia congenita. In their series of five cases the first two patients were brother and sister, and there had been another brother in the family who had died of a progressive wasting disorder, diagnosed as tabes dorsalis, but considered by Batten and Gibb to have been the same condition as that of his sibs. The living brother, aged 40, gave a three-year history of progressive difficulty in walking, with weakness of the legs and of grip. He had noticed wasting of his forearm and leg muscles, and admitted to difficulty in relaxing his grip for at least ten years before the onset of other symptoms. Batten and Gibb noted the myotonia of grip and commented on the striking lack of expression, due to a generalised weakness of the facial muscles. They found complete atrophy of the sternomastoids, contrasting with normal bulk of the other neck muscles. The features in the 46 year old sister were similar; she also had noticed difficulty in relaxing her grip for as long as she could remember.

Batten and Gibb described three other unrelated patients, all adult males, with what they considered to be the same disorder. All showed the same combination of a characteristic pattern of muscle weakness and wasting with myotonia. Their case 5 is shown in Figure 1-1, and illustrates the characteristic facies and sternomastoid atrophy. Batten and Gibb reviewed the earlier literature and found 15 cases, including those already mentioned, which they believed represented "myotonia atrophica", rather than Thomsen's disease.

With the publication of Steinert's and Batten and Gibb's papers, the foundations for the study of myotonic dystrophy had been thoroughly laid and it soon became clear that this new disease was, in fact, considerably

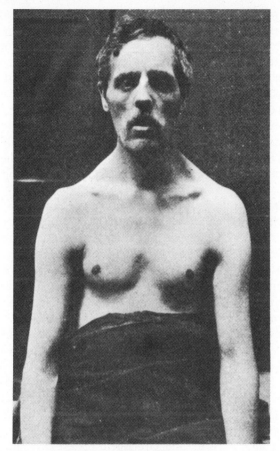

Figure 1-1. The earliest published photograph of a patient with myotonic dystrophy (case 5 of Batten and Gibb, 1909).

more common than the classical myotonia congenita or "Thomsen's disease" of which it had originally been considered a variant. A further major advance soon came with the recognition of cataract as a feature of myotonic dystrophy. This was first described by Greenfield (1911) in a large family of 13 sibs of whom five had myotonic dystrophy. Three of these had cataract, as did two of the apparently unaffected sibs, one of whom was examined by Greenfield. Later that year Kennedy and Obendorf (1911) described an American patient with both myotonic dystrophy and cataract, and it speaks for the rapidity of scientific publication at the time that they were able to provide a full discussion of Greenfield's paper, published in the same year.

The significance of cataract as a systemic feature of myotonic dystrophy was recognised by Curschmann (1912), who considered this and the occurrence of testicular atrophy to be indicators of a generalised endocrine disturbance, and that myotonic dystrophy should be classed as a generalised disorder rather than simply a muscular one (Curschmann, 1925, 1936). The subject of cataract in myotonic dystrophy is considered more fully in Chapter 8, but after some initial doubts whether the relationship was more than coincidental, the extensive work of Fleischer (1918) provided conclusive evidence. He described 35 patients with both myotonic dystrophy and cataract, and in a number of families noted the occurrence of cataract alone in previous generations, linking the affected members.

The time of World War I corresponds to the end of the initial period of our knowledge of myotonic dystrophy, and the studies of the subsequent 30 years, although contributing a large amount of detailed information, did not essentially alter the framework that had been established. Many of the specific discoveries are considered in later chapters, but some of the major contributions are mentioned here, and can be taken in two groups, those dealing with clinical and pathological aspects, and those concerned with the hereditary nature of the disease.

Following the recognition of gonadal atrophy and cataract, the next major extramuscular feature to be linked conclusively with myotonic dystrophy was the occurrence of mental changes (see Chapter 7). Curschmann (1912, 1925) noted his patients to have an abnormal personality and low intelligence, and Rohrer (1916) found some of them to be apathetic. However, since many of the patients were disabled and living in poor circumstances socially and economically, it is not surprising that some authors such as Adie and Greenfield (1923) attributed the mental changes to these factors. The finding of mental subnormality, sometimes severe enough to result in institutional care, led to the reassessment of this view, and Maas and Paterson (1937) were able to document it in a large series of patients, finding reduced intelligence in 17 out of 29 patients and lack of initiative in a number of others. Thomasen (1948) paid particular attention to these aspects in his extensive and thorough study of 100 Danish patients. The findings, discussed fully in Chapter 7, confirmed the high frequency of both low intelligence and abnormal personality, and carried added weight from being based on observations made in the patients' homes. In addition, his monograph conveys the impression of an understanding and sympathetic person, not inclined to judge his patients harshly, in contrast to some of the earlier investigators who regarded "unwillingness to submit to special investigations" as evidence of an abnormal personality!

As the body of clinical material accumulated, it began to be realised that many patients were dying from cardiorespiratory problems, some of them sudden deaths, others in connection with surgery. The earliest case reports, including that of Steinert (1909), noted bradycardia, and an extreme case was that of Griffith (1911) who found a pulse rate of 36 in a man reported as having myotonia congenita, but in fact with typical features of myotonic dystrophy. Few patients had cardiac symptoms, however, and it was not until the electrocardiogram came into regular use that cardiac involvement was found to be frequent. The first full study was that of Evans (1944), which was followed by an extensive review by De Wind and Jones (1950), conduction defects being the principal abnormality found, as discussed in Chapter 5.

These and other clinical studies received support from the growing body of pathological evidence based on autopsy studies and, in the case of muscle itself, from biopsies. The early studies of Rossolimo and Rohrer have already been mentioned; material from Rohrer's patients was studied by Heidenhain (1918), both working in Heidelberg, so that the microscopic changes were rapidly documented by what then were advanced techniques (see Fig. 1–2). Perhaps the most important result of this was the realisation that the muscle changes of myotonic dystrophy, with fibre degeneration, internal nuclei in chains and inequality of fibre size, were distinct from those seen in myotonia congenita, at least of the classical type, in which hypertrophy of fibres was the principal feature. Subsequently, there was little advance until the arrival of histochemistry and electron microscopy (Chapter 12).

The autopsy studies provided valuable evidence on the change in other organs. Among the larger series were those of Black and Ravin (1947) and Thomasen (1948), and the entire literature was collected in a valuable review by Berthold (1958). These studies confirmed the clinical finding of testicular atrophy, and showed it to result from a diffuse tubular atrophy and fibrosis. More widespread, although less constant changes were also shown in other endocrine glands, such as the pituitary and adrenal. The autopsy studies also provided firm evidence that both cardiac and smooth muscle were involved by the disease, and that no gross abnormalities were constantly found in peripheral nerves to account for the muscular degeneration.

The hereditary aspects of myotonic dystrophy, fully considered in Chapters 10 and 11, received attention from the earliest description of the disease, and have to be seen in the context of Thomsen's original description of myotonia congenita being already well-known. Thus, the point which perplexed authors such as Batten and Gibb and Steinert was not that some of their cases were familial — both series contained affected sibs — but that most of their cases appeared to be isolated ones. In particular, the regular transmission from parent to child seen in Thomsen's family did not appear to occur in myotonic dystrophy, and it was not until later that it became clear that mild involvement of the parent was the rule rather than the exception.

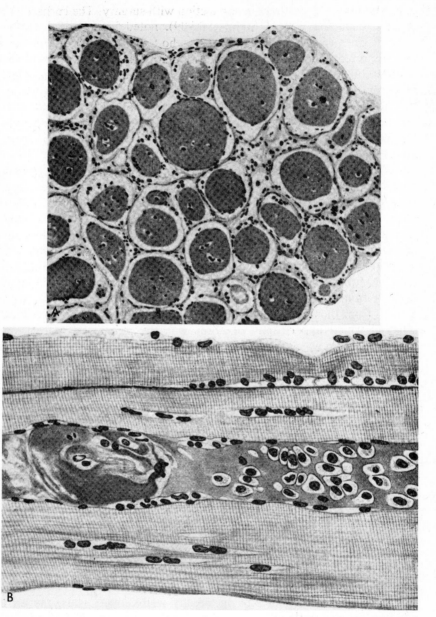

Figure 1–2. EARLY PATHOLOGICAL STUDIES IN MYOTONIC DYSTROPHY (FROM ROHRER, 1916).

47 year old man with moderately severe myotonic dystrophy.

A, Biopsy from right forearm (flexor digitorum sublimis) showing increased internal nuclei.

B, Biopsy from right pectoralis major showing arrangement of central nuclei in chains.

Rohrer (1916) was the first person to look systemically at the genetic aspects of myotonič dystrophy, finding that 43 of the cases were familial and 49 non-familial. From this he concluded, democratically but not very logically, that in most cases the disease was not hereditary in nature. This view was soon refuted by the work of Fleischer (1918) who, as already mentioned, showed that cataract, as well as the fully developed neurological disorder, had to be considered, and that this could provide the connection, particularly in the parental generations, between apparently unrelated cases. By the time that Adie and Greenfield reviewed the subject in 1923, they were convinced that myotonic dystrophy should be classified among the hereditary neurological degenerative diseases, along with such disorders as Friedreich's ataxia and Huntington's chorea. They discussed the problem of apparently isolated cases of the disease and concluded that the existence of these was not in itself an argument against its hereditary nature, and their scepticism towards many of these supposedly sporadic cases can be seen in a comment that remains apposite to investigators of myotonic dystrophy today. They quote the instance of a patient

"who went so far as to deny that he had any brothers and persisted in his denials until he was confronted with a photograph of himself and two brothers that had been taken at the hospital some years before".

Despite the general agreement by this time that myotonic dystrophy was hereditary, the precise mode of inheritance remained in doubt for much longer. This was in part because the extreme degree of variation in the clinical expression of the disease was not yet fully appreciated, and partly because the collections of scattered cases had not been systematically investigated and were not suitable for a critical genetic analysis. As described in Chapter 10, this had to await the more detailed studies of Julia Bell (1948) and Thomasen (1948), and even after this the disease has continued to produce a number of confusing problems, such as that of "anticipation" and the maternal inheritance of the congenital disease, that have provided scope for disagreement among both clinicians and geneticists up to the present.

A surprising development during the 1930s, which in retrospect seems more of a step backwards, was the questioning whether myotonic dystrophy was indeed a specific disease, separate from myotonia congenita, and the proposition that all the features of each disease were common to both. The importance of this question to the genetic and biochemical basis is obvious, and is discussed in Chapter 10. Among the workers who considered myotonic dystrophy and myotonia congenita to be identical were Rouquès (1931) in France and Maas in London, who in a series of papers (Maas, 1937; Maas and Paterson, 1939, 1950) upheld the unitary view with increasing vigour. A similar view was still being taken as late as 1963 by Caughey and Myrianthopoulos, but has since largely disappeared in the face of the overwhelming evidence that almost all genetic diseases are much more heterogeneous than was previously believed.

The supposed identity of the two conditions was based largely on the occurrence of cases intermediate between the classical picture of myotonia congenita and that of myotonic dystrophy, and also on patients who initially were typical of the former but later developed dystrophic features. In retrospect it seems likely that the large family of Dr. Julius Thomsen and the recognition of myotonia congenita prior to that of myotonic dystrophy misled later workers into overestimating the relative frequency of myotonia congenita, and that many of the early cases of this were in fact myotonic dystrophy. It is perhaps relevant that Maas had never seen a case of myotonia congenita, and workers such as Thomasen (1948), who had extensive experience of both conditions, were never in any doubt that they were dealing with two distinct disorders.

The subsequent chapters of this book will consider in more detail some of the features that have been outlined here. The next two chapters are essentially practical, dealing with the main neurological features of myotonic dystrophy and the diagnosis of the disease in relation to other muscle dystrophies and myotonic disorders. Myotonia congenita is considered only as part of this differential diagnosis, and no attempt has been made to give it equal treatment to that of myotonic dystrophy. Not only has the author limited experience of myotonia congenita, but a thorough review of it and the related non-dystrophic myotonias has recently been produced by Becker (1977), whose personal experience of these disorders is unrivalled. Chapters 4 to 8 of the present book develop the theme of myotonic dystrophy as a generalised disease, dealing in turn with the various systems involved by it. Chapter 9 is a more personal account of myotonic dystrophy in childhood, a subject hardly touched on in the previous major works on the subject, and one which the author has found particularly fascinating. The subsequent two chapters are likewise based to a considerable extent on personal studies of the genetic basis of the disease, although it is hoped that these will not have provided too unbalanced an account in relation to the work of others in the field. In the final sections, recent experimental studies in the areas of muscle pathology, electrophysiology and biochemistry are emphasised, and it is in these fields that the most rapid developments are being seen, not only in myotonic dystrophy itself, but in Duchenne dystrophy and other muscle diseases.

REFERENCES

Adie W. J. and Greenfield J. G. (1923): Dystrophia myotonica (myotonia atrophica). Brain 46:73–127.
Batten F. E. and Gibb H. P. (1909): Myotonia atrophica. Brain 32:187–205.
Becker P. E. (1977): Myotonia Congenita and Syndromes Associated with Myotonia. Thieme, Stuttgart.
Bell J. (1948): Dystrophia myotonica and allied diseases. In Treasury of Human Inheritance 4. Cambridge University Press.

Berthold H. (1958): Zur pathologischen Anatomie der Dystrophia Myotonica (Curschmann-Steinert). Dtsch. Z. Nervenheilkd. *178*:394–412.

Black W. C. and Ravin A. (1947): Studies in dystrophia myotonica. VII. Autopsy observations in five cases. Arch. Pathol. *44*:176–191.

Caughey J. E. and Myrianthopoulos N. C. (1963): Dystrophia myotonica and related disorders. Charles C Thomas, Springfield, Ill.

Curschmann H. (1906): Demonstration eines Falles Thomsen'scher Krankheit mit ausgedehnten Muskelatrophien. München Med. Wochenschrift *53*:1281.

Curschmann H. (1912). Über familiare atrophische Myotonie. Dtsch. Z. Nervenheilkd. *45*:161–202.

Curschmann H. (1925): Zur Nosologie und Symptomatologie der myotonischen Dystrophie. Dtsch. Arch. Klin. Med. *149*:129–144.

Curschmann H. (1936): Myotonische Dystrophie (atrophische Myotonie). *In* Handbuch der Neurologie (Eds: Bumke and Foerster). Berlin, pp. 465–485.

Dana C. L. (1888): An atypical case of Thomsen's disease (myotonia congenita). Medical Record (New York) *33*:433–435.

De Wind L. T. and Jones R. J. (1950): Cardiovascular observations in dystrophia myotonica. J.A.M.A. *144*:299–303.

Erb W. (1886): Die Thomsen'sche Krankheit (Myotonia congenita). Leipzig.

Evans W. (1944): The heart in myotonia atrophica. Br. Heart J. *4*:41–47.

Fleischer B. (1918): Über myotonische Dystrophie mit Katarakt. Albrecht von Graefes Arch. Klin. Ophthalmol. *96*:91–133.

Fürnrohr W. (1907): Myotonia Atrophica. Deutsch. Z. Nervenheilkd. *33*:25–44.

Greenfield J. G. (1911): Notes on a family of "myotonia atrophica" and early cataract, with a report on an additional case of myotonia atrophica. Rev. Neur. Psych. (Edin.) *9*:169–181.

Griffith T. W. (1911): On myotonia. Q. J. Med. *5*:229–248.

Heidenhain H. (1918): Über progressive Vererbung der Muskulatur bei Myotonia Atrophica. Beitr. Pathol. *64*:198–225.

Hoffmann J. (1896). Ein Fall von Thomsen'scher Krankheit, complizirt durch Neuritis Multiplex. Dtsch. Z. Nervenheilkd. *9*:272–278.

Hoffmann J. (1900): Zur Lehre von der Thomsen'schen Krankheit mit besonderer Berucksichtigung des dabei vorkommenden Muskelschwandes. Dtsch. Z. Nervenheilkd. *18*: 197–216.

Kennedy F. and Obendorf C. P. (1911): Myotonia atrophica, with a report of two cases. J.A.M.A. *57*:1117–1118.

Maas O. (1937): Observations on dystrophia myotonica. Brain *60*:498–524.

Maas O. and Paterson A. S. (1937): Mental changes in families affected by dystrophia myotonica. Lancet *1*:21–23.

Maas O. and Paterson A. S. (1939): The identity of myotonia congenita (Thomsen's disease), dystrophia myotonica (myotonia atrophica) and paramyotonia. Brain *62*:198–212.

Maas O. and Paterson A. S. (1950): Myotonia congenita, dystrophia myotonica and paramyotonia; reaffirmation of their identity. Brain *73*:318–336.

Nonne (1905): Combination von Myotonie und Dystrophia muscular. Neurol. Zentralb. *24*:142.

Pässler (1906): Zwei Brüder mit amyotrophischer Myotonie. Neurol. Zentralb. *25*:1064–1066.

Rohrer K. (1916): Ueber Myotonia Atrophica (Dystrophia Myotonica). Dtsch. Z. Nervenheilkd. *55*:242–304.

Rossolimo G. (1902): Atrophische form der Thomsen'schen Krankheit. Neurol. Zentralb. *21*:135–136.

Rossolimo G. (1902): De la myotonie atrophique.Nouv. Iconog. Salpetrière *15*:63–77.

Rouquès L. (1931): La myotonie atrophique (maladie de Steinert): thesis. Paris.

Steinert H. (1909): Myopathologische Beiträge. 1. Über das klinische und anatomische Bild des Muskelschwunds der Myotoniker. Dtsch. Z. Nervenheilkd. *37*:58–104.

Steinert H. (1910): Ein neuer Fall von atrophischer Myotonie; ein Nachtag zu meiner Arbeit in Bild 37. Dtsch. Z. Nervenheilkd. *39*:168–173.

Thomasen E. (1948): Myotonia. Universitetsforlaget, Aarhus.

Thomsen J. (1876): Tonische Krampfe in willkurlich beweglichen Muskeln infolge von erebter psychischer Disposition (Ataxia muscularis). Arch. Psychiatr. Nervenkr. *6*:702–718.

CHAPTER TWO

Myotonic Dystrophy – the Clinical Picture

THE PATTERN OF MUSCLE INVOLVEMENT

Myotonic dystrophy is rarely a difficult diagnosis to make, provided that the possibility is in the mind of the clinician who sees the patient. Despite this, it is surprising how late many cases of myotonic dystrophy receive a correct diagnosis; in part this reflects the uncomplaining nature of many patients, amounting to a positive avoidance of doctors in some instances; in part it is the result of patients presenting not with neuromuscular symptoms, often existing but uncomplained of, but with such disorders as cataract, dysphagia and other abdominal symptoms, and respiratory difficulties. Clinicians concentrating on these immediate problems may easily overlook or misinterpret a degree of myotonia and muscle weakness that would have been obvious if specifically sought.

The finding of myotonia, in conjunction with progressive muscle weakness and wasting, allows the confident diagnosis of myotonic dystrophy to be made in a high proportion of cases, but the diagnosis may often be clear from the characteristic distribution of muscle involvement before a formal neurological examination has been performed, or myotonia has been elicited. None of the other inherited myopathies of adult life show the same combination of facial weakness, involvement of the jaw and anterior neck muscles, and distal weakness of the limbs; of the acquired myopathies, only myasthenia gravis shows more than a superficial resemblance.

Table 2–1 summarises the distribution of muscle involvement in the disease, and Table 2–2 compares the main clinical features with those of other muscle dystrophies seen in adult life. Although it is probably true to state that all muscles may show some degree of involvement in myotonic dystrophy, major clinical changes follow a characteristic pattern in most patients.

14

Table 2-1. MUSCULAR INVOLVEMENT IN MYOTONIC DYSTROPHY

Muscles Most Prominently Affected
Superficial facial muscles
Levator palpebrae superioris
Temporalis
Sternomastoids
Distal muscles of forearm
Dorsiflexors of foot
Other Muscles Commonly Affected
Quadriceps
Diaphragm and intercostals
Intrinsic muscles of hands and feet
Palate and pharyngeal muscles
Tongue
External ocular muscles
Muscles Frequently Spared
Pelvic girdle
Hamstrings
Soleus and gastrocnemius

Facial Weakness

This is one of the earliest and most constant features of myotonic dystrophy, and its diagnostic importance is enhanced by its faithful recording in family photographs, which may show it to be present many years before the diagnosis was made (Fig. 2–1) or in relatives no longer living.

Table 2-2. MUSCLE INVOLVEMENT IN MYOTONIC DYSTROPHY AND OTHER ADULT MYOPATHIES

	Myotonic Dystrophy	Facio-scapulo-humeral Dystrophy	Autosomal Recessive Limb-girdle Dystrophy	Becker Dystrophy
Facial weakness	++	++	+	−
Ptosis	++	++	−	−
Jaw muscles	++	+	−	−
Sternomastoids	++	+	±	±
Shoulder girdle	±	++	+	+
Pelvic girdle	±	+	++	++
Proximal limb muscles	+	+	++	++
Distal limb muscles	++	±	+	+
Myotonia	++	−	−	−
Pseudohypertrophy	±	−	±	++

++ prominent feature
+ may occur
± inconsistent or late feature
− absent

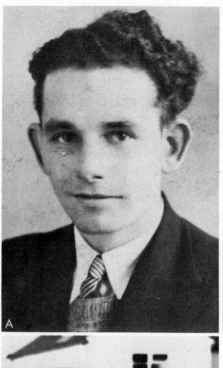

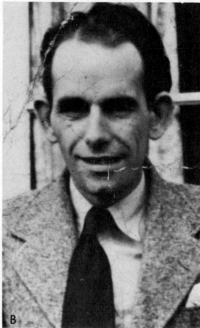

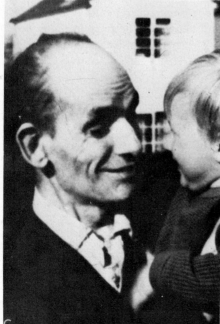

Figure 2–1. Evolution of facial appearance of myotonic dystrophy documented by family photographs: patient J.G.J.)

A, Aged 17 years: no facial weakness.

B, Aged 30 years: slight facial weakness and ptosis detectable.

C, Aged 44 years: the facial features are now obvious, but the patient had no symptoms at this time.

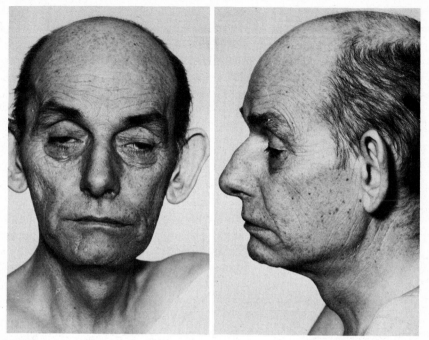

Figure 2–2. FACIAL WEAKNESS IN MYOTONIC DYSTROPHY.

Further views of patient J.G.J., aged 56 years at time of first diagnosis, to show ptosis and facial weakness. He also showed marked weakness and wasting of sternomastoids and distal limb muscles, together with active and percussion myotonia, widespread external ocular muscle weakness, cataract and retinal degeneration (see Chapter 8). Symptoms were limited to visual deterioration and non-specific tiredness of two years' duration.

The author, like others seeing numerous patients and their families, has found that one becomes sensitised to very minor degrees of the abnormal facial appearance. The composite picture of facial involvement results from a general weakness and immobility of the superficial muscles, along with ptosis, and weakness and wasting of the jaw muscles. Formal examination shows diminished power of eye closure from weakness of the orbicularis oculi muscles, along with inability to whistle and to retain air in the cheeks. The appearance is more vividly illustrated by pictures than by words (Fig. 2–2 and 2–3). In adults the facial weakness is rarely as marked as is seen in patients with facio-scapulo-humeral dystrophy, and much less than in some neurogenic facial palsies. In children with congenital myotonic dystrophy, however, it may be a most striking feature (Chapter 9). Conversely, some mildly affected patients, particularly those presenting late in life with cataract, may have an entirely normal facial appearance. Figure 2–5 demonstrates this variation within a single family.

Ptosis

Ptosis, generally symmetrical, forms an integral part of the abnormal facies (Fig. 2–2), and like the other facial features can often be recognised from old photographs. Although sometimes sufficient to cause a compensatory tilting of the head, it is more often mild, and is less marked than in isolated congenital ptosis (also dominantly inherited). The variability characteristic of myasthenia gravis is absent.

Extraocular Muscles

The involvement of extraocular muscles is described in Chapter 8 along with other ocular problems. Formal testing shows them to be frequently involved, but symptoms directly attributable to extraocular muscle weakness, such as diplopia, are uncommon.

Jaw Muscles

Hollowing of the temples from wasting of the temporalis muscles is a prominent early feature of myotonic dystrophy (Fig. 2–4). With more severe weakness the jaw may hang open, and this is particularly characteristic of those patients with congenital onset (Fig. 2–6). Mouth breathing is common in such children. Temporo-mandibular dislocation is well-documented. Gold (1966) studied the jaw movements of 15 affected patients and found six with symptoms of temporo-mandibular dislocation. Recurrent locking of the jaw, difficulty in chewing and frequent clicks were the main complaints. Ten patients showed radiographic abnormalities of the temporo-mandibular joint. An example of the problem is shown in Figures 2–3 and 2–7.

Text continued on page 22

Figures 2–3 and 2–4. FACIAL FEATURES OF MYOTONIC DYSTROPHY.

Patient K.A., aged 52. Progressive weakness noticed for three years; myotonia of grip and percussion. Cataracts were diagnosed at age 32 years and extracted at age 39, but myotonic dystrophy was not diagnosed until the age of 51. The photographs show the characteristic facies resulting from facial weakness, ptosis, and wasting and weakness of the jaw muscles.

See illustration on opposite page

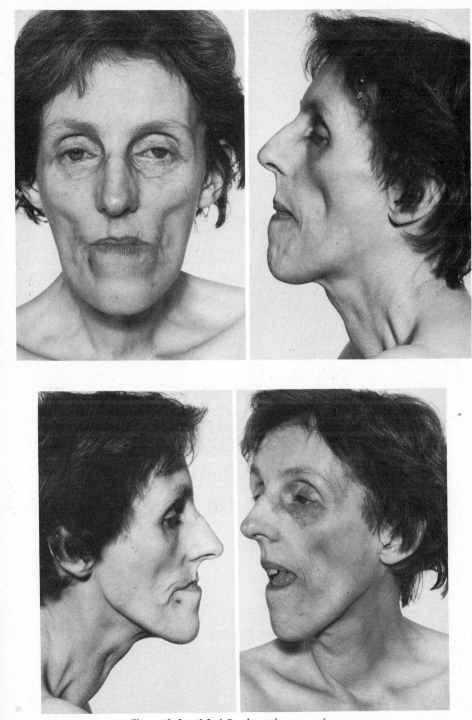

Figures 2–3 and 2–4 *See legend on opposite page*

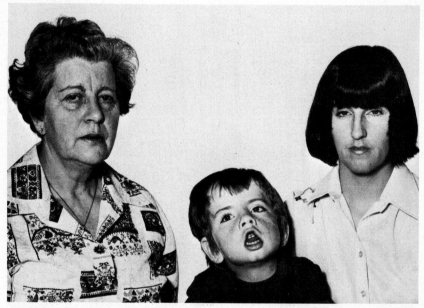

Figure 2–5. Variation of facial appearance within a single family with myotonic dystrophy (see Chapter 9 for detailed case history). The grandmother (*left*) had bilateral cataract extractions at age 40 and shows percussion myotonia on examination; muscle symptoms are entirely absent and she shows no facial weakness. Her daughter (*right*) had no symptoms until after the birth of her severely affected child; examination shows moderate facial weakness and ptosis, with active and percussion myotonia; lens opacities were noted on first examination and cataract extraction has subsequently been performed. The child (*centre*) has congenital myotonic dystrophy, and shows marked facial diplegia and jaw weakness, present from birth.

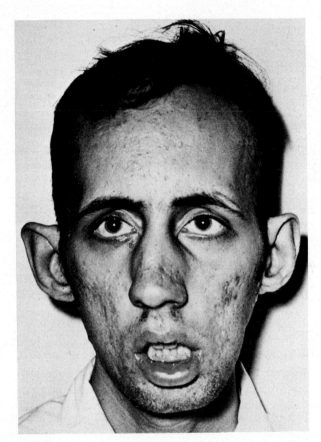

Figure 2–6. JAW AND FACIAL WEAKNESS IN MYOTONIC DYSTROPHY.

28 year old mentally retarded male diagnosed after 11 years in a hospital for the mentally subnormal. The patient had no muscle symptoms but showed marked myotonia of grip and percussion in addition to the characteristic facies. A brother was similarly affected. (Patient studied by courtesy of Dr. V. A. McKusick, Baltimore.)

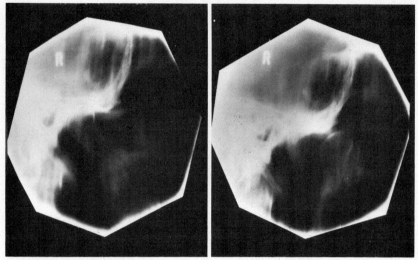

Figure 2–7. Temporo-mandibular dislocation in myotonic dystrophy.

Patient K.A. (see Fig. 2–3).
A, Jaw closed.
B, Jaw open. An abnormal range of movement of the head of the mandible is seen. The patient has repeated episodes of temporary inability to close the jaw after yawning, and a loud click was audible on opening the jaw.

Larynx

Laryngeal involvement is common in patients with advanced muscle disease, but is unusual as an early symptom. It was first noted in Steinert's original description (1909), and both Thomasen (1948) and Caughey and Myrianthopoulos (1963) noted vocal cord paralysis, although this rarely seems to be complete or to be a major factor in speech disturbance in comparison with facial and palatal weakness.

Palate and Tongue

Weakness of the palate is of considerable importance. It contributes to the nasal, indistinct speech that may trouble adults with advanced muscle disease, and may hinder speech development in young children. Incompetence of the palate predisposes to aspiration of material into the bronchial tree, and together with involvement of tongue and jaw provides an abnormal start to the swallowing process, which may be further aggravated by involvement of the pharyngeal and oesophageal musculature (see Chapter 4). Patients with early onset of the disease frequently show a narrow, high arched palate; this may itself result from longstanding weakness of the palatal muscles.

Sternomastoids

Wasting and weakness of the sternomastoids and adjoining anterior muscles of the neck is often marked (Fig. 2–8), and this may occur at a stage when the involvement of most other muscles is relatively mild (Fig. 2–9). Inability to raise the head while in bed is a frequent complaint. By contrast the extensors of the neck and the shoulder girdle muscles are not involved early, providing a contrast with facio-scapulo-humeral dystrophy (Fig. 3–6). In affected children the degree of sternomastoid involvement may be extreme, and like the facial involvement appears to result from intrauterine abnormality of development rather than from subsequent progressive atrophy.

Limb Weakness

Early involvement of distal limb muscles is usual (Fig. 2–10), and provides one of the major distinguishing features from the other principal dystrophies including Duchenne, Becker, autosomal limb-girdle and facio-scapulo-humeral dystrophies, in which the proximal limb muscles are principally involved.

The rare form of distal myopathy and such neuropathic disorders as peroneal muscular atrophy lack the associated central muscle involvement of face, jaw and neck, as well as the myotonia. Distal muscle wasting in myotonic dystrophy is less marked than in these disorders, and pseudohypertrophy of the calves likewise is not seen in myotonic dystrophy, although occasional early patients with severe myotonia may show a general hypertrophy of muscle build. Early symptoms in the hands result more often from myotonia than from weakness, but loss in power at the wrist is seen early, along with weakness of dorsiflexion of the foot, which may result in tripping and stumbling. Wasting of intrinsic hand muscles is frequent (Fig. 2–11), but occurs later and less prominently than wasting of the long flexors and extensors of the fingers; claw hand and pes cavus are not seen, in contrast with peroneal muscular atrophy and similar neuropathic disorders. As the disease progresses more general limb weakness occurs, but severe weakness of the weight-bearing muscles remains rare; in contrast to the limb-girdle dystrophies in which an otherwise well-preserved patient may be wheelchair-bound for many years, those with myotonic dystrophy are mostly able to maintain a limited mobility within the house at an advanced stage of general muscle weakness.

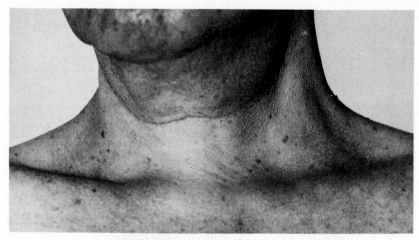

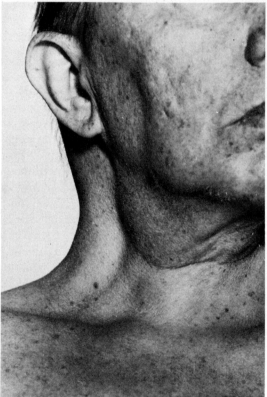

Figure 2–8. STERNOMASTOID WASTING IN MYOTONIC DYSTROPHY.

Patient W.R., a 56 year old man with advanced myotonic dystrophy. There is near-total atrophy of the sternomastoid muscles, and the patient was unable to raise his head against gravity while supine.

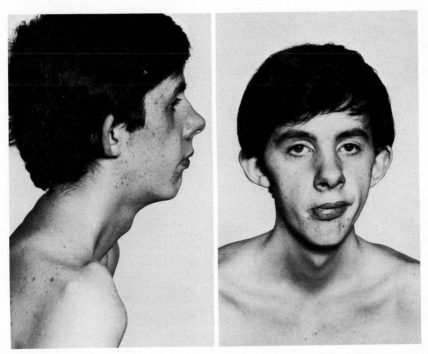

Figure 2–9. STERNOMASTOID WASTING IN MYOTONIC DYSTROPHY.

Patient A.R., aged 19, with no symptoms of muscle weakness but obvious ptosis, facial weakness and wasting of anterior neck muscles. Severe smooth muscle involvement in this patient is discussed in Chapter 4.

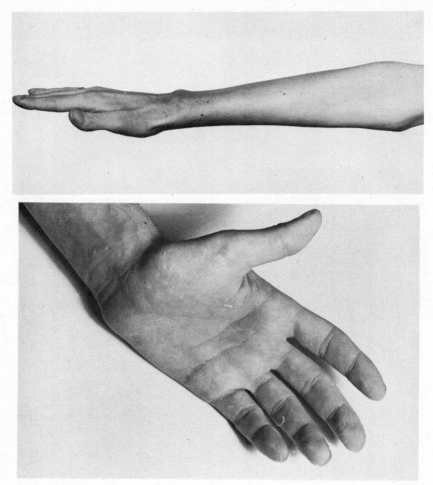

Figures 2–10 and 2–11.   Distal limb involvement in myotonic dystrophy.

Patient A.R., aged 19 years. Figure 2–10 shows wasting of forearm muscles; Figure 2–11 wasting of intrinsic hand muscles.

Myotonia

This phenomenon, the hallmark of myotonic dystrophy, can be elicited in almost every symptomatic patient with the disease, and also is probably the single most valuable sign of the disorder in presymptomatic individuals bearing the abnormal gene. Myotonia is best tested in the hand muscles where, following a forceful grip, there is a delayed ability to relax the grip. The characteristic posture of the hand as the patient attempts to overcome this is seen in Figure 2–12. As is frequent with neurological

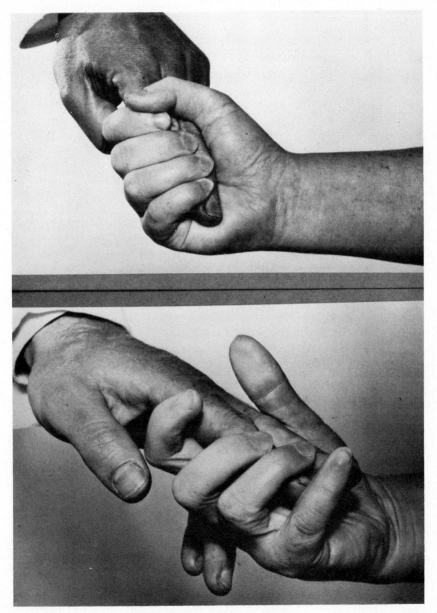

Figure 2–12. MYOTONIA OF GRIP.

The hand is shown (*A*) during and (*B*) immediately after forceful gripping of the examiner's hand. Attempted relaxation produces the position shown. Patient is a 43 year old female with minimal muscle weakness but severe active and percussion myotonia.

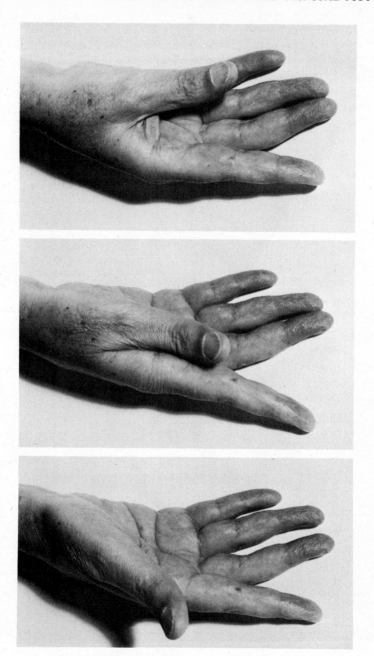

Figure 2–13. PERCUSSION MYOTONIA OF THE HAND.

    Sequence to show position of hand at two-second intervals following forceful percussion of the thenar eminence. Following percussion the thumb is drawn across the hand, remains in this position for several seconds, and gradually returns to its original state.

disabilities, patients may attempt to overcome or conceal the abnormality by gripping weakly in the first instance, or by pulling the arm away rather than relaxing the grip, factors that the examiner should guard against. Repeated contraction and relaxation may diminish myotonia, as may warmth, and the overheated state of many hospitals may be a factor contributing to myotonia being overlooked.

Some patients in whom active myotonia of grip is slight or absent will nevertheless show definite myotonia on percussion of the thenar muscles. A firm blow with the patellar hammer on the thenar eminence is required; a gentle tap is generally unrevealing. Figure 2–13 shows the characteristic sequence of movements as the thumb is drawn across the hand, remains adducted for several seconds, and then slowly returns to its former position. Percussion myotonia may also be elicited in the tongue (Fig. 2–14), but the author has rarely found this to be helpful. The symptoms resulting from myotonia are varied. Some patients specifically complain of inability to relax grip, with difficulty in releasing such objects as door handles, cups and tools. The literature abounds in descriptions of occupational hazards of comparable origin: soldiers unable to release the trigger of their gun, drivers unable to let go of the steering wheel of vehicles, etc.

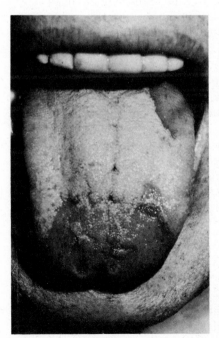 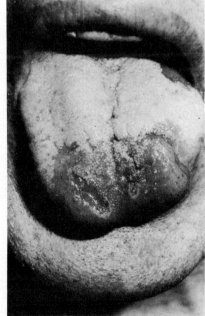

Figure 2–14. PERCUSSION MYOTONIA OF THE TONGUE.

After percussion of the left side, prolonged contraction can be seen of the percussed area.

Aggravation by cold weather is commonly noted. Some patients, particularly the elderly, may interpret their muscle stiffness as "arthritis"; others again may not realise that their myotonic symptoms are in any way abnormal. Thus, one patient of the author, a woman aged 35, had noted stiffness of grip since early childhood but had considered it normal; she only sought medical advice 20 years later because of the development of muscle weakness, and was surprised to be told that her myotonia was an abnormality related to this.

Severe clinical problems arising directly from myotonia are rare in myotonic dystrophy, and in this respect there is a marked contrast with myotonia congenita, in which the myotonia is often severe. However, myotonia of the facial muscles, eyelid spasm, and stiffness and slowness of the tongue and jaw muscles during speech or eating may all occur on occasions, although episodes in which generalised myotonia causes falling are rare.

Myotonia as a clinical finding is commonly most marked in those patients with relatively minor muscle weakness and wasting, and may be difficult to elicit in advanced cases with severe wasting. At the other extreme of life likewise it is not a feature of infants with congenital myotonic dystrophy. Although careful EMG studies may show myotonic potentials to be present in the first year of life, clinical myotonia was not found under the age of 2 years in the author's study (Harper, 1975a), although it had invariably developed by the age of 10 years. A history of myotonia dating from infancy should suggest the diagnosis of myotonia congenita, not myotonic dystrophy.

In general the most remarkable feature of myotonia in myotonic dystrophy is the lack of complaint by the patient concerning it. Although drug treatment may improve it considerably (Chapter 15), few patients are prepared to continue with this; enquiry as to why treatment was stopped usually elicits the not unreasonable reply that it was weakness, not myotonia, about which the patient had complained in the first instance. The author has seen patients with florid myotonia categorically deny its existence, and it must be emphasised that no family member should be considered unaffected until thoroughly examined, however asymptomatic he may be.

NATURAL HISTORY

Few published works on myotonic dystrophy give an adequate conception of the immense range of variability of this remarkable disorder. Indeed, variability, even between members of the same family, is one of the main hallmarks of the condition, and is of diagnostic, prognostic and theoretical importance. The theoretical considerations of possible genetic heterogeneity and the basis of "anticipation" are dealt with later, but the overall pattern of variability is considered here in the context of the clinical features.

One factor that applies to myotonic dystrophy more than most other disorders is that the impression of severity and age at onset, as well as the type of symptoms, depend to a large extent on the nature of the observer. Thus, neurologists usually encounter myotonic dystrophy as a progressive neuromuscular disorder of adult life, which in its later stage may be extremely disabling, and which requires distinction from a variety of related conditions. The paediatrician, by contrast, if he recognises it at all, encounters it as a cause of respiratory distress in the newborn, or as a hypotonic infant with developmental delay. The ophthalmologist generally sees the condition in later life presenting with cataract, and with the muscle involvement often minimal. The medical geneticist is likely to gain a more complete picture of the overall pattern of disease by actively investigating family members regardless of age or the nature of their complaints. The author's own surveys have led him to the conclusion that the extremes of the disease are likely to be missed by hospital clinicians; the mildly affected may never seek medical attention, and the severe neonatal cases in the past have frequently died in infancy without a specific diagnosis being made.

Age at Onset

This may be difficult to document precisely, and considerable variation will result depending on whether age at diagnosis or age at first symptoms is taken as the starting point. Some patients seen because of muscle weakness in middle age give a history of myotonia dating from adolescence, but which has not caused them to seek medical attention. Others are more definite in the onset of their disease and in the lack of previous symptoms. Bearing in mind these limitations it is still possible to construct a table of age at onset, and Figure 2–15 shows data from various studies, those of the author being given separately in Figure 2–15A.

The data agree closely in showing a median age at onset of around 20 to 25 years, but vary more considerably in the proportion of patients with onset after 30 years, a point of importance in deciding how confidently one can reassure individuals at risk in this age group that they are unlikely to develop the disorder later. It is perhaps surprising that the different curves agree so closely, but this is likely to reflect the fact that these data come from genetic studies of entire families rather than from patients presenting with a specific set of symptoms. Even so, it is likely that these curves underestimate the number of severe neonatal cases, which have been fully recognised only in the last few years (see Chapter 9). The

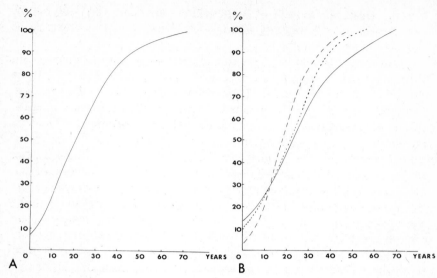

Figure 2–15. AGE AT ONSET IN MYOTONIC DYSTROPHY.

Cumulative frequency curve showing age at onset of first symptoms.
A, Data of the author (from Harper, 1977).
B, Other published data (Bell, 1947; Thomasen, 1948; Klein, 1958).

curves also give a misleading appearance in reaching 100 percent manifestation by old age — since the data are for confirmed cases it is obvious that they cannot reveal anything about the proportion of patients who are never diagnosed and who thus are unrecorded. This problem is considered further in Chapter 10.

Age at Death

Data on age at death in myotonic dystrophy are less adequate than are data on age at onset, and are equally subject to bias. Thomasen (1948) found the mean age at death of 24 patients to be 43.5 years; Bell (1948) found that of 85 published cases to be almost identical — 44.7 years, compared with approximately 60 years for the population as a whole over the same period. A confusing finding was that unaffected sibs of patients had an even earlier age at death (36.5 years, omitting deaths under the age of 5 years) than the affected members; this may have resulted in part from the social and occupational background of the families under study, and illustrates the caution needed in interpreting the data. The correlation of age at death within sibships was very low (0.079). Klein recorded a somewhat higher mean age at death (50.6 years), which may reflect the generally improved life expectation since the collection of Bell's data (Klein, 1958).

It is likely that the distribution of age at death is considerably wider than indicated by these figures. In particular, the high neonatal mortality of the congenital form does not appear in these data, and it is equally likely that there is under-ascertainment of mildly affected individuals with little or no muscle involvement.

Degree of Disability

This can give a guide to the severity of the muscle disease and was investigated by Thomasen (1948) in his 101 patients. He found 26 with no significant muscle disability and a further 36 with only slight disability, whereas only 18 had severe disability (working ability reduced to less than one-third). Despite this apparently benign picture, a much higher proportion (61 percent) were not actually working, a fact attributed by Thomasen to social and mental deterioration (discussed more fully in Chapter 7). Unfortunately, Thomasen's data did not relate disability to duration of muscle disease. Klein (1958) found 31 percent of his patients to have working capacity reduced to less than one-third, but did not differentiate between muscle disease and other factors as the cause of disability.

Prognosis

It is clear from the data presented here that to give an accurate prognosis in myotonic dystrophy is no easy task. In contrast to a disorder such as Duchenne dystrophy, in which the severity, steady progression and eventually fatal course can be predicted with depressing certainty, one is faced in myotonic dystrophy with almost every degree of severity, and no clear guide to the age when symptoms will develop. In a patient with established disease some help can be gained from the previous course of the illness, for there is rarely any great variation in speed of deterioration, nor is true remission seen, although progression may be extremely slow. A further clue is the pattern of the disease in other family members, but this has to be interpreted with caution in view of Bell's finding of both low parent-child correlation for age at onset and low correlation between sibs for age at death (Bell, 1948). The work of Bundey and Carter (1972) suggests a somewhat greater intra-family correlation, and the genetic aspects of this are discussed more fully in Chapter 10. The relevant point to be considered here is that mild disease in one family member does not exclude severe disease in another. The strongest correlation is probably for the congenital form of the disease, in which the author's study (Harper, 1975b) found a high proportion of sibs also to show this severe form.

SYSTEMIC ASPECTS

The occurrence of a variety of abnormalities outside muscle is perhaps the most characteristic feature of myotonic dystrophy, and these abnormalities are both a help in diagnosis and also a problem when they are the presenting feature rather than an accompanying one. The systemic difficulties are also of major importance in management and in prognosis, and in many patients are of considerably greater importance than the muscular aspects. The various systems that may be affected are considered in detail in subsequent chapters, but are introduced briefly at this point to emphasise that myotonic dystrophy must be seen as a generalised disorder, with muscle involvement merely one of a number of manifestations of the abnormal gene. Table 2–3 summarises the principal extramuscular abnormalities.

Although one can document accurately the various abnormalities in this way, it is considerably more difficult to assess their relative frequency and importance. Thus, the frequency of an abnormality such as cataract depends on the age group studied, on whether the study is being per-

**Table 2–3.   SYSTEMIC INVOLVEMENT IN
MYOTONIC DYSTROPHY**

System	Principal Involvement
Smooth muscle	Oesophagus, colon, uterus (other sites may also be affected)
Heart	Conduction defects, in particular heart block, atrial arrhythmias; less commonly, cardiomyopathy
Lungs	Aspiration pneumonia from oesophageal and diaphragmatic involvement, hypoventilation
Peripheral nerve	Variable and rarely clinically significant; minor sensory loss may occur
Brain	Severe involvement in congenital form; mild mental deterioration frequent in adults; hypersomnia
Endocrine	Testicular tubular atrophy; diabetes (rarely clinically significant); sometimes abnormalities of growth hormone and other pituitary functions
Eye	Cataract, retinal degeneration, ocular hypotonia, ptosis, extraocular weakness
Skeletal	Cranial hyperostosis, air sinus enlargement; jaw and palate involvement; talipes (childhood cases); scoliosis (uncommon)
Skin	Premature balding; calcifying epithelioma

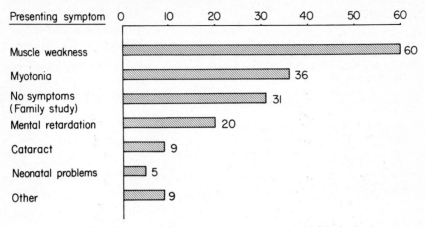

Figure 2–16. Frequency of presenting symptoms in myotonic dystrophy.

formed by a neurologist or an ophthalmologist, and on whether abnormalities are being sought in all patients or only in those with specific eye symptoms. Many patients have clinical abnormalities of several systems at the time of diagnosis, and the symptom that the patient considers most important may not be the one that leads to diagnosis. The author's own data on 170 patients studied personally are shown in Figure 2–16. The patients were all studied in the USA (Harper, 1972) and were studied as complete families at home, without deliberate selection for age or mode of presentation. The presenting symptom is considered to be that which initially brought the patient to medical attention, regardless of whether or not the diagnosis of myotonic dystrophy was made at that time. As expected, muscle weakness and myotonia predominated, but mental retardation was a prominent feature in view of the fact that the childhood form of the disease was not under special study. Even more noteworthy was the discovery of 31 patients who had not come to medical attention prior to the family study, but who had definite clinical abnormalities; some of these were genuinely symptom-free, others had simply avoided doctors.

The nine patients grouped as "other" provide an illustration of the diverse ways in which myotonic dystrophy may present. These include dysphagia, dysarthria, writing difficulty, behaviour problems at school, tiredness, unexplained somnolence, post-anaesthetic respiratory problems and talipes. Any of these symptoms could have numerous causes, and a clinician in almost any branch of medicine could have been faced with making the diagnosis.

REFERENCES

Bell J. (1948): Dystrophia myotonica and allied diseases. *In* Treasury of Human Inheritance 4, Part V. Cambridge University Press.

Bundey S. and Carter C. O. (1972): Genetic heterogeneity for dystrophia myotonica. J. Med. Genet. *9*:311–315.

Caughey J. E. and Myrianthopoulos N. C. (1963): Dystrophia myotonica and related disorders. Charles C Thomas, Springfield, Ill.

Gold G. D. (1966): Temporomandibular joint dysfunction in myotonic dystrophy. Neurology *16*:212–216.

Harper P. S. (1972): Genetic studies in myotonic dystrophy: thesis. University of Oxford.

Harper P. S. (1975a): Congenital myotonic dystrophy in Britain. 1. Clinical Aspects. Arch. Dis. Child. *50*:505–513.

Harper P. S. (1975b): Congenital myotonic dystrophy in Britain. 2. Genetic basis. Arch. Dis. Child. *50*:514–521.

Harper P. S. (1977): Phenotypic variation in myotonic dystrophy: causes and consequences. *In* Pathogenesis of Human Muscular Dystrophies (Ed.: L. P. Rowland). Excerpta Medica, Amsterdam, pp. 705–712.

Klein D. (1958): La dystrophie myotonique (Steinert) et la myotonie congénitale (Thomsen) en Suisse. J. Genet. Hum. (Suppl.) *7*:1–328.

Steinert H. (1909): Über das klinische und anatomische Bild des Muskelschwunds der Myotoniker. Dtsch. Z. Nervenheilkd. *37*:38–104.

Thomasen E. (1948): Myotonia. Universitetsforlaget, Aarhus.

CHAPTER THREE

The Differential Diagnosis of Myotonic Dystrophy: Other Dystrophies and Myotonic Disorders

Myotonic dystrophy is a member of a large group of disorders that traditionally have been regarded as primary inherited diseases of muscle. Even though our concepts of pathogenesis have been modified by experimental studies (see Chapter 14) and there is increasing evidence to suggest that many are more generalised conditions, these diseases still form a natural group that has to be considered in relation to myotonic dystrophy, both as regards aetiology and in the more practical matter of differential diagnosis. Among the primary inherited myopathies are three principal groups, and myotonic dystrophy could equally well be placed in any or all of them:

1. The muscular dystrophies, characterised by progressive muscle degeneration, with wasting and weakness.

2. The myotonic syndromes, which have the phenomenon of myotonia as their common feature; several other disorders that give muscle stiffness clinically resembling myotonia can usefully be considered with them.

3. The non-progressive myopathies, particularly those with congenital onset; these require consideration in the diagnosis of congenital myotonic dystrophy and are discussed with this in Chapter 9.

Not all the primary myopathies are discussed here, and those that are are considered principally in relation to myotonic dystrophy. There are a number of excellent reviews, some of which cover the entire field of muscle disease (Walton, 1974), while others deal in detail with specific groups such as the non-progressive myotonias (Becker, 1977), paramyotonia congenita (Becker, 1970), the inherited myopathies of childhood (Gardner-Medwin, 1977; Dubowitz, 1978) and basic research in muscle dystrophies (Rowland, 1977).

THE MUSCULAR DYSTROPHIES

The classification of the muscular dystrophies is not a fixed system, but has evolved over the years with our understanding of their basis. Clinical, genetic and pathological classifications have all been used, but in general they agree well and there has been remarkably little change since the foundations of the subject were laid by Walton and Nattrass (1954). Table 3–1 lists only the principal forms of muscular dystrophy now recognised, and it should be emphasised that a number of families exist who do not fit readily into any of these types; it also remains possible, indeed likely, that further work will show some of the individual types to be heterogeneous. Among the principal types the two major changes since the original classification of Walton and Nattrass have been the realisation that: (1) the X-linked Duchenne and Becker forms are distinct entities; and (2) many cases thought to represent the autosomal recessive limb-girdle form are in fact due to anterior horn cell disease of the spinal cord.

Myotonic dystrophy is the only muscular dystrophy in which myotonia is a feature, and if this has been recognised, other dystrophies pose no problem in its differential diagnosis. Frequently, however, patients with myotonic dystrophy present as cases of progressive muscle weakness alone, and myotonia may be inconspicuous or overlooked; the other muscular dystrophies then require careful consideration, and the distinguishing features of the five principal types are given in Table 3–2. It can be seen that, if the clinical features, inheritance and time course of the

Table 3-1. THE PROGRESSIVE MUSCULAR DYSTROPHIES

Duchenne dystrophy Becker dystrophy } Emery-Dreifuss type	X-linked recessive
Early-onset "Duchenne-like" girdle dystrophy } Limb-girdle dystrophy (Erb)	autosomal recessive
Facio-scapulo-humeral Distal } Oculo-pharyngeal	autosomal dominant
Myotonic dystrophy	autosomal dominant

disorder are carefully documented, there should rarely be confusion with myotonic dystrophy, and equally the distinction between the other forms can usually be made with confidence on these grounds, reinforced by measurement of serum creatine kinase (SCK) activity, electromyography and muscle biopsy. The importance of an accurate diagnosis is self-evident, not only to give as clear guidance as possible to prognosis, but in the genetic counselling of affected individuals and other family members.

Duchenne Dystrophy

This X-linked disorder (Fig. 3–1), relentlessly progressive and invariably fatal in its course, is the commonest and most extensively studied of all the muscular dystrophies. The incidence in Western Europe and America is around 1 in 3,500 male births. First clearly described by Duchenne (1868), the principal features are progressive weakness and wasting of proximal muscles, particularly the pelvic girdle and lower limbs, with later involvement of all muscle groups. Onset is commonly at age 2 to 4 years, and most patients are severely disabled by 12 years; progressive scoliosis with associated respiratory difficulties may be a serious problem. Death usually occurs in the early 20s and reproduction has not been recorded. Pseudohypertrophy of the calf muscles is a prominent feature; muscle biopsy shows intense degenerative and (less often) inflammatory changes, along with fatty and fibrous infiltration (Dubowitz and Brooke, 1973). The changes are compared with those of myotonic dystrophy in Chapter 12. Cardiac involvement is common, although general loss of mobility minimises its clinical effects. The ECG is almost always abnormal by late childhood (Emery, 1972). Mental retardation, static in nature, is also frequent (Dubowitz, 1965), and the overall intelligence distribution of affected patients is reduced to an extent that cannot be explained adequately by the physical handicap. In affected males the SCK activity is exceptionally high (commonly over 1,000 IU/l) and this elevation is seen in preclinical cases; early recognition of this may help to prevent the subsequent birth of further affected male sibs (Gardner-Medwin et al, 1978). A normal or only moderately elevated level should lead to reconsideration of the diagnosis. Newborn screening for Duchenne dystrophy using the SCK level on a filter-paper bloodspot has been advocated (Zellweger and Antonik, 1975) and appears feasible, but is of doubtful justification in the absence of treatment.

The X-linked recessive mode of inheritance confines the disorder to males, although occasional instances of girls with early-onset girdle dystrophy have been reported (Fig. 3–3) in whom the precise nature of the disorder is uncertain (Gardner-Medwin, 1970). The XO (Turner) chromosome constitution may result in a phenotypic female being affected.

Table 3–2. MUSCULAR DYSTROPHIES:
DISTINGUISHING FEATURES

	Myotonic Dystrophy	*Duchenne Dystrophy*
INHERITANCE	Autosomal dominant	X-linked recessive
AGE AT ONSET	Exceptionally variable; commonly 20-40, but may be at any age, including infancy	Early childhood, commonly 2 to 5 years
PROGRESSION	Variable; severe disability rare before 35 years; muscle involvement may remain minimal	Steadily progressive; severe disability usual by 12 years; death by early 20s
PATTERN OF MUSCLE INVOLVEMENT	Face, jaw, neck, with distal limb involvement	Proximal muscle weakness; pelvic girdle first affected
OTHER MUSCLE ABNORMALITIES	Myotonia; muscle hypertrophy may occur	Pseudohypertrophy of calves common
CARDIAC INVOLVEMENT	Common, particularly conduction defects and arrhythmias	ECG commonly abnormal; clinical cardiomyopathy rarer
OTHER SYSTEMS INVOLVED	Numerous, including central nervous system, eye, smooth muscle, endocrine glands, *testes*	Mental retardation frequent

c Plc   *minimal*   *↑↑*
cancer   *normal*   *70% ↑ c Plc, minor*
PDL   *membrane abnl*
                  myotonia congenita
                      thomsen's disease
                  periodic paralysis
                  paramyotonia congenita
                  acquired - drug
                          malignancy

**Table 3–2. MUSCULAR DYSTROPHIES:
DISTINGUISHING FEATURES (Continued)**

Becker Dystrophy	Autosomal Recessive Limb-girdle Dystrophy	Facio-scapulo-humeral Dystrophy
X-linked recessive	Autosomal recessive	Autosomal dominant
Late childhood and adolescence, commonly 6 to 16 years	Late childhood to early adult life	Adolescence and early adult life; sometimes late childhood
Slowly progressive; disability rarely severe before adult life; death commonly in 40s	Variable; disability rare in childhood but lifespan generally shortened	Very slow; disability rarely significant before middle age; lifespan commonly normal
Proximal muscle weakness; pelvic girdle first affected	Proximal muscle weakness with pelvic girdle usually first affected; shoulder girdle and facial muscles usually involved later	Face, neck, shoulder girdle; pelvic girdle and other proximal muscles involved later
Pseudohypertrophy of calves often striking	Pseudohypertrophy unusual	Congenital absence of muscles frequent
Usually normal	Usually normal	Normal
Occasional mental retardation; otherwise normal	No	No

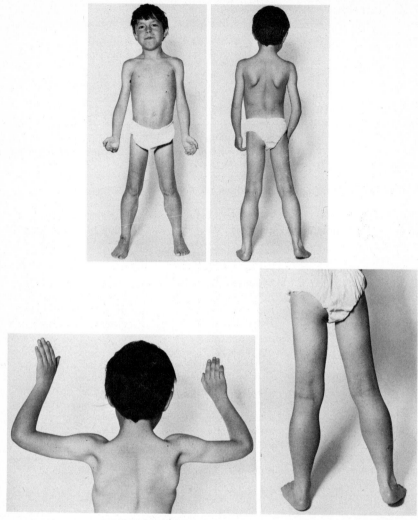

Figure 3–1. DUCHENNE MUSCULAR DYSTROPHY.

Patient P.J., aged 9 years. Early development normal but slow to walk (20 months), with abnormal gait suspected by parents from age 2 years. Duchenne dystrophy diagnosed at age 4 years; proximal muscle weakness and pseudohypertrophy of calves noted at that time. SCK grossly elevated (over 2,000 mu/ml). Subsequent steady deterioration and now largely confined to wheelchair. The photographs show the proximal muscle wasting of upper and lower limbs, shoulder and pelvic girdles, with pseudohypertrophy of the calves. There is no significant facial weakness. Intelligence is in the low normal range.

Carrier women may show a variety of minor muscle abnormalities and are occasionally symptomatic (Moser and Emery, 1974); such a patient is shown in Figure 3–2. SCK levels show a variable elevation, being consistently normal in some but markedly raised in others. Increased accuracy in predicting the carrier state can be obtained by deriving specific risk estimates for values within the normal range of creatine kinase (Wilson et al, 1965) and by the combined use of genetic and biochemical information (Emery, 1969).

Carrier detection is particularly problematical in the mothers of isolated cases. Genetic theory (Haldane, 1935) predicts that one-third of

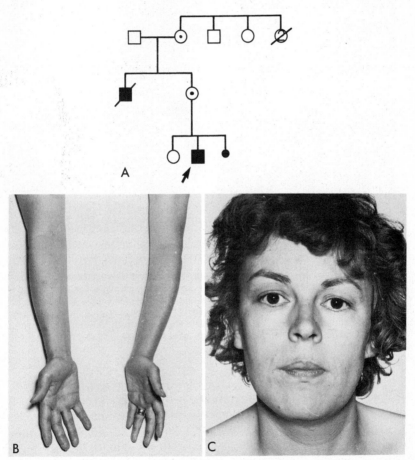

Figure 3–2. Muscle weakness in an obligatory carrier of Duchenne muscular dystrophy.

Patient M.J., mother of the patient in Figure 3–1, also had an affected brother, and is therefore an obligatory carrier (see pedigree, *A*). She had noted since childhood that her left arm was smaller than the right (*B*), and at age 30 years developed slowly increasing weakness of the left arm. There is no detectable generalized weakness; no pseudohypertrophy of calves; equivocal facial weakness. SCK 2,300 mu/ml; electromyography showed changes of primary muscle disease confined to the left arm.

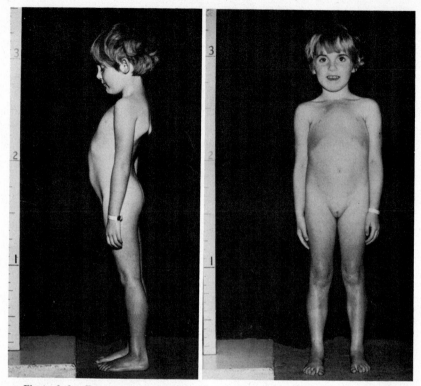

Figure 3-3. EARLY ONSET AUTOSOMAL GIRDLE DYSTROPHY RESEMBLING DUCHENNE
DYSTROPHY.

B. T., proposita, born 20 December 66. This girl was first seen aged 4 years because of
an abnormal gait and difficulty climbing stairs; she had been normal in infancy but did not
walk unaided until 17 months old. The main clinical abnormalities were waddling gait, increased lumbar lordosis, pelvic girdle weakness and early Achilles tendon contractures.
CPK was greatly elevated (1620 mu/ml). There has been steady subsequent clinical deterioration. One healthy young brother and both parents showed normal CPK levels (33.39
and 34 mu/ml respectively).

these should represent new mutations, with no risk of recurrence in the
family. This agrees well with the distribution of creatine kinase levels in
isolated cases (Gardner-Medwin, 1971; Sibert et al, 1978), but studies
using red blood cell protein kinase assays (Roses et al, 1976; see Chapter
14) have suggested that cases representing new mutations may be relatively rare, although this is not generally accepted. At present the basic
biochemical defect is entirely unknown; better understanding of this may
lead to more satisfactory carrier detection and possibly to prenatal diagnosis. Fetal sex determination is feasible to discover whether a pregnancy
is at risk, but there is no established direct method of prenatal diagnosis
at present, although this may become possible as a result of improved

techniques of fetal blood sampling or the detection of consistent abnormalities in the cultured cell. The possible use of fetal blood SCK is under experimental study at present.

Duchenne dystrophy should rarely be confused with myotonic dystrophy, even in childhood. The pattern of muscle weakness, the lack of myotonia and the mode of inheritance are but a few of the major differences between the conditions. Unfortunately the lay public, as well as many clinicians, still tend to equate all dystrophies with the Duchenne form, with resulting misinformation regarding inheritance, carrier status and prognosis for families with other types of dystrophy.

Becker (Benign X-linked) Dystrophy*

Becker and Kiener (1955) were the first investigators clearly to recognise this disorder as being distinct from Duchenne dystrophy, and it has been further delineated in reports by Becker (1957, 1963), Zellweger and Hanson (1967) and Emery (1968). Emery and Skinner (1976) in an extensive study of 67 patients have analysed the main distinctions and similarities with Duchenne dystrophy. The clinical evidence for the distinct nature of the two conditions is supported by genetic linkage data showing that the Becker locus is linked to that for deutan colour-blindness (Skinner et al, 1974), whereas the locus for Duchenne dystrophy is not. An interesting suggestion has been made by Lyon (1975) that the two loci may have evolved by gene duplication from a single original locus, and that this pattern may also hold for other pairs of X-linked loci such as those for colour-blindness and haemophilia A and B.

Like Duchenne dystrophy, the Becker type affects mainly the limb girdles and proximal limb muscles, the lower limbs being affected first. Distal muscles are involved late, and facial muscles are generally spared. Pseudohypertrophy of the calves is a prominent feature (Fig. 3–4) and may antedate onset of weakness. Onset is generally later than in Duchenne dystrophy. Emery and Skinner found a mean onset of 11 years with a range of 2.5 to 21 years. Mean age at death was 42 years (range 23 to 63), and the mean age for becoming chair-bound was 27 years. These last two features were found to be more accurate means of distinction from Duchenne dystrophy than was age at onset. Further distinctions are lack of ECG or other cardiac changes, and comparative rarity of mental retardation. The SCK may be greatly raised in affected males, but is able to detect fewer carrier females than in Duchenne dystrophy.

The X-linked recessive inheritance of Becker dystrophy means that it is confined to males; in contrast to Duchenne dystrophy reproduction

---

*See Figure 3–4.

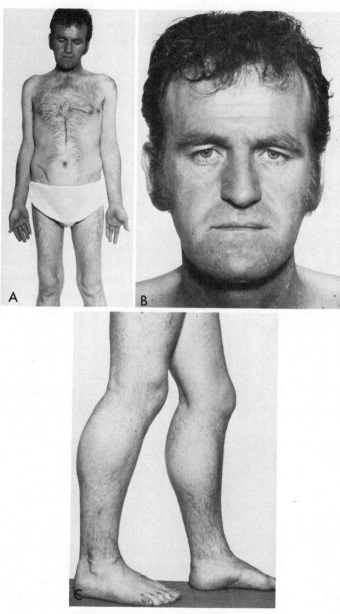

Figure 3–4. *See legend on opposite page.*

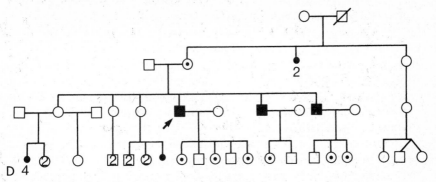

Figure 3-4. BECKER (LATE ONSET X-LINKED) MUSCULAR DYSTROPHY.

A to *C*, 40 year old man with onset of progressive muscle weakness around age 18 years. Now moderately disabled, with marked weakness of proximal limb muscles and pelvic girdle, but strong distal muscles in both upper and lower limbs and no facial weakness. Note pseudohypertrophy of calves. SCK 530 mu/ml.

D, Pedigree. The patient was the eldest of three affected brothers, all of whom were married, with a total of ten healthy children. The six daughters are obligatory carriers, regardless of results of carrier testing, and have a 50 per cent risk of their own sons being affected. The three sisters of the affected males have a 50 per cent risk of being carriers, a risk modified by the outcome in their own offspring and by their SCK levels.

This family illustrates how the relatively benign nature of this disorder allows greater multigeneration transmission than is common in Duchenne dystrophy, and underlines the need for genetic counselling of known and potential carriers.

frequently occurs, all daughters of an affected male being obligatory carriers, whatever level of creatine kinase they show.

Diagnosis is rarely difficult when a characteristic X-linked pedigree pattern is present, with late surviving relatives allowing exclusion of Duchenne dystrophy. The distinction is less easy in isolated cases detected early, and neither SCK estimations nor muscle biopsy appearance provide conclusive evidence. In families containing only two affected brothers it may be difficult to exclude the autosomal recessive form of limb-girdle dystrophy. Lack of pseudohypertrophy and more marked upper girdle involvement favour this diagnosis; the SCK in general is only moderately elevated in affected individuals and is not elevated in carriers (both parents) of the autosomal form.

Becker dystrophy should not be confused with myotonic dystrophy: not only is myotonia absent, but the pattern of muscle weakness is entirely different, with the proximal muscles most involved and the distal muscles, sternomastoids and facial muscles spared, in contrast to their early involvement in myotonic dystrophy. The characteristic extramuscular features of myotonic dystrophy are likewise absent.

Autosomal Recessive Limb-girdle Dystrophy*

Both the Duchenne and Becker forms of X-linked muscular dystrophy are "limb-girdle dystrophies", but the existence of a distinct dystrophy of relatively late onset affecting both sexes has been recognised for many years. First described clearly by Erb (1884), its clinical and genetic differences from other dystrophies were established by Walton and Nattrass (1954).

Onset of weakness is usually in late childhood or adolescence, but in some cases weakness may develop earlier, with significant disability during childhood, whereas others may not present until early adult life. Lifespan is significantly shortened in many patients, with severe disability common by early middle age and frequently before this. The development of weakness may begin in either the shoulder or pelvic girdle, both showing early involvement, in contrast to the sparing of the pelvic girdle usual in the early stages of facio-scapulo-humeral dystrophy; the X-linked dystrophies likewise show more selective involvement of the pelvic girdle. As the disease progresses, proximal limb weakness increases, with consequent restriction of mobility, but distal power is usually spared even when patients are confined to a wheelchair. Facial weakness is variable, but is much less prominent than in facio-scapulo-humeral dystrophy, and may be entirely absent. Cardiac and other systemic involvement is not seen, and myotonia is absent.

Before this form of dystrophy is diagnosed, a number of other disorders must be carefully excluded. The late-onset Kugelberg-Welander form of spinal muscular atrophy may closely mimic it clinically (Kugelberg and Welander, 1956), and will require electromyography and muscle biopsy to show features of denervation. Metabolic myopathies secondary to thyrotoxicosis or Cushing's syndrome may produce a similar pattern of muscle involvement, as may chronic polymyositis. Even when such disorders are excluded one is left with a wide range of variability that makes it highly likely that this is still a heterogeneous disorder.

Further problems result from the fact that many cases, as is to be expected with autosomal recessive inheritance, are isolated. Genetic counselling in such instances is difficult, particularly when the clinical features are atypical. If the disorder occurs in an isolated male or in two brothers, distinction from Becker dystrophy may be difficult or impossible, yet the importance of separating the two is great since the healthy sisters or daughters of patients with the X-linked Becker type may be at risk of their own sons being affected, whereas this is most unlikely in the autosomal recessive limb-girdle dystrophy. Helpful points are the prominence of calf pseudohypertrophy in Becker dystrophy and the generally

---

*See Figure 3–5.

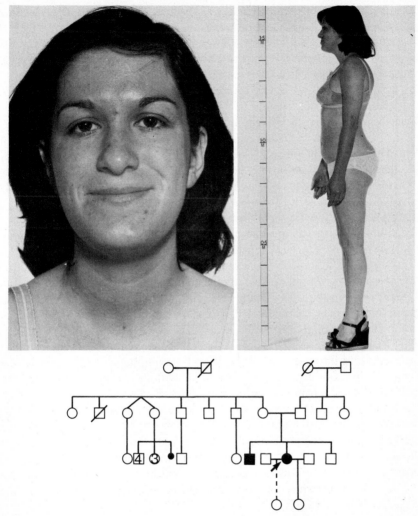

Figure 3–5. LIMB GIRDLE MUSCULAR DYSTROPHY (AUTOSOMAL RECESSIVE INHERITANCE).

S. J., proposita, born 22 January 55. Normal infancy and motor landmarks. Waddling gait was noted at age 3 years, with slowly progressive difficulty in walking over subsequent 15 years; she is now moderately disabled but can type and drive an adapted car. Marked weakness and wasting of proximal limb muscles, pelvic and shoulder girdle and neck muscles; minimal facial weakness. Distal muscles of limbs and intrinsic hand muscles of normal power. Normal intelligence; no cardiac defect. SCK 350 mu/ml; EMG (1970) changes of primary muscle disease, with polyphasic and low amplitude potentials, absence of spontaneous activity at rest, and normal nerve conduction velocity.

One elder brother is affected and is now confined to a wheelchair; there is one healthy younger brother. Parents are healthy and unrelated. Two children of the proposita are clinically normal at present and would not be expected to be affected.

greater elevation of creatine kinase, particularly in early cases. A further guide is the absence of elevation of SCK activity in the carrier parents of the autosomal recessive form, whereas Becker carrier women commonly show elevated levels (Emery and Skinner, 1976). Histological changes in muscle are compared in Chapter 12.

Facio-scapulo-humeral Dystrophy*

The pattern of muscle involvement in this disorder is superficially similar to that of myotonic dystrophy, but the absence of myotonia provides a ready means of distinction. The facial muscles are prominently involved, with inability to smile or whistle, weak eye closure and ptosis giving a characteristic facial appearance (Fig. 3–6). The involvement of facial muscles is usually more severe and more generalised than in myotonic dystrophy. The neck muscles and shoulder girdle are involved early; winging of the scapula is often seen in asymptomatic individuals, and the sternomastoids are not so selectively involved as in myotonic dystrophy. Distal power in the upper limbs is spared, although foot drop may occur. Some muscles, in particular the pectoralis major, may show a partial or complete congenital absence.

Onset is commonly in adolescence, although symptoms may be minimal or absent into early adult life. Careful examination may show minor signs of the condition in asymptomatic children, and changes can be confirmed by electromyography. SCK is rarely elevated presymptomatically. Deterioration in most patients is extremely slow, and severe disability rare before late middle age; lifespan is commonly normal and no cardiac or other abnormalities have been noted. Inheritance is autosomal dominant, and since the gene is expressed by adult life it is usually possible to give a confident reassurance regarding the risk of transmitting the disorder to a family member showing no clinical abnormality.

---

*See Figure 3–6.

Figure 3–6. FACIO-SCAPULO-HUMERAL MUSCULAR DYSTROPHY.

P.B., propositus, born 7 October 51. This 22 year old music student had a normal infancy and childhood and played games normally at school. Apart from minimal symptoms of muscle weakness in arms he had no complaints and was seen primarily for genetic counselling. Definite weakness of face, sternomastoids and shoulder girdle muscles; no pelvic girdle or lower limb weakness. SCK normal (67 mu/ml). EMG: changes of primary muscle disease, with excessive small amplitude polyphasic potentials, but no myotonia and no spontaneous fibrillation or other changes of denervation.

One sister, the mother and the maternal grandmother were all affected; the mother was only moderately disabled at age 59, and the grandmother had lived until 83 years of age.

See illustration on opposite page

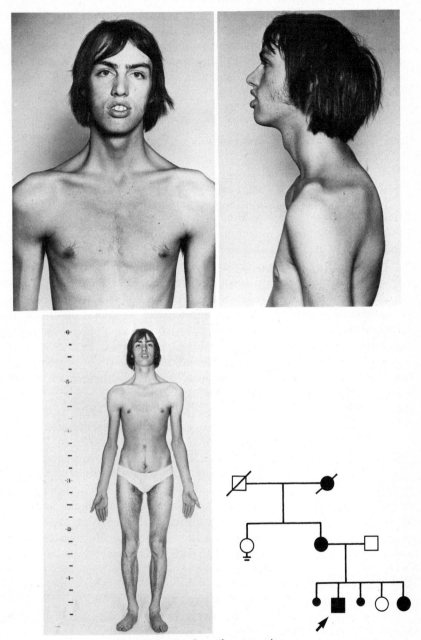

Figure 3–6. *See legend on opposite page*

Although the prognosis in facio-scapulo-humeral dystrophy is normally benign in comparison with that in other forms of dystrophy, caution is made necessary by the likelihood of heterogeneity in this condition. Not only are occasional families seen with early onset and rapid progression, but histology shows great variability of changes, some cases revealing only minor degrees of fibre atrophy and hypertrophy, and others showing a prominent inflammatory response (Dubowitz and Brooke, 1973).

Other Forms of Muscular Dystrophy

DISTAL MYOPATHY

Most patients with progressive weakness and wasting confined to the distal limb muscles prove to have neurogenic disorders such as Charcot-Marie-Tooth disease (peroneal muscular atrophy), itself a heterogeneous disorder; a few patients with a similar pattern of weakness prove to have a primary myopathy that appears to be distinct from other forms of muscle disease. The onset of this disorder is generally late, and symptoms may not develop until after 40 years of age. Progression is slow and extension to proximal muscles late and minor in degree. Although the distal limb involvement may suggest myotonic dystrophy as a diagnosis, this is readily excluded by the lack of facial muscle involvement and of myotonia, and the other major dystrophies of adult life show proximal limb involvement. The main diagnostic problem is to distinguish the disorder from primary neuropathic processes, and electromyography and muscle biopsy are essential for this.

Most cases reported have shown a clear autosomal dominant inheritance, in particular the extensive families studied in Sweden by Welander (1957), where possible homozygous cases resulting from marriage of affected individuals were found, being more severely affected. The rarity of the disorder in most countries makes it uncertain whether sporadic cases represent new mutations for this condition or whether at least some of them represent different conditions. Since the proportion of new mutations would be expected to be low in such a late-onset benign disorder, it would seem likely that the second possibility is correct.

OCULAR MYOPATHIES*

This confusing group of disorders contains two major categories, although a number of patients are not readily classified.

---

*See Figure 3–7.

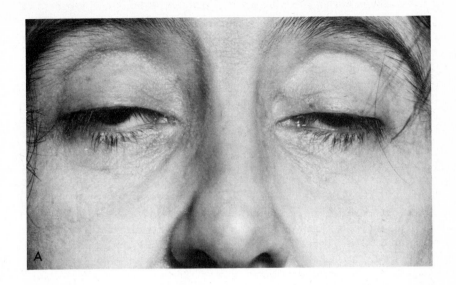

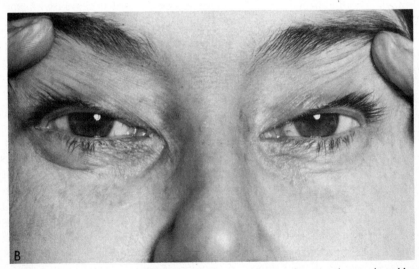

Figure 3–7. 49 year old woman with eight-year history of progressive ptosis and loss of eye movements, and with episodic choking attacks for one year. No other affected family members. The main features on examination were complete bilateral ptosis, total external ophthalmoplegia, mild facial weakness and slight wasting of sternomastoid, shoulder girdle and deltoid muscles. Intelligence was normal and there was no retinopathy or features of CNS disease. Serum SCK 60 mu/ml (normal 0 to 110). No response to Tensilon. EMG (R. triceps) showed minor myopathic changes; biopsy (R. triceps) was essentially normal, with no "ragged red" fibres. *A*, Severe bilateral ptosis. The patient is attempting to open her eyes to the maximal extent. *B*, Complete ophthalmoplegia. The patient's eyelids are supported and she is attempting to look to the left.

1. *Oculopharyngeal muscular dystrophy.* Ptosis and progressive external ophthalmoplegia are the initial features, with onset in adult life, frequently not until middle age. Difficulty in swallowing may occur later and is variable in severity, and weakness of facial, jaw and neck muscles, as well as a degree of more general involvement, may also be seen. The ophthalmoplegia may become total and is a distinguishing feature from facio-scapulo-humeral dystrophy. An early stage of the disorder could be confused with myotonic dystrophy, but myotonia is lacking in oculopharyngeal dystrophy, and ocular muscle involvement in early myotonic dystrophy is rarely severe. Inheritance is autosomal dominant in some families, but a number of cases are isolated and the overall pattern is not clear. Biopsy of a limb muscle often shows variation in fibre size, with marked vacuolation (Dubowitz and Brooke, 1973).

2. *Kearns-Sayre type ophthalmoplegia.* In this disorder the ophthalmoplegia develops early, usually in childhood or adolescence, and is associated with variable extramuscular features, in particular retinitis pigmentosa, ataxia and sometimes mental retardation. Biopsy shows a fragmented and vacuolated appearance, staining red with trichrome stain (the "ragged red" fibre). Electron microscopy shows this to be due to increased and morphologically abnormal mitochondria (Dubowitz and Brooke, 1973).

THE MYOTONIC SYNDROMES

Myotonic dystrophy is not the only disorder characterised by myotonia, but it is by far the most common, and is the only myotonic disorder in which progressive muscle weakness and wasting occur to a significant degree, and the only one in which extramuscular features are seen. Most patients with myotonic dystrophy therefore do not present a problem of confusion with other myotonic disorders, particularly when the full features of the disease are present in other family members. Difficulties can arise, however, with early cases of myotonic dystrophy in which myotonia may be the only obvious clinical abnormality, and in which no significant progression of muscle weakness may be evident over a number of years. Likewise, a mild degree of weakness may be seen in essentially non-progressive disorders such as myotonia congenita, especially the recessive form, and may lead to an erroneous diagnosis of myotonic dystrophy. Such confusion is minimised if a careful study of the family is made, together with slit-lamp examination of the lenses for the specific early changes in myotonic dystrophy; electromyography and muscle biopsy examination may also provide evidence of dystrophic changes. The fact that occasional patients may prove almost impossible to distinguish is not surprising; this is usually resolved by the passage of time.

In view of the general acceptance now that myotonic dystrophy and myotonia congenita are distinct entities, clinically and genetically, it is surprising to see how recently their unity was upheld, and how much controversy revolved around this point. The constancy of the clinical picture of myotonia congenita in Dr. Julius Thomsen's own family might have been thought to have resolved the matter from the outset, and most early investigators were clear that the two conditions were distinct (as discussed in the introduction), but the strongly expressed views of Maas and Paterson (1939, 1950) revived the question, and were supported in part by Walton and Nattrass (1954). Caughey and Myrianthopoulos (1963) took the even more extreme view that a "spectrum" of disease existed linking all the myotonic syndromes, and that all were essentially one disorder.

All these views were based on the existence of a degree of overlap between the different myotonic disorders, and they show a complete misconception of the essential nature of disorders following mendelian inheritance, where a single and unique primary defect must exist, even if the phenotype overlaps. As McKusick (1975) has cogently argued, genetic diseases are either distinct disorders or not; to talk of a "spectrum" of disease is meaningless in genetic terms and distinctly unhelpful even at the clinical level, since the aim of classification is to delineate entities that can be shown to be consistent clinically, pathologically, genetically and, ultimately, at the molecular level. With these problems in mind, the various conditions other than myotonic dystrophy in which myotonia occurs can now be discussed.

Table 3–3 summarises the principal myotonic syndromes, and it is clear that they form a heterogeneous group. As discussed in Chapters 13 and 14, myotonia is essentially a response of the muscle which may arise from a variety of different mechanisms and underlying causes, and heterogeneity is thus to be expected. Most of the myotonic disorders apart

Table 3–3. THE MYOTONIC SYNDROMES

	Inheritance
Myotonic dystrophy	Autosomal dominant
Myotonia congenita (a) Thomsen's disease	Autosomal dominant
(b) recessive type	Autosomal recessive
(c) with painful cramps	Autosomal dominant
Paramyotonia congenita	Autosomal dominant
Periodic paralysis (a) hypokalaemic	Autosomal dominant
(b) normo/hyperkalaemic	Autosomal dominant
(adynamia episodica)	
Chondrodystrophic myotonia	Autosomal recessive
(Schwartz-Jampel syndrome)	
Acquired myotonia (a) drug-induced	
(b) associated with malignancy	

from myotonic dystrophy are rare or very rare, and it should again be stressed that the great majority of patients with myotonia will prove to have myotonic dystrophy.

Myotonia Congenita

DOMINANTLY INHERITED MYOTONIA CONGENITA (THOMSEN'S DISEASE)

This disorder, the first of all the myotonic disorders to be delineated, was put on record by Dr. Julius Thomsen in 1876 in his classic paper: "Tonische Krämpfe in Wilkürlich beweglichen Muskeln infolge bei von ererbter psychischer Disposition (Ataxia muscularis?)". Thomsen was himself affected, and as a physician was able to give a precise account of the symptoms. He noted the hypertrophy of muscular development as well as the stiffness and impaired relaxation of voluntary muscles, and

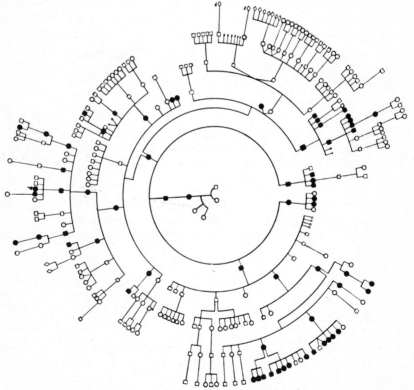

Figure 3–8.   Myotonia congenita in the family of Dr. Julius Thomsen showing autosomal dominant inheritance (after Becker, 1971, courtesy of Professor P. E. Becker).

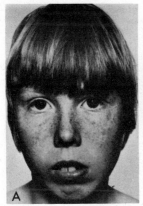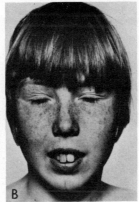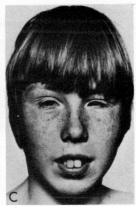

Figure 3–9. BLEPHAROSPASM IN MYOTONIA CONGENITA.

Patient J.M., an 8 year old boy with moderately severe generalised myotonia since 4 years old; no muscle weakness or other features of myotonic dystrophy. Well-built but without definite muscle hypertrophy. Father similarly affected. The photographic sequence shows the patient's attempts to open his eyelids after forceful closure of the eyes. The persistent myotonic spasm can be seen.
   A, Immediately before eye closure.
   B, Approximately 5 seconds later.
   C, After approximately 10 seconds.

clearly recognised the unique nature of the condition. However, he believed that the cause of the disturbance lay in the brain, and associated it with the tendency to psychosis shown by some members of the family in previous generations.

It is of interest that Thomsen was only provoked into publishing his account by the refusal of the Prussian authorities to believe that his son, also affected, had a genuine medical reason for avoiding conscription. He traced the disorder in his family back to 1742, and subsequent descendants have been documented by Nissen (1923), himself a family member, Thomasen (1948) and Becker (1971) down to the present time (Fig. 3–8). Thomsen, although Danish by birth, lived in the part of Schleswig that was ceded to Prussia; thus, some of his descendants are in Denmark, others in Germany.

Myotonia is the principal feature of Thomsen's disease, and its severity may be considerable, in contrast to most patients with myotonic dystrophy, in whom it is rarely disabling. Not only the hands but the face and eyelids may be affected. Blepharospasm may be troublesome (Fig. 3–9, and myotonia of jaw and tongue may produce difficulty of speech and of swallowing and chewing. Sudden episodes of generalised myotonia may result in falling to the ground in rigid positions; they may be precipitated by a sudden noise or fright, and should be distinguished from the longer-lasting episodes of flaccid weakness seen in the periodic paralyses. Myotonia on examination is readily elicited by both grip and thenar

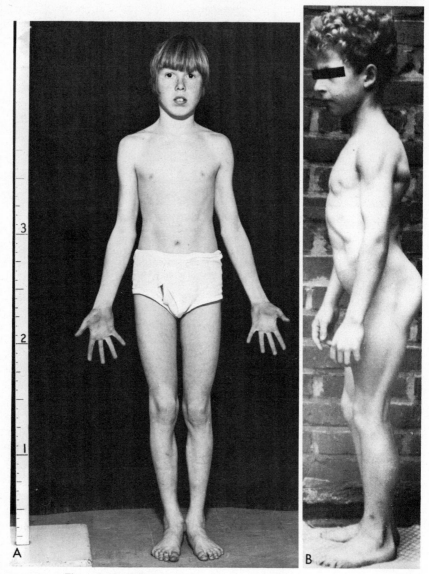

Figure 3–10. MUSCLE HYPERTROPHY IN MYOTONIA CONGENITA

Although muscle hypertrophy is a prominent feature of some patients, it is frequently slight or absent. It tends to be more marked in patients with recessively inherited myotonia congenita, as shown in these illustrations of boys of comparable age.

A, Patient J.M., aged 8 years. Dominantly inherited myotonia congenita. Muscle development is essentially normal.

B, Patient with recessively inherited myotonia congenita, showing marked muscle hypertrophy. A sister was similarly affected (from Becker, 1977 by permission of Professor P.E. Becker and the publishers).

Table 3–4. MYOTONIC DYSTROPHY AND MYOTONIA CONGENITA: CLINICAL FEATURES IN ADULT LIFE

	Myotonia Congenita	*Myotonic Dystrophy*
ONSET OF MYOTONIA	Infancy or early childhood	Late childhood to adult life
SEVERITY OF MYOTONIA	Often severe, generalized	Usually moderate or slight
MUSCLE WEAKNESS	Slight; non-progressive	Very variable–may be severe; progressive
CARDIAC AND SMOOTH MUSCLE INVOLVEMENT	Absent	Common
CATARACT	Absent	Diagnostic
OTHER SYSTEMIC ABNORMALITIES	Absent	Widespread
INHERITANCE	Autosomal dominant or recessive types; sporadic cases frequent	Autosomal dominant; sporadic cases rare

percussion, and frequently by percussion of other muscle groups. Muscle hypertrophy is particularly marked in males, but is not invariable (Fig. 3–10).

Electromyography shows abundant myotonic discharges without the reduced voltage potentials and other dystrophic changes commonly seen in myotonic dystrophy. The changes noted on muscle biopsy are slight (*see below*).

The question of the distinction between myotonia congenita and myotonic dystrophy has already been discussed, but the main relevant features are summarised in Table 3–4.

The natural history of Thomsen's disease is essentially benign. The careful studies of Thomasen (1948) on the descendants of Dr. Julius Thomsen and on other affected families leave no doubt that lifespan is unaffected, that significant progressive muscular weakness does not occur, and that the systemic features of myotonic dystrophy are not seen. Patients investigated by slit-lamp examination have been either normal or at most had a few atypical opacities; no cardiac or endocrine abnormalities have been found, and intelligence is normal. The original suggestion of an association with mental instability was re-examined by Thomasen, who found no consistent correlation between these features and the occurrence of muscle disease in members of the Thomsen family.

Thomasen noted that almost all the propositi in his and in previously studied families were men (145 out of 157 total propositi). He rightly suspected that this reflected the more severe muscle hypertrophy and myotonia in males, and the greater likelihood of its interfering with work. When the propositi were discounted the sex ratio was found to be nearly equal (53 percent males), illustrating the importance of recognising the ascertainment bias that results if such propositi are included in genetic analysis.

RECESSIVELY INHERITED MYOTONIA CONGENITA

The clear-cut dominant inheritance shown by some families with myotonia congenita, including Thomsen's own family, obscured for many years the existence of a form showing different inheritance. The recognition of this syndrome is largely due to the painstaking work of Becker (1966, 1971, 1977), who managed to study the remarkable number of 125 kindreds with non-dystrophic myotonia congenita in the Federal Republic of Germany. His patients included many of Dr. Thomsen's descendants, but in only 24 kindreds were two or more generations found to be affected. In a further 39 kindreds sibs were affected but not parents, and 62 cases were sporadic. These findings suggested that a recessively inherited disorder was accounting for a considerable proportion of the

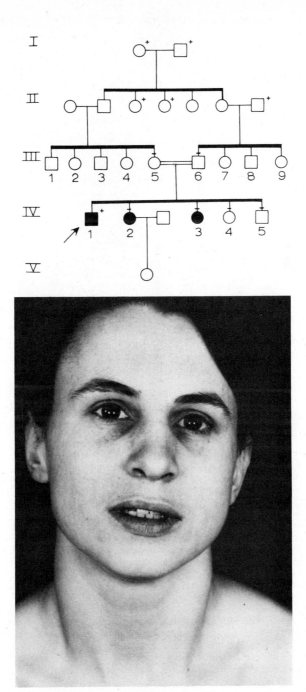

Figures 3–11 and 3–12. *See legend on following page.*

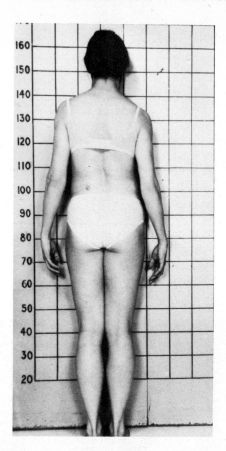

Figures 3–11 and 3–12. Recessively inherited myotonia congenita.*

The pedigree of this white American family is shown in Figure 3–11.

IV-1, (not examined personally). This boy developed stiffness of the legs at age 6 years and was found at that time to have muscle hypertrophy and myotonia; myotonia congenita was diagnosed. Myotonic symptoms steadily increased until his death in an automobile accident at age 19 years.

IV-2, This 25 year old girl was first noted to have myotonia at age 3 years, when examined together with her affected older brother, but symptoms did not begin until she was 6 years old. Stiffness of the legs progressively developed from 6 to 12 years of age, but subsequently remained static. Examination showed severe generalised myotonia, confirmed by EMG. Slight weakness of sternomastoids, biceps, wrist flexors and iliopsoas was present. Muscle hypertrophy was pronounced, particularly in neck muscles (Fig. 3–12*A*) and in calves (Fig. 3–12*B*). No other abnormalities were found, in particular no lens opacities on slit-lamp examination.

IV-3, Symptoms developed around 6 years of age, but became more severe than in her sister, with frequent falls in a rigid posture and myotonia affecting legs, tongue, jaw, face and hands. When examined aged 20 years, clinical and electromyographic findings were similar to those of her sister.

The parents were first cousins, and were normal on examination. No myotonic potentials were found on EMG. The child of *IV-2* was adopted in infancy but is not known to be affected.

*From Harper and Johnston, 1972.

affected kindreds, and this view was supported by the finding of a tenfold increase in cousin marriages.

Becker compared the clinical features of the families showing a clearly dominant inheritance with those containing multiple affected sibs but normal parents, suggesting recessive inheritance. He found the recessive form to show distinct overall differences, though with considerable overlap. Symptoms of myotonia tended to be absent in infancy and early childhood, but became progressively more severe, being accompanied by definite weakness in some instances; progressive weakness and wasting as in myotonic dystrophy were never seen, nor were extramuscular features such as cataract or cardiac involvement present. However, some dystrophic fibres were seen on muscle biopsy.

Becker estimated that two-thirds of cases of myotonia congenita were of this recessively inherited form, and since the subject has received little attention outside the German literature it may be asked whether Germany is atypical in this respect. Evidence against this can be seen in Thomasen's (1948) collected data. He found 157 kindreds in the world literature of which only 34 showed more than one generation affected — findings very similar to Becker's. Thomasen raised the question of recessive inheritance but rejected it because he felt that inadequate documentation of many families made it likely that an affected parent had existed in most cases.

In the author's experience myotonia congenita, whether dominant or recessive, is extremely rare in comparison with myotonic dystrophy. One American family (Harper and Johnston, 1972) showed clear-cut recessive inheritance, with three affected sibs, consanguinity present, and complete absence of clinical and EMG abnormalities in either parent. This family is illustrated in Figures 3–11 and 3–12. Of three British families studied subsequently, one showed dominant inheritance, one recessive inheritance, and a third case was isolated. In such isolated cases the mode of inheritance is of considerable consequence for genetic counselling: if it is recessive, and the parents of an affected child are normal, they have a 1 in 4 chance of a subsequent child being affected, compared with a negligible chance if the child represents a new dominant mutation. Conversely, the risk for offspring of an affected person is minimal with recessive inheritance, but 50 per cent with dominant inheritance.

FURTHER HETEROGENEITY IN MYOTONIA CONGENITA

Apart from the recessively inherited form it is likely that the dominant form of myotonia congenita is itself heterogeneous. Becker (1971) recognised a family in whom myotonia was accompanied by painful cramps, and further families have been well documented by Stohr et al

(1975), Torbergsen (1975) and Sanders (1976). The characteristic finding has been that the painful and prolonged muscle cramps are electrically silent, although patients also show electrical myotonia similar to that of classical Thomsen's disease. No specific biochemical cause has yet been identified. Becker (1977) has suggested that classical Thomsen's disease may contain further separate entities; although this may indeed prove to be the case, it seems premature to split the disorder further without firmer evidence. Genetic linkage data would be of value here, especially for the large, individual dominantly inherited families. The only published data are those of Mohr (1954) on the original Thomsen kindred.

Muscle histology in myotonia congenita has been studied by several investigators, although it is not always made clear whether the patient had the dominant or recessive form. Most reports have shown only minimal changes (Norris, 1962; Engel and Brooke, 1966). Even electron microscopy has revealed few changes, Fisher et al (1975) finding no alteration in sarcolemma, sarcoplasmic reticulum or transverse tubular system. Histochemical studies, however (Dubowitz and Brooke, 1973; Crews et al, 1976), have suggested that the fibre type designated IIB on the basis of the myosin ATPase reaction is completely absent in both recessive and dominant forms. All reports agree that dystrophic changes such as are seen in myotonic dystrophy are almost completely absent, nor is there selective loss of type I fibres. Becker (1977) has recently argued, however, that in recessively inherited myotonia congenita a few patients may show mild but definite dystrophic changes on muscle biopsy, with some increase in internal nuclei. A certain distinction from myotonic dystrophy in such patients would be extremely difficult.

Paramyotonia Congenita

This uncommon condition, first described by Eulenburg (1886), shows a number of distinctive features and has proved hard to classify among the myotonic disorders. At various times it has been considered to be identical to myotonia congenita (Caughey and Myrianthopoulos, 1963), to hyperkalaemic periodic paralysis and even to myotonic dystrophy, but the major features are sufficiently different from any of these disorders to justify its recognition as a separate entity. Although the number of families studied has not been large the clinical picture has been relatively constant, and is summarised in Table 3–5.

The characteristic clinical abnormality seen in paramyotonia is a prolonged myotonic reaction related to cold. In contrast to the myotonic reaction seen in myotonic dystrophy and myotonia congenita, where the muscle has usually relaxed fully within 30 seconds of the contraction, the cold-induced reaction in paramyotonia may last several minutes, and may

Table 3–5. PARAMYOTONIA: MAJOR FEATURES

Prolonged "myotonic" reaction to cold, progressing to weakness
Episodic flaccid weakness, usually related to cold
Myotonic lid-lag
Myotonia of grip and facial muscles, often increased by repetitive movement
Muscle hypertrophy
No progressive weakness or wasting

progress to marked weakness lasting for up to half-an-hour. Local cooling of hand or face will frequently induce the response in the cooled region. Some patients may also experience episodes of flaccid weakness similar to those seen in periodic paralysis, but the cold-related and prolonged rigid contractions of paramyotonia are quite unlike the minor myotonic symptoms seen in periodic paralysis, nor have changes in serum potassium ever been shown in paramyotonia.

Myotonic lid-lag is common in paramyotonia, and myotonia of grip and percussion may be seen unrelated to cold, although not in all families (Thrush et al, 1972). Myotonia may be paradoxical, i.e., worsened, not improved by repetitive movements. Muscle hypertrophy is usual, and as with the other non-dystrophic myotonias there is essentially no progressive weakness, although minor degrees of distal limb weakness may be seen. Cataract and other systemic features of myotonic dystrophy are absent. The inheritance is autosomal dominant, and the thorough studies of Becker (1970, 1977) in Germany have suggested that mutation is a rare event. Starting with 23 propositi Becker managed to study the remarkable total of 308 patients affected with paramyotonia. All his families were localised in one area of Germany, and most could be related to a single common ancestor. No family members showed features of Thomsen's disease or myotonic dystrophy, supporting the distinct identity of paramyotonia.

Muscle biopsy has shown changes more marked than those seen in myotonia congenita (Thrush et al, 1972). There was an increased variation in fibre diameter, with both hypertrophic and atrophic fibres, and histochemically there was a lack of differentiation into type I and II fibres. Central nuclei were seen as in myotonic dystrophy, and the terminal nerve fibres stained with methylene blue showed elongation and expansion. Electrical studies have been reported by Haynes and Thrush (1972), including recording of end-plate potentials at biopsy. Typical myotonic runs were found, particularly on moving the electrode, but the cold-induced "myotonia" was found to be electrically silent, in this respect resembling the contraction seen in McArdle's disease and in the families of myotonia congenita with painful but electrically silent cramps.

Thus, paramyotonia appears to be an example of a true myotonic disorder in which a non-myotonic muscular reaction may occur; the underlying biochemical basis for the abnormal sensitivity to cold is completely unknown.

The Periodic Paralyses and Adynamia Episodica Hereditaria

This confusing group of disorders, in which the principal feature consists of episodes of flaccid paralysis of varying degrees of severity, contains at least two separate disorders. In the first form, accompanied by hypokalaemia, and in which administration of potassium may relieve an attack, myotonia is rarely seen. Myotonic lid-lag has been described in three patients (Resnick and Engel, 1967) but no clinical or electrical myotonia could be shown elsewhere. In the form accompanied by normal or elevated potassium, also termed "adynamia episodica hereditaria" (Gamstorp, 1956), myotonia may be present both in and between attacks of weakness, although it rarely causes serious symptoms. Myotonia has been recorded in the eyelids, facial muscles and hands (McArdle, 1962; Danowski et al, 1975). Clinically the muscles most severely involved in the episodes of weakness in both forms are the limb muscles, especially the proximal muscles of the lower limbs. The ocular, bulbar and respiratory muscles are generally spared except in the severest attacks, accounting for the rarity of death in attacks. The episodes may last for a few hours or for several days, and rarely have defined precipitating factors.

Distinction from myotonic dystrophy is readily made by the lack of serious progressive dystrophic features and by the episodic attacks of weakness; where these are few or absent, as in some members of the family shown in Fig. 3–13, the condition may be confused with myotonia congenita. This family was also noteworthy for the extreme elevation of SCK despite the benign course, with total absence of progressive dystrophy. In most patients the differential diagnosis is not from other myotonic disorders but from such conditions as myasthenia gravis or psychiatric disorders, and knowledge of the family history is an important aid. Demonstration of hypokalaemia in attacks will confirm the diagnosis of this form, but a raised serum potassium is seen much less regularly in most patients with the hyper- or normokalaemic type, and failure to demonstrate electrolyte abnormalities is not incompatible with the diagnosis.

Ultrastructural studies have shown a consistent dilatation of the sarcoplasmic reticulum in both hypokalaemic and hyper/normokalaemic forms (Danowski et al, 1975), but other changes are lacking. Inheritance in all reported families is autosomal dominant.

No evidence exists from linkage or other genetic studies as to whether the disorders are allelic with each other, or with other myotonic disorders.

The Schwartz-Jampel Syndrome (Chondrodystrophic Myotonia)

In 1962 Schwartz and Jampel described a brother and sister with a remarkable disorder in which blepharophimosis and generalised muscle stiffness were accompanied by an unusual facial appearance, joint contractures and a chondrodystrophy. The same patients were restudied by Aberfeld et al (1965), and a number of subsequent case reports have appeared (Huttenlocher et al, 1969; Fitch et al, 1971; Saadat et al, 1972; Cadhilac et al, 1975). A particularly thorough study by Fowler et al (1974) has given details of electromyographic and ultrastructural changes in the muscles, and both the muscle and the skeletal abnormalities were studied by Aberfeld et al (1965, 1970) in biopsies and in post mortem material from one of their patients who died accidentally. Considering its extreme rarity the condition has been well documented; the main features are outlined below and are summarised in Table 3-6.

The affected children usually present with abnormal muscle stiffness in the first weeks of life, which may cause feeding problems. A weak cry is characteristic and the voice is later high-pitched and nasal. Mental development is normal but motor landmarks are delayed, and progressive limitation of joint movements occurs during childhood, along with spasm of the orbicularis oculi and other facial muscles, resulting in the characteristic "pinched" facial features (Fig. 3-13). Generalised muscle spasms, frequently painful, may occur and the stiffness persists during sleep. The muscles appear hypertrophied. Most patients have been dwarfed, with x-ray appearances said to resemble those of the Morquio syndrome, though with no evidence of abnormal mucopolysaccharide metabolism from study of urine or of cultured skin fibroblasts (Fowler et al, 1974). Unfortunately, full skeletal x-ray details have rarely been given and the changes seen to vary between cases, so the nature of the skeletal abnormality at present cannot be classified with confidence.

Electromyography has shown features of myotonia in some cases but in others has been characterised by continuous muscle fibre activity (*see*

Table 3–6.   SCHWARTZ-JAMPEL SYNDROME: PRINCIPAL FEATURES

Muscle stiffness
Muscle hypertrophy
Weak, nasal speech
Unusual facial appearance
Blepharospasm and blepharophimosis
Clinical and electromyographic myotonia
Short stature
Progressive joint contractures
X-ray evidence of bone dysplasia
Autosomal recessive inheritance

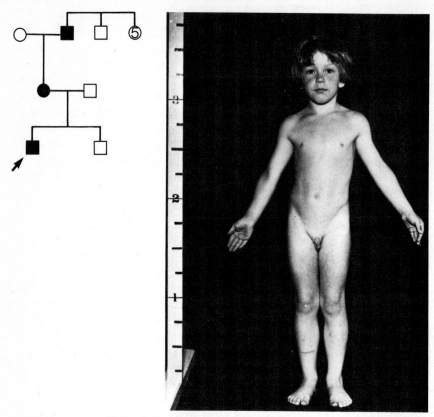

Figure 3–13. Myotonic periodic paralysis.

The propositus was first seen aged 6 years with a two-year history of episodic weakness, attacks occurring almost monthly, and lasting one to two days. General health was otherwise entirely normal. Examination showed bulky muscles, with no weakness or active myotonia; slight thenar percussion myotonia was elicited. No abnormality of serum potassium was found in or between attacks, but SCK was repeatedly greatly elevated (over 1,000 mu/ml).

The mother admitted to stiffness of the hands since the age of 17 years and had two episodes of weakness during pregnancy. She also showed slight percussion myotonia. Electromyography on the propositus, mother and maternal grandfather showed profuse myotonic discharges in all three. Although the grandfather (aged 48) had clinical myotonia of grip he denied episodic weakness.

below). Fowler et al found that the activity was blocked by curare but persisted during general anesthesia, in contrast to true myotonia. Although histological changes in the muscles were minimal, they found an increase in the distribution of acetylcholinesterase over the muscle fibres, and suggested that the disorder resulted from a failure of the normal process of localisation of activity of this enzyme to the end-plate region that occurs in fetal life. It is also of interest to ask how the neuromuscular abnormality might be related to the skeletal defect: although a primary metabolic abnormality affecting both muscle and skeletal development cannot be excluded, it seems distinctly plausible that the bony abnormalities are the direct result of the continuous neuromuscular activity. This view, if confirmed, would have important implications for our concepts of interaction between neural and skeletal development; the Schwartz-Jampel syndrome thus seems likely to be another example of the light thrown on normal processes by rare disorders. Finally, it should be noted that although the inheritance is probably autosomal recessive, there may well be heterogeneity between the cases reported. In particular the sibs described by Mereu et al (1969) appear to be a different clinical entity.

Acquired Myotonia

The subject of drug-induced myotonia is fully discussed in Chapter 13. The drug that causes it most readily, the cholesterol-lowering agent diazacholesterol, was rapidly withdrawn after reports of myotonia induced by it (Burns et al, 1965), but more recently myotonia has been reported in response to the widely used drug clofibrate, Atromid-S (Dromgoole et al, 1975). Apart from drug-induced myotonia, true acquired myotonia is extremely rare, most apparent instances proving to be some other neuromuscular disturbance when investigated electromyographically. In some cases of polymyositis myotonic runs may be seen, but clinical myotonia has not been noted and is certainly not a diagnostic problem. So far no case of myotonia in association with a neoplasm has been fully published, although a single instance of bronchial carcinoma producing myotonia has been reported in brief (Humphrey et al, 1976). If this is confirmed it will have important theoretical implications for the basis of myotonia, as has already been the case for the myasthenic disorders associated with neoplasia. In the meantime the rarity of myotonia in acquired neuromuscular diseases should always raise the suspicion that myotonia found along with such a disorder may be due to coincidental myotonic dystrophy, and this possibility must be firmly excluded before the diagnosis of acquired myotonia can be accepted.

Muscle Stiffness Mimicking Myotonia

Not all delayed relaxation of muscle is the result of myotonia, and a number of conditions exist that may be considered on clinical grounds to show this but in which the underlying electrophysiological defect is either distinct, or in which no electrical abnormality is seen. The main disorders

Table 3–7.   CAUSES OF MUSCLE STIFFNESS RESEMBLING MYOTONIA

McArdle syndrome (glycogenosis type V)
Hoffmann syndrome (hypothyroidism with muscle rigidity)
Continuous muscle fibre activity (neuromyotonia)
Stiff man syndrome
Hyperpyrexic myopathy
Tetanus
Tetany

that must be considered are listed in Table 3–7, and the importance of careful electromyographic studies in any suspected myotonic disorder cannot be overemphasised.

McARDLE'S DISEASE (GLYCOGENOSIS TYPE V)

This disorder, originally described by McArdle (1951), is unlikely to be confused with myotonic dystrophy, but has to be considered in the differential diagnosis of the non-progressive myotonic disorders. It is a benign disorder, characterised by muscle stiffness and cramps, particularly on exertion. Symptoms are rare in infancy and frequently do not begin until adolescence. Weakness may occur, but is rarely progressive, and muscle stiffness may actually improve with increasing age in some patients. Hypertrophy is not seen.

McArdle's disease is due to a deficiency of muscle phosphorylase (Schmid and Mahler, 1959) and it remains one of the few primary disorders of muscle of which the biochemical basis is understood. The glycogen content of muscle is increased, and it cannot be converted to lactic acid during exercise — hence the exercise-related nature of the symptoms. Despite the superficial similarity of the muscle stiffness to myotonia, no electrical evidence of myotonia is seen on electromyography: the cramps are electrically silent.

A similar clinical picture is seen in another rare form of glycogenosis (type VII) due to deficiency of muscle phosphofructokinase (Tarui et al, 1965). It is also likely that McArdle's disease is itself genetically heterogeneous (Dimauro et al, 1977), since some families appear to show immunological activity for phosphorylase whereas others do not. Both type V and type VII disease follow autosomal recessive inheritance. The only other glycogenosis that needs to be considered in relation to myotonic dystrophy is type II (acid maltase deficiency) which may present with generalised hypotonia in infancy and be confused with congenital myotonic dystrophy (Chapter 9). The fact that cardiac involvement and cerebral involvement may also occur in both conditions is further reason for excluding acid maltase deficiency in this diagnostic situation.

"MYOTONIA" IN HYPOTHYROIDISM; HOFFMANN'S SYNDROME

Although occasional patients with coexisting myotonic dystrophy and hypothyroidism have been described, there is no convincing evidence that the two are causally related. A distinct though rare syndrome undoubtedly exists, however, in which hypothyroidism is accompanied by muscular stiffness closely resembling myotonia, and by muscular hypertrophy. Hoffmann gave a clear description of the syndrome in 1897 in a man of 18, and subsequent cases have been reported in both adults and children, including some infants with congenital hypothyroidism (De Lange, 1934; Debré and Semelaigne, 1935). Thomasen (1948) thoroughly reviewed the disorder in his monograph, and Waldstein et al (1957) investigated the electromyographic aspects.

The principal clinical feature is the muscle stiffness, often accompanied by painful cramps. Muscle hypertrophy may be conspicuous, and a "myotonic" reaction, with contraction followed by delayed relaxation, may result from direct percussion of muscles. This must be distinguished from the slow relaxation of a reflex contraction which is almost invariable in hypothyroidism. Although the clinical picture might fairly be classed as myotonia, electromyography of most cases has not shown typical myotonic potentials, but rather an increased irritability with prolongation of both contraction and relaxation. Repetitive discharges occurred after reflex stimulation, and polyphasic potentials were frequent (Waldstein et al, 1957).

All authors agree that response to adequate thyroxine therapy is prompt and generally complete. In one patient with myotonic dystrophy and hypothyroidism, thyroxine treatment also produced reduction in myotonic symptoms, although thyroxine has not been found generally effective in treating myotonia.

Hoffmann's syndrome therefore appears not to be a myotonic disorder in the strict sense, but it certainly needs to be considered in the clinical differential diagnosis of myotonia, in particular because of its treatable nature.

CONTINUOUS MUSCLE FIBRE ACTIVITY (NEUROMYOTONIA)

This phenomenon, in which muscle rigidity is accompanied by electrical evidence of continuous activity, may be mistaken clinically for myotonia, although there are fundamental differences at both a clinical and a physiological level. Originally reported by Isaacs (1961), patients have been described with onset at a variety of ages, from birth (Black et al, 1972) to middle age, and it is likely that the syndrome may have multiple causes, mostly not hereditary. The principal symptom is muscle stiffness, which is generally constant and, unlike true myotonia, persists during sleep and anaesthesia. Muscle relaxation is delayed but there is no percussion myotonia, and on electromyography the pattern of activity is entirely different from that seen in myotonia (see Chapter 13). A further distinction is its abolition by curarisation, indicating its dependence on neuromuscular transmission, in contrast to true myotonia.

STIFF MAN SYNDROME

In this disorder, first described by Moersch and Woltman (1956), progressive but episodic muscle stiffness occurs, with onset usually in adult life and no obvious genetic basis (Gordon et al, 1967). The muscle spasms are painful and may be seriously disabling; they are commonly accompanied by profuse sweating, tachycardia and other features of autonomic overactivity. In contrast to continuous muscle fibre activity the stiffness is abolished during sleep, and by spinal and general anaesthesia. Electromyography shows continuous tonic contraction of the muscles, but action potentials are entirely normal. No abnormalities have been found in the muscle itself on biopsy. Autopsy evidence is scanty, but changes in the spinal cord, possibly virally-induced, were noted in one case (Kasperek and Zebrowski, 1971). The muscle stiffness may be mistaken for myotonia in the early stages of the disorder, but confusion with tetanus and tetany is more likely, and patients not infrequently may be labelled as "hysterical".

MALIGNANT HYPERPYREXIA

The dramatic and often fatal muscle rigidity and hyperpyrexia that occur in this disorder in response to anaesthetics and muscle relaxants can hardly be mistaken for myotonia, and it has already been mentioned that a hyperpyrexic response is not usually a feature of myotonic dystrophy nor of other true myotonic disorders. Nevertheless, the condition may require distinction from myotonia congenita, for most patients with malignant hyperpyrexia have a mild, subclinical, non-progressive, dominantly inherited myopathy (Denborough et al, 1962; Isaacs and Barlow, 1973), and as in myotonia congenita frequently show muscle hypertrophy. Myotonia is not present in hyperpyrexic myopathy, either clinically or electromyographically, and the muscles in contracture are electrically silent.

TETANUS AND TETANY

It is to be hoped that the muscle spasms of tetanus will not be confused with myotonia, but the author has seen myotonia mistaken for tetany, and the position assumed by the hand after thenar percussion or active grip is not unlike that found in alkalotic or hypocalcaemic tetany, both of which are electrically silent, however. One patient seen by the author had been misdiagnosed as having hypoparathyroidism on the basis of cataract and "tetany", which was in fact myotonia.

Other Neurological Disorders Mimicking Myotonic Dystrophy

Although it is possible to confuse almost any disorder characterised by progressive muscle wasting and weakness with myotonic dystrophy, this usually occurs because the possibility of myotonic dystrophy has not been considered, myotonia has not been looked for, and a careful family history has not been documented. Most erroneous diagnoses are soon resolved when these basic steps have been taken, but a few disorders remain which are still readily confused despite a fundamental lack of similarity in their pathogenesis, and these are mentioned briefly here. Paradoxically it is easier to confuse them with the advanced case of myotonic dystrophy, in which wasting is marked and myotonia inconspicuous, than with earlier stages of the disease. However, the uncomplaining nature of many patients with myotonic dystrophy frequently delays their coming to medical attention and makes such confusion more likely.

MYASTHENIA GRAVIS

The finding of myotonia, the absence of fatigue of contraction and the lack of response to cholinergic drugs should readily exclude myasthenia gravis, but the author has seen several patients with myotonic dystrophy in whom myasthenia gravis has been the initial erroneous diagnosis. The facial weakness and ptosis common to both conditions may give a similar facial appearance. The converse situation, in which myasthenia gravis is erroneously labelled as myotonic dystrophy, is uncommon but even more important to avoid, since myasthenia is a much more treatable disorder.

The aetiology of myasthenia gravis has been the subject of a large amount of work that has been well reviewed (Simpson, 1974) and will not be discussed here. The role of autoimmune processes (Feltkamp et al, 1974) and the lack of mendelian inheritance in most instances make it unlikely that there is any close relationship of aetiology, but some similarities nevertheless exist. In particular the phenomenon of congenital myasthenia suggests a parallel to congenital myotonic dystrophy, although, as discussed in Chapter 9, its transient nature and the independence of the genotype are major differences; the demonstration of circulating antibodies to the acetylcholine receptor of the neuromuscular junction (Almon and Appel, 1974) provides an example of one type of humoral factor that might be involved in myotonic dystrophy, although this has been looked for and excluded (Drachman and Famborough, 1976).

POLYMYOSITIS

This is a second acquired disorder that may cause diagnostic confusion (Walton and Adams, 1958; Devere and Bradley, 1975). Not all patients have the acute features of muscle pain and tenderness, and although a raised creatine kinase, high ESR and other evidence of disturbed immunity are common, some patients present as a chronic, progressive muscle degeneration. Myotonia is not seen clinically, but "pseudomyotonic" high frequency discharges may be noted on electromyography (see Chapter 13). Muscle biopsy usually provides confirmation of the diagnosis, with changes of necrosis, regeneration and inflammatory infiltration quite unlike any of the muscular dystrophies of adult life.

MOTOR NEURON DISEASE

Although the more rapid downhill course, bulbar symptoms and clear evidence of neuropathic changes in most cases of motor neuron disease are unlikely to result in confusion with myotonic dystrophy, there is great variability in the pattern of expression, and a patient with rapidly progressive myotonic dystrophy and no symptomatic myotonia could readily be mistaken for a rather benign case of amyotrophic lateral sclerosis. Motor neuron disease frequently produces muscle pain and cramps, but clinical myotonia is not seen, and electromyography will clearly show predominantly denervating changes (although there may be pseudomyotonic discharges). Familial aggregations of motor neuron disease are unusual and no clear pattern of mendelian inheritance is seen.

PERONEAL MUSCULAR ATROPHY (CHARCOT-MARIE-TOOTH DISEASE)

This heterogeneous disorder contains at least three subgroups on genetic grounds, autosomal dominant, autosomal recessive and X-linked recessive patterns all having been described. Clinical and nerve conduction features fall into two broad groups, one having the properties of a peripheral neuropathy, the other of an anterior horn cell disorder. All have in common distal wasting and weakness of the legs and to a lesser extent the hands, but the early involvement of intrinsic hand and foot muscles, loss of tendon reflexes, and absence of facial and sternomastoid involvement should provide a ready distinction from myotonic dystrophy, which can be confirmed by electrophysiological investigations.

When investigating a confusing diagnostic situation it is as well to remember that more than one neurological disease may occur in the same family, and even in the same patient. Caughey and Myrianthopoulos (1963) record two large families with myotonic dystrophy, in one of which motor neuron disease occurred, and in the other peroneal muscular atrophy. In the first family at least one individual appeared to have both conditions; in the second the two genes segregated independently. The author encountered this latter family in his genetic linkage study of myotonic dystrophy (Harper, 1972) and found that the two disorders had been transmitted from separate parents rather than by the same individual as was thought likely by Caughey and Myrianthopoulos.

A similar coexistence of myotonic dystrophy and dominantly inherited myotonia congenita has also been seen in a single family (Busch, 1978, personal communication). So far no unusually severe "compound" disorder has been noted in this family to suggest that the two disorders are allelic to each other.

REFERENCES

Aberfeld D. C., Hinterbuchner L. P. and Schneider M. (1965): Myotonia, dwarfism, diffuse bone disease and unusual ocular and facial abnormalities (a new syndrome). Brain 88:313–22.

Aberfeld D. C., Namba T., Vye M. V. and Grob D. (1970): Chondrodystrophic myotonia: report of two cases. Arch. Neurol. 22:455–462.

Almon R. R. and Appel S. H. (1974): Serum antibodies against the acetyl choline receptor in myasthenia gravis. In Recent Advances in Myology (Eds.: W. G. Bradley, D. Gardner-Medwin and J. N. Walton). Excerpta Medica, Amsterdam.

Becker P. E. (1957): Zur Frage der Heterogenie der Erblichen Myotonien. Nervenarzt 28:455–460.

Becker P. E. (1963): Two new families of benign sex-linked recessive muscular dystrophy. Rev. Can. Biol. 21:551–66.

Becker P. E. (1966): Zur Genetik der Myotonien. In Progressive Muskeldystrophie, Myotonie, Myasthenie. Springer, Berlin, pp. 247–255.

Becker P. E. (1970): Paramyotonia Congenita (Eulenberg). Thieme, Stuttgart.

Becker P. E. (1971): Genetic approaches to the nosology of muscular disease: myotonias and similar diseases. Birth Defects Original Article Series 7, 52–62.

Becker P. E. (1977): Myotonia congenita and syndromes associated with myotonia. Thieme, Stuttgart.

Becker P. E. (1977): Syndromes associated with myotonia: clinical, genetic. In Pathogenesis of the Human Muscular Dystrophies (Ed.: L. P. Rowland). Excerpta Medica, Amsterdam.

Becker P. E. and Kiener R. (1955): Eine neue X-chromosomale Muskeldystrophie. Arch. Psychiatr. Nervenkr. *193*:427–448.

Black J. T., Garcia-Mullin R., Good E. and Brown S. (1972): Muscle rigidity in a new-born due to continuous peripheral nerve hyperactivity. Arch. Neurol. *27*:413–425.

Burns T. W., Dale H. E. and Langley P. L. (1965): The lipid and electrolyte composition of plasma of the erythrocyte of the myotonic goat. Clin. Res. *13*:235.

Cadhilac J., Baldet P., Greze J. and Duday H. (1975): E. M. G. studies of two family cases of the Schwartz and Jampel syndrome. Electromyogr. Clin. Neurophysiol. *15*:5–12.

Caughey J. E. and Myrianthopoulos N. E. (1963): Dystrophia Myotonica and Related Disorders. Charles C Thomas, Springfield, Ill.

Crews J., Kaiser K. K. and Brooke M. H. (1976): Muscle pathology of myotonia congenita. J. Neurol. Sci. *28*:449–457.

Danowski T. S., Fisher E. R., Vidalon C., Vester J. W., Thompson R., Nolans, S. T. and Sunder J. H. (1975): Clinical and ultrastructural observations in a kindred with normo-hyperkalaemic periodic paralysis. J. Med. Genet. *12*:20–28.

Davie A. M. and Emery A. E. H. (1978): Estimation of proportion of new mutants among cases of Duchenne muscular dystrophy. J. Med. Genet. *15*:339–345.

Debré R. and Sémelaigne G. (1935): Syndrome of diffuse muscular hypertrophy in infants causing athletic appearance. Am. J. Dis. Child. *50*:1351–1361.

Denborough M. A., Forster J. F. A., Lovell R. R. H., Maplestone P. A. and Villiers J. D. (1962): Anaesthetic deaths in a family. Br. J. Anaesth. *34*:395–396.

Devere R. and Bradley W. G. (1975): Polymyositis: its presentation, morbidity and mortality. Brain *98*:637–666.

DiMauro S., Mehler M., Arnold S. and Miranda A. (1977): Genetic heterogeneity of glycogen diseases. *In* Pathogenesis of Human Muscular Dystrophies (Ed.: L. P. Rowland). Excerpta Medica, Amsterdam.

Drachman D. B. and Famborough D. M. (1976): Are muscle fibers denervated in myotonic dystrophy? Arch. Neurol. *33*:485–488.

Dromgoole S. H., Campion D. S. and Peter J. B. (1975): Myotonia induced by clofibrate and sodium chlorophenoxyisobutyrate. Biochem. Med. *14*:238–240.

Dubowitz V. (1965): Intellectual impairment in muscular dystrophy. Arch. Dis. Child. *40*:296–301.

Dubowitz V. (1978): Muscle Disorders in Childhood. W. B. Saunders Co., London, Philadelphia.

Dubowitz V. and Brooke M. H. (1973): Muscle Biopsy: A Modern Approach. W. B. Saunders Co., London, Philadelphia.

Duchenne G. B. (1868): Récherches sur la paralysie musculaire pseudohypertrophique ou paralysie myosclérosique. Arch. Gen. Med. *11*:5, 179, 305, 421, 552.

Emery A. E. H. (1968): Benign X-linked muscular dystrophy. *In* Research in Muscular Dystrophy. Pitman, London.

Emery A. E. H. (1969): Genetic counselling in X-linked muscular dystrophy. J. Neurol. Sci. *8*:579–87.

Emery A. E. H. (1972): Abnormalities of the electrocardiogram in hereditary myopathies. J. Med. Genet. *9*:8–11.

Emery A. E. H. and Skinner R. (1976): Clinical studies in benign (Becker type) X-linked muscular dystrophy. Clin. Genet. *10*:189–201.

Engel W. K. and Brooke M. H. (1966): Histochemistry of the myotonic disorders. *In* Symposion über Progressiven Muskeldystrophie (Ed.: E. Kuhn). pp. 203–222.

Erb W. (1884): Über die "juvenile form" der progressiven Muskelatrophie ihre Beziehungen zur sogennanten Pseudohypertrophie der Muskeln. Dtsch. Arch. Klin. *34*:467.

Eulenburg A. (1886): Über eine familiäre, durch 6 Generationen verfolgbare Form congenitaler Paramyotonie. Neurol. Centralbl. *5*:265.

Feltkamp T. E. W., van den Berg-Lodnen P. M., Oosterhuis H. J. G. H., Nijenhuis L. E., Engelfriet C. P., van Rossum A. L. and van Loghem J. J. (1974): Myasthenia gravis, histocompatibility antigens and autoimmunity. *In* Recent Advances in Myology (Eds. W. G. Bradley, D. Gardner-Medwin and J. N. Walton). Excerpta Medica, Amsterdam.

Fisher E. R. et al (1975): Electron microscopical study of a family with myotonia congenita. Arch. Pathol. *99*:607–610.

Fitch N., Karpati G. and Pinsky L. (1971): Congenital blepharophimosis, joint contractures and muscular hypotonia. Neurology (Minneap.) *21*:1214–1220.

Fowler W. M., Layzer R. B., Taylor R. G., Eberle E. D., Sims G. E., Munsat T. L., Philippart M. and Wilson B. W. (1974): The Schwartz-Jampel syndrome. Its clinical, physiological and histological expression. J. Neurol. Sci. *22*:127–146.

Gamstorp I. (1956): Adynamia episodica hereditaria. Acta Paediatr. (Uppsala) *45* (Suppl. 108):1–126.

Gardner-Medwin D. (1970): Muscular dystrophy in young girls. Br. Med. J. *4*:51–52.

Gardner-Medwin D. (1971): Mutation rate in Duchenne type of muscular dystrophy. J. Med. Genet. *7*:334–337.

Gardner-Medwin D. (1977): Children with genetic muscular disorders. Br. J. Hosp. Med. *17*:314–316, 321–324, 326.

Gardner-Medwin D., Bundey S. and Green S. (1978): Early diagnosis of Duchenne muscular dystrophy. Lancet *2*:1102.

Gordon E. E., Januszko D. M. and Kaufman L. (1967): A clinical survey of the stiff man syndrome. Am. J. Med. *42*:582–599.

Haldane J. B. S. (1935): The rate of spontaneous mutation of a human gene. J. Genet. *31*:317–326.

Harper P. S. (1972): Calcifying epithelioma of Malherbe: association with myotonic muscular dystrophy. Arch. Dermatol. *106*:41–44.

Harper P. S. and Johnston D. M. (1972): Recessively inherited myotonia congenita. J. Med. Genet. *9*:213–215.

Haynes J. and Thrush D. C. (1972): Paramyotonia congenita: an electrophysiological study. Brain *95*:553–558.

Humphrey J. G., Hill M. E., Gordon A. S. and Kalow W. (1976): Letter: Myotonia associated with small cell carcinoma of the lung. Arch. Neurol. *33*:375–376.

Huttenlocher P. R., Landwirth J., Hanson V., Gallagher B. B. and Bensch K. (1969): Osteo-chondro-muscular dystrophy. A disorder manifested by multiple skeletal deformities, myotonia and dystrophic changes in muscle. Pediatrics *44*:945–958.

Isaacs H. (1961): A syndrome of continuous muscle-fibre activity. J. Neurol. Neurosurg. Psychiatry *24*:319–325.

Isaacs H. and Barlow M. B. (1973): Malignant hyperpyrexia. J. Neurol. Neurosurg. Psychiatry *36*:228–243.

Kasperek S. and Zebrowski S. (1971): Stiff-man syndrome and encephalitis. Arch. Neurol. *24*:22–30.

Kugelberg E. and Welander M. (1956): Heredofamilial juvenile muscular atrophy simulating muscular dystrophy. Arch Neurol. Psychiatr. *75*:500.

Lyon M. F. (1975): Mechanisms and evolutionary origins of variable X-chromosome activity in mammals. Proc. R. Soc. Lond. (Biol.) *187*:243–268.

Maas O. and Paterson A. S. (1939): The identity of myotonia congenita (Thomsen's disease), dystrophia myotonica (myotonia atrophica) and paramyotonia. Brain *62*:198–212.

Maas O. and Paterson A. S. (1950): Myotonia congenita, dystrophia myotonica and paramyotonia; reaffirmation of their identity. Brain *73*:318–336.

McArdle B. (1951): Myopathy due to a defect in muscle glycogen breakdown. Clin. Sci. *10*:13–35.

McArdle B. (1962): Adynamia episodica and its treatment. Brain *85*:121.

McKusick V. A. (1972): Heritable Disorders of Connective Tissue, 4th ed. C. V. Mosby Co., St. Louis.

McKusick V. A. (1975): Mendelian inheritance in man. Johns Hopkins University Press, p. xv.

Mereu T. R., Porter I. H. and Hug G. (1969): Myotonia, shortness of stature, and hip-dysplasia. Am. J. Dis. Child. *117*:472–478.

Moersch F. P. and Woltman H. W. (1956): Progressive fluctuating muscular rigidity and spasm ("stiff man" syndrome). Mayo Clin. Proc. *31*:421–427.

Mohr J. (1954): A Study of Linkage in Man. Munksgaard, Copenhagen.

Moser H. and Emery A. E. H. (1974): The manifesting carrier in Duchenne muscular dystrophy. Clin. Genet. *5*:271–284.

Nissen K. (1923): Congenital myotonia. Z. Klin. Med. *97*:58–93.

Norris F. H. (1962): Electroencephalog. Clin. Neurophysiol. *14*:197.

Resnick J. S. and Engel W. K. (1967): Myotonic lid lag in hypokalaemic periodic paralysis. J. Neurol. Neurosurg. Psychiatry *30*:47–51.

Roses A. D., Roses M. J., Miller S. E., Hull K. L. and Appel S. H. (1976): Carrier detection in Duchenne muscular dystrophy. N. Engl. J. Med. *294*:193–198.

Rowland L. P. (1977): Pathogenesis of Human Muscular Dystrophies. Excerpta Medica, Amsterdam.

Saadat M. L., Mokfi H., Vakil H. and Ziai M. (1972): Schwartz syndrome: myotonia with blepharophimosis and limitation of joints. J. Pediatr. *81*:348–350.

Sanders D. B. (1976): Myotonia congenita with painful muscle contractions. Arch. Neurol. *33*:580–582.

Schmid R. and Mahler R. F. (1959): Chronic progressive myopathy with myoglobinuria. Demonstration of a glycogenolytic defect in the muscle. J. Clin. Invest. *38*:2044–2058.

Schwartz O. and Jampel R. S. (1962): Congenital blepharophimosis associated with a unique generalized myopathy. Arch. Ophthalmol. *68*:52.

Sibert J. R., Harper P. S. and Thompson R. J. (1978): Carrier detection in Duchenne muscular dystrophy: evidence from the study of obligatory carriers and mothers of isolated cases. *In* The Biochemistry of Myasthenia Gravis and Muscular Dystrophy (Eds.: G. G. Lunt and R. M. Marchbanks). Academic Press, New York, pp. 239–243.

Simpson J. A. (1974): Myasthenia gravis and the myasthenic syndromes. *In* Disorders of Voluntary Muscle (Ed.: J. N. Walton). Churchill Livingstone, London. pp. 653–692.

Skinner R., Smith C. and Emery A. E. H. (1974): Linkage between the loci for benign (Becker types) X-borne muscular dystrophy and deutan colour-blindness. J. Med. Genet. *11*:317–320.

Stohr M., Schlote W., Bundschu H. D. and Reichenmiller H. E. (1975): Myopathia myotonica. J. Neurol. *210*:41–66.

Tarui S., Okuno G., Ikura Y., Tanaka T., Suda M. and Nishikawa M. (1965): Phosphofructokinase deficiency in skeletal muscle: a new type of glucogenosis. Biochem. Biophys. Res. Commun. *19*:517–523.

Thomasen E. (1948): Myotonia. Universitetsforlaget Aarhus.

Thrush D. C., Morris C. J. and Salmon M. V. (1972): Paramyotonia congenita: a clinical histochemical and pathological study. Brain *95*:537–552.

Torbergsen T. (1975): A family with dominant hereditary myotonia, muscular hypertrophy and increased muscular irritability, distinct from myotonia congenita (Thomsen). Acta Neurol. Scand. *51*:225–232.

Waldstein S. S., Bronsky D., Shrifter H. B. and Oester Y. T. (1957): The electromyogram in myxedema. Arch. Intern. Med. *101*:97–102.

Walton J. N. (1974): Disorders of Voluntary Muscle. Little, Brown & Co., Boston, Mass.

Walton J. N. and Adams R. D. (1958): Polymyositis. Livingstone, Edinburgh.

Walton J. N. and Nattrass F. J. (1954): On the classification, natural history and treatment of the myopathies. Brain *77*:169–231.

Welander R. L. (1957): Homozygous appearance of distal myopathy. Acta Genet. Med. *7*:321–325.

Wilson K. M., Evans K. A. and Carter C. O. (1965): Creatine kinase levels in women who carry genes for three types of muscular dystrophy. Br. Med. J. *1*:750–753.

Zellweger H. and Antonik A. (1975): Newborn screening for Duchenne muscular dystrophy. Pediatrics *55*:30–34.

Zellweger H. and Hanson J. W. (1967): Slowly progressive X-linked recessive muscular dystrophy (type III b). Arch. Intern. Med. *120*:525–535.

CHAPTER FOUR

Smooth Muscle in Myotonic Dystrophy

The involvement of smooth muscle as well as striated muscle in myotonic dystrophy has been recognised for a number of years, and provides some of the major clinical features of the disease, which on occasion may be the presenting problem at a stage when involvement of skeletal muscle is giving minimal symptoms. The frequency of clinical involvement varies considerably from organ to organ, being seen most constantly in the pharynx and oesophagus; function of such organs as the bladder and the small gut is affected relatively rarely. The nature of the smooth muscle involvement may also vary according to the stage of the disease; most of the evidence is of loss of smooth muscle function in patients with advanced disease, but more recently it has become clear that smooth muscle may show a myotonic abnormality akin to that of striated muscle, at a stage when its function is otherwise little impaired. Table 4–1 summarises the systems in which involvement of smooth muscle has been documented.

GASTROINTESTINAL TRACT

The main sites affected are listed in Table 4–2.

Pharynx and Oesophagus

Involvement of these organs has been shown to be a constant feature by a number of studies. Dysphagia occurs as a symptom in most patients, and a combination of the four major series shows it to be present in 33 out

79

Table 4-1.   SMOOTH MUSCLE INVOLVEMENT IN
MYOTONIC DYSTROPHY

Gastrointestinal tract	Widespread involvement, particularly of pharynx and oesophagus
Gallbladder	Delayed emptying; high incidence of stones
Urinary bladder	Probably unaffected
Ureter	Isolated instances of dilatation
Uterus	Incoordinate contraction in labour and in vitro
Eye	Ciliary body affected; low intraocular tension

of 50 patients studied (Hughes et al, 1965; Schuman et al, 1965; Pifaretti and Todorov, 1966; Garrett et al, 1969). Dysphagia and abdominal pain were the presenting complaints in the 58 year old man described by Maze et al (1973), who had no neuromuscular complaints at the onset of his gastrointestinal symptoms.

The nature of the swallowing defect in myotonic dystrophy has been thoroughly investigated by a variety of techniques, including barium studies, cineradiography, and oesophageal pressure measurements, and these have made it clear that abnormalities occur in both pharynx and oesophagus.

Kelley (1964) demonstrated reduced oesophageal pressure and failure of peristalsis in a patient with dysphagia, and Harvey et al (1965) found reduced amplitude of contraction of the upper oesophagus in 11 out of 12 patients studied, the lower oesophagus being affected in six of the 12. Garrett et al (1969) found similar abnormalities in all of 13 patients studied, and also documented a reduced resting pressure at the gastrooesophageal junction. Siegel et al (1966) performed detailed pressure measurements at 1-cm intervals along the oesophagus; in addition to the reduced amplitude of pressure waves they noted prolonged contractions and a prolonged relaxation phase, suggesting that myotonia of the oesophageal muscle was involved as well as simple failure of its action. Harvey et al (1965) noted marked exacerbation of its effect by giving the

Table 4-2.   GASTROINTESTINAL TRACT INVOLVEMENT
IN MYOTONIC DYSTROPHY

Pharynx	Delayed relaxation, retention of bolus; frequent tracheal aspiration
Oesophagus	Reduced motility and pressure; dilatation; dysphagia frequent
Stomach	Dilatation, food retention (rare)
Small bowel	Usually normal; occasionally malabsorption
Colon	Megacolon, faecal impaction, symptoms of "spastic colon"; rarely volvulus
Anal sphincter	Myotonia demonstrable

patients iced water to drink, which correlates with the known effects of cold on striated muscle myotonia.

Radiological studies have shown dilatation of the oesophagus with hold-up of barium at the cardiac sphincter as prominent abnormalities (Hughes et al, 1965; Pifaretti and Todorov, 1966). Cineradiography has contributed particularly to detailed study of the pharyngeal region and initiation of swallowing. The most constant findings here are retention of barium in the pharynx after swallowing, with pooling in the vallecula and frequent aspiration into the trachea. Pierce et al (1965) showed the cricopharyngeal sphincter to be flaccid, with no definable sphincter region separating pharynx from oesophagus, and free flow of air in and out of the oesophagus. Bosma and Brodie (1969) studied mildly affected patients and showed that abnormalities were present that were masked in more advanced stages of the disease. Their detailed cine studies showed a myotonic abnormality of the muscles suspending the hyoid, with delayed return of the hyoid to its normal position. There was loss of the normal channelling of contrast, resulting in an abnormally-shaped bolus being presented to the pharynx. These studies make it clear that at least part of the swallowing abnormality results from defective function of the striated muscles involved in initiation of swallowing, in addition to the smooth muscle abnormality of the lower pharynx and oesophagus. Cine studies of the middle and lower oesophagus may be entirely normal in some patients, but in others there may be delay or complete absence of peristalsis. Figure 4–1 shows the changes in the pharynx and oesophagus in a severely affected patient.

The major clinical problem resulting from defective swallowing in myotonic dystrophy, as in other neuromuscular disorders, is the danger of aspiration of material into the trachea and bronchial tree. This, in conjunction with weakened respiratory muscles, results in pneumonic lung changes which are seen in most severely affected patients (Garrett et al, 1969), and which are frequently the cause of death. Reduced pressure at the cardiac sphincter provides a further risk from regurgitation of gastric contents. The high frequency of aspiration of contrast medium is repeatedly emphasised in the radiological studies discussed above, and two practical examples of the severe clinical problems that may result are given in Figures 4–2 and 5–2. In both instances the patients presented as acute medical emergency admissions rather than as neurological problems.

The abnormalities of swallowing are not confined to adult life. Pruzanski and Profis (1966) found abnormal pharyngeal barium retention in all of five childhood cases examined; two had dysphagia as a presenting complaint. The occurrence of hydramnios in pregnancies that produce an infant with the congenital form of myotonic dystrophy, discussed in Chapter 9, is likely to arise from failure of the fetus to swallow effectively,

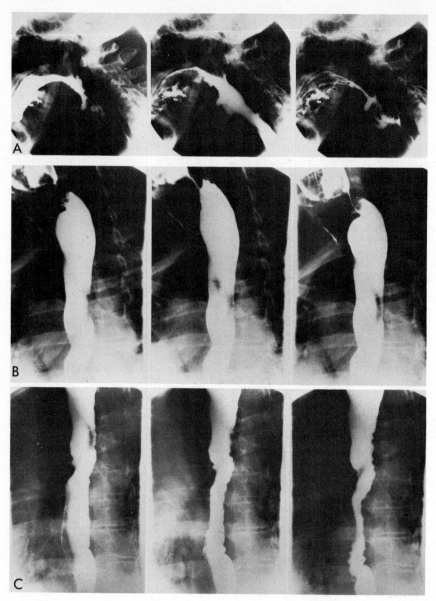

Figures 4–1 and 4–2. ABNORMALITIES OF SWALLOWING IN MYOTONIC DYSTROPHY.

Patient W.R., a 56 year old man with severe myotonic dystrophy. Initial symptom myotonia at age 25 years, followed by slowly progressive muscle weakness. Now severely disabled with generalised weakness. No complaint of dysphagia. Admitted as an emergency with breathlessness and chest pain; signs of right-sided consolidation. History of recurrent similar episodes over the preceding two years. Rapid response to physiotherapy and antibiotic therapy; no further episodes over the succeeding year following introduction of measures to minimize bronchial aspiration. The cine study was performed two months after recovery from the acute aspiration pneumonia.

4–1*A*, Cine study of pharynx and upper oesophagus. There was retention of contrast medium in the vallecula (frames taken at one-second intervals after swallow). No myotonia of hyoid was seen in this study.

82

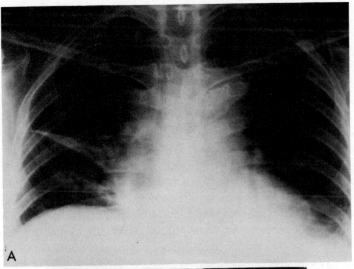

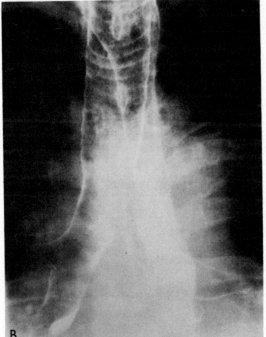

Figures 4–1 and 4–2 *Continued*

4–1*B* and *C*, There was complete absence of normal peristaltic waves throughout the oesophagus, but non-propulsive, tertiary contractions were seen in the lower two-thirds (*C*).

4–2, Radiographs following administration of small quantity of Dionosil during acute admission with aspiration pneumonia. Contrast is outlining the right main bronchus and its branches as well as passing down the oesophagus.

A, Plain chest film on admission.

B, After swallowing contrast medium.

Radiological studies performed by Dr. Brian Lawrie, University Hospital of Wales.

and it is distinctly possible that some of the neonatal deaths in this form of the disease result from aspiration. One neonate in the author's series (family 22 in Harper, 1975a) showed an atonic oesophagus on barium swallow.

Stomach and Small Bowel

Significant symptomatic involvement of these organs in myotonic dystrophy is rare in comparison with the oesophageal and pharyngeal changes. Kuiper (1971) reported a 51 year old woman with myotonic dystrophy who showed dilatation and diminished peristalsis of the stomach, and who had multiple food concretions initially thought to be a gastric carcinoma. The patient's edentulous state and therapy with procainamide were queried as contributing factors. Schuman et al (1965) found normal gastric emptying in all of ten patients studied.

Several cases of malabsorption associated with myotonic dystrophy have been reported, but the great majority of the patients whose small bowel function has been studied have been normal, and diarrhoea in this disorder appears to be more related to colonic than to small bowel abnormality. Kaufman and Heckert (1954) described a man with myotonic dystrophy who developed rapid onset of severe diarrhoea with greatly elevated faecal fats and other evidence of malabsorption. Multiple dilated loops of small bowel and delayed motility were found, but small bowel biopsy was not done. This patient would seem to have had a blind-loop syndrome with bacterial contamination, rather than malabsorption resulting directly from the myotonic dystrophy. Similarly, the case of Lups (1941), a 29 year old man with longstanding malabsorption, may have been coincidental. Most systemic studies have been negative. Harvey et al (1965) found increased faecal fat in only one of 16 patients; jejunal biopsy was normal, as it was in the case of Goldberg and Sheft (1972). The most extensive study has been that of Sjaastad (1975) on 44 patients, which was essentially negative.

Colon

Colicky abdominal pain is a frequent complaint of patients with myotonic dystrophy, particularly in younger age groups. The clinical picture may be that of "spastic colon", with accompanying constipation or diarrhoea, and although no radiological abnormality may be seen in some cases, in others the changes may be gross. Colonic dilatation was first noted in five patients by Bertrand (1949), and Kohn et al (1964) described two patients with frank megacolon. One of Bertrand's patients, as well as the patient of Greenstein and Kark (1972), developed a sigmoid volvulus in association with a dilated colon. The degree of colonic dilatation that may occur is illustrated by patient A. N., who was found to have gross megacolon at the time of his emergency admission with aspiration pneumonia (Fig. 4–3). Chronic constipation had been present since early childhood, regular enemas still being required at the age of 14 years. Aspiration of liquid paraffin, given since infancy, may have contributed to this patient's bronchiectasis, and is contraindicated in myotonic dystrophy in which minor episodes of aspiration are extremely frequent. In young children faecal soiling may be a prominent complaint. This was encountered in several of the author's series of children with congenital myotonic dystrophy, and has been attributed to psychogenic factors; these may have contributed to the problem, but it seems more likely that organic colonic involvement is the major factor in such cases, as discussed in Chapter 9.

Reduced motility is the likely cause of the colonic defect, and was documented in the 21 year old man studied by Goldberg and Sheft (1972)

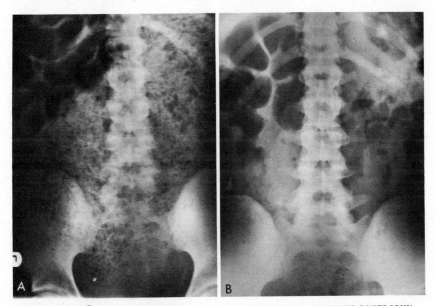

Figure 4–3. COLONIC AND OESOPHAGEAL INVOLVEMENT IN MYOTONIC DYSTROPHY.

Patient A.N. (UHW 178911), born 22 April 57. Constipation was noted from infancy, with liquid paraffin administered regularly over many years. In addition he had recurrent chest infections throughout childhood, with chronic productive cough, and had been mildly mentally retarded (IQ 72 in 1964; 56 in 1968). Equinus deformities of the feet developed at age 11 years and were corrected surgically. Myotonic dystrophy was diagnosed at this time on the basis of grip and percussion myotonia with slight muscle weakness; his mother was also noted to be affected. Aged 18 years he was admitted as an emergency having collapsed following vomiting. He was moribund, with unrecordable blood pressure and profuse coarse crepitations over the lung fields; the abdomen was grossly distended, and plain abdominal film showed a massive collection of faeces in the distal colon (A) which had largely disappeared at the time of discharge (B). *Illustration continued on following page.*

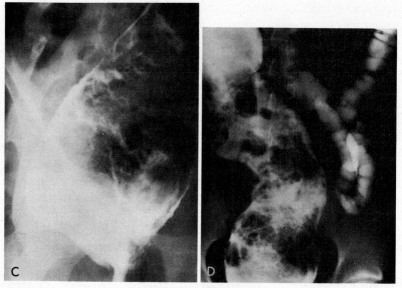

Figure 4–3. (*Continued*)

Aspiration pneumonia was diagnosed, and following prolonged resuscitative measures he recovered. Administration of contrast medium by mouth showed bronchial aspiration with bronchiectatic changes demonstrated. Prolonged colonic washouts were required and were continued at home; barium enema two years subsequently still showed severe dilatation and distention of the rectum and distal sigmoid colon with faeces (*C* and *D*). Following discontinuation of liquid paraffin and regular physiotherapy no further episodes of aspiration have occurred; cine studies showed failure of peristalsis in the upper oesophagus but normal peristaltic activity in the lower oesophagus.

A, Plain abdominal film on admission.
B, Plain abdominal film after repeat washout.
C, Limited contrast study after two years.
Radiological studies performed by Dr. Brian Lawrie, University Hospital of Wales.

whose primary complaint was lower abdominal pain. No haustra could be demonstrated in the colon, and the colonic pressure did not change. Rectal biopsy showed not only a normal mucosa but normal ganglion cells. No instances of an aganglionic segment comparable to Hirschsprung's disease have been noted. By contrast, Orndahl et al (1973) could find no evidence of abnormal colonic function in nine patients studied by pressure measurements, indicating that colonic involvement is not an invariable feature of the disease.

Anal Sphincter

A final feature to be mentioned in the gastrointestinal changes of myotonic dystrophy is involvement of the anal sphincter, which has not escaped the attention of gastroenterologists. Schuster et al (1965), using pressure balloons in the anal canal and rectum, showed a myotonic reaction in both external and internal sphincters, induced by mechanical distension. The response of the internal sphincter, composed of smooth muscle, was more delayed and more prolonged than that of the striated muscle external sphincter.

GALLBLADDER

A high incidence of gallstones has frequently been stated to be a feature of myotonic dystrophy, but without reference to control series. Chiu and Englert (1962) found eight out of 34 patients (mean age 44 years) to have stones. Robert et al (1972) noted gallstones or their complications in six of 32 patients, five of the six being males in contrast to the normal female predominance of gallbladder disease.

Stone formation could be related to defective gallbladder function or could result from a more fundamental metabolic disturbance involving cholesterol and its precursors (see Chapter 14). Harvey et al (1965) found an abnormal response to intravenous injection of cholecystokinin in nine of 12 patients. The autopsied case of Pruzanski and Huvos (1967) showed a thinned gallbladder wall as well as gallstones.

Cholecystectomy should not be undertaken lightly in patients with myotonic dystrophy; this operation is prominent in case reports of post-operative fatalities (see Chapter 5) and seems particularly to be associated with respiratory problems, although precise data are lacking.

OTHER SMOOTH MUSCLE ABNORMALITIES

By comparison with the gastrointestinal tract, abnormalities of smooth muscle function in other systems are relatively minor. Sciarra and Steer (1961) studied the response of isolated strips of uterine muscle as well as its function in the parturient patient; both were abnormal, and are discussed along with the complications of myotonic dystrophy in pregnancy in Chapter 6.

The urinary tract is generally unaffected by the disease, although Bundschu et al (1975) have described brothers with myotonic dystrophy who showed dilatation of the ureters and renal pelvis. Bladder function was studied by Orndahl et al (1973), using cystometrograms, and found to be normal in nine patients. Harvey et al (1965) reviewed material from a previous autopsy case and found only slight vacuolisation of the bladder smooth muscle syncytium.

Involvement of the ciliary muscle of the eye is discussed in Chapter 8 as the probable cause of the low intraocular tension characteristic of myotonic dystrophy, and has been documented histologically in an autopsy study (Manschot, 1968).

The Histological Basis of Smooth Muscle Changes

Few studies on the histology of smooth muscle in myotonic dystrophy have been undertaken, in comparison with the numerous biopsy and autopsy reports on skeletal muscle. The existing knowledge is derived mostly from autopsy material, and although suction biopsy specimens give little information on the muscle of the bowel, it is disappointing that the not infrequent abdominal operations undertaken in these patients have not been utilised to obtain material for study.

The first report came from Kerschner and Davison (1933) who found degeneration and fatty replacement in muscle of the small intestine. Pruzanski and Huvos (1967) studied two further autopsy cases, and demonstrated degeneration in the muscle of both small and large bowel, as well as in the urinary bladder. The gallbladder wall was abnormally thin. One case also showed fatty infiltration of the stomach wall, with disorganisation of the muscle layers, but since the patient died from a bleeding gastric ulcer too much empahsis cannot be placed on these changes.

A third report is that of Jéquier and Todorov (1967), who examined oesophageal muscle in a patient with severe dysphagia, and documented abnormalities of motility. In this case there was marked atrophy of striated muscle but relatively few changes in smooth muscle. Unfortunately the exact site of the sample and how it was obtained were not mentioned.

Smooth muscle from the appendix of a case of childhood myotonic dystrophy has recently been studied by Lenard et al (1977); the clinical aspects of their patients with colonic involvement are discussed in Chapter 9. The muscle layers of the appendix were well-preserved but showed separation of the muscle fibres by bands of collagen.

From what has been reviewed here it is clear that the abnormalities of smooth muscle function in myotonic dystrophy need much more study, particularly to relate the functional aspects with adequate histological studies. Assessment of the effects of drugs might well prove rewarding for the patient; involvement of oesophagus and colon are of major importance in some patients, and their dysfunction may possibly be more amenable to treatment than many other aspects of myotonic dystrophy.

REFERENCES

Bertrand L. (1949): Le mégacolon dans la maladie de Steinert. Rev. Neurol. 81:480–486.
Bosma J. F. and Brodie D. R. (1969): Cineradiographic demonstration of pharyngeal area myotonia in myotonic dystrophy patients. Radiology 92:104–109.

Bundschu H. D., Hauger W., and Lang H. D. (1975): Myotonische Dystrophie Curschmann-Steinert. Urologiche Besonderheiten und histochemische Befunde an der Muskalatur. Dtsch. Med. Wochenschr. *100*:1337–1341.

Chiu V. S. W. and Englert E. (1962): Gastrointestinal disturbances in myotonia dystrophica. Gastroenterology *42*:745–746.

Garrett J. M., Dubose T. D., Jackson J. E. and Norman J. R. (1969): Esophageal and pulmonary disturbances in myotonia dystrophica. Arch. Intern. Med. *123*:26–32.

Goldberg H. I. and Sheft D. J. (1972): Esophageal and colon changes in myotonia dystrophica. Gastroenterology *63*:134–139.

Greenstein A. S. and Kark A. E. (1972): Sigmoid volvulus in myotonic dystrophy. Am. J. Gastroenterol. *57*:571–577.

Harper P. S. (1975): Congenital myotonic dystrophy in Britain. 1. Clinical aspects. Arch. Dis. Child. *50*:505–513.

Harvey J. C., Sherbourne D. H. and Siegel C. I. (1965): Smooth muscle involvement in myotonic dystrophy. Am. J. Med. *39*:81–90.

Hughes D. T., Swann J. C., Gleeson J. A. and Lee F. I. (1965): Abnormalities in swallowing associated with dystrophia myotonica. Brain *88*:1037–1042.

Jéquier M. and Todorov A. (1967): Aspects nouveaux de la maladie de Steinert. Rev. Otoneuroophtalmol. *39*:108–112.

Kaufman K. K. and Heckert E. W. (1954): Dystrophia myotonica with associated sprue-like symptoms. Am. J. Med. *16*:614–616.

Kelley M. L. (1964): Dysphagia and motor failure of the oesophagus in myotonia dystrophica. Neurology *14*:955–960.

Kerschner M. and Davison C. (1933): Dystrophia myotonica. Arch. Neurol. Psychiatr. *30*:1259.

Kohn N. N., Faires J. S. and Rodman T. (1964): Unusual manifestation due to involvement of involuntary muscles in dystrophia myotonica. N. Engl. J. Med. *271*: 1179–1183.

Kuiper D. H. (1971): Gastric bezoar in patients with myotonic dystrophy. Am. J. Dig. Dis. *16*:529–534.

Lenard H. G., Goebel H. H. and Wiegel W. (1977): Smooth muscle involvement in congenital myotonic dystrophy. Neuropaediatrie *8*:42–52.

Lups S. (1941): Dystrophia myotonica mit steatorrhoe. Acta. Med. Scand. *106*:557–578.

Manschot W. A. (1968): Histological findings in a case of dystrophia myotonia. Ophthalmologica (Basel) *155*:294–296.

Maze M., Novis B. H., Lurie B. D. and Bank S. (1973): Involuntary muscle involvement in dystrophia myotonica. S. Afr. Med. J. *47*:1947–1950.

Örndahl G., Kock N. G. and Sundin T. (1973): Smooth muscle activity in myotonic dystrophy. Brain *96*:857–860.

Pierce J. W., Creamer B. and MacDermot V. (1965): Pharynx and oesophagus in dystrophia myotonica. Gut *6*:392–395.

Pifaretti P. G. and Todorov A. (1966): Les troubles de motilité pharyngooesophagienne dans la maladie de Steinert. Rev. Med. Suisse Romande *86*:666–690.

Pruzanski W. (1966): Variants of myotonic dystrophy in pre-adolescent life. Brain *89*:563–568.

Pruzanski W. and Huvos A. G. (1967): Smooth muscle involvement in primary muscle disease. 1. Myotonic dystrophy. Arch. Pathol. *83*:229–233.

Pruzanski W. and Profis A. (1966): Dysfunction of the alimentary tract in myotonic dystrophy. Isr. J. Med. Sci. *2*:59–64.

Robert J. M., Pernod J., Plauchu M., Chollet A. and Paffoy J. C. (1972): Maladie der Steinert et Lithiase. Lyon Med. *227*:762–763.

Schuman B. M., Rinaldo J. A. and Darnley J. D. (1965): Visceral changes in myotonic dystrophy. Ann. Intern. Med. *63*:793–799.

Schuster M. M., Tow D. E. and Sherbourne D. H. (1965): Anal sphincter abnormalities characteristic of myotonic dystrophy. Gastroenterology *49*:641–648.

Sciarra J. J. and Steer C. M. (1961): Uterine contractions during labor in myotonic muscular dystrophy. Am. J. Obstet. Gynecol. *82*:612–615.

Siegel C. I., Hendrix T. R. and Harvey H. C. (1966): The swallowing disorder in myotonia dystrophica. Gastroenterology *50*:541–550.

Sjaastad O. (1975): Intestinal absorption in myotonic dystrophy. Acta Neurol. Scand. *51*: 59–73.

CHAPTER FIVE

Cardiorespiratory Problems

THE HEART IN MYOTONIC DYSTROPHY

For many years cardiac abnormalities, notably arrhythmias, have been recognised to occur as a complication of myotonic dystrophy, and there has been considerable debate as to their degree of clinical importance, their underlying basis and their relationship to the disease as a whole. The subject has been thoroughly reviewed by Caughey and Myrianthopoulos (1963) and Church (1967) among others, but the development of a variety of new cardiological techniques has provided fresh evidence since this time. In addition some unresolved questions will be examined here, in particular the occurrence of cardiac abnormalities in individuals without muscle symptoms as a potential aid in early diagnosis, and the possible association of childhood myotonic dystrophy with heart disease.

Clinical Aspects

Cardiac involvement in myotonic dystrophy was first noted by Griffith (1911) who reported extreme bradycardia in a 48 year old man. Electrocardiographic evidence of impaired cardiac conduction was documented early (Maas and Zondek, 1920; Guillain et al, 1932), and Evans (1944) found delayed conduction to be common in a series of patients, with probable Stokes-Adams attacks in one patient. Hypotension was reported to be a consistent feature by Waring et al (1940) and Evans (1944), but no characteristic clinical abnormalities were noted in the early studies other than those arising from conduction problems.

All studies agree that only a minority of patients with myotonic dystrophy have cardiac symptoms, in contrast with the high proportion who can be shown to have cardiac abnormalities on investigation. The most extensive overall study has been that of Church (1967), who investigated the cardiac abnormalities in 17 patients and reviewed the cardiac aspects of 300 cases previously reported in the literature. Only 16 per cent of patients had cardiac symptoms, which were attributable to arrhythmias in half the cases. The great majority of patients were normotensive, contradicting the earlier view of Evans (1944) that significant hypotension was a characteristic feature. The incidence of angina was not mentioned, but other studies have shown it to be rare (Thomasen, 1948; Fearrington et al, 1964).

A clinical picture of cardiac failure due to myocarditis in the absence of arrhythmia (Holt and Lambert, 1964; Casas, 1973), although well-documented, is also uncommon, in distinction to some other disorders such as Friedreich's ataxia, in which cardiac failure and cardiomegaly are frequently a major clinical problem.

Abnormalities of the electrocardiogram (ECG) are, by contrast, extremely common in myotonic dystrophy, regardless of the presence or absence of symptoms. Church (1967) found the ECG to be abnormal in 202 out of 236 cases, although a bias towards including abnormal results in published reports may make this an overestimate. The main ECG abnormalities, based on Church's data, are shown in Table 5-1. The commonest abnormality was first-degree heart block, followed by varying degrees of

Table 5-1. ELECTROCARDIOGRAPHIC ABNORMALITIES
IN MYOTONIC DYSTROPHY*

	Number
Total studied	222
Abnormal	192
Conduction defects:	
Prolonged PR interval (>0.20 sec)	84
Prolonged QRS (>0.08 sec)	48
Bundle-branch block	23
Complete heart block	1
Arrhythmias:	
Atrial flutter	16
Atrial fibrillation	4
Atrial ectopic beats	3
Ventricular ectopic beats	8
Ventricular arrhythmias	2
Other changes:	
ST and T-wave abnormalities	37
Left axis deviation	41
Left ventricular hypertrophy	9
Right axis deviation	4
Right ventricular hypertrophy	1

*After Church, 1967.

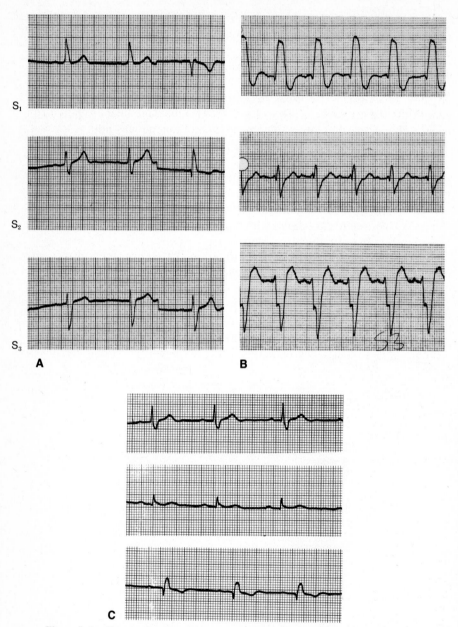

Figure 5-1. ELECTROCARDIOGRAPHIC ABNORMALITIES IN MYOTONIC DYSTROPHY

Electrocardiograms (standard leads 1–3) of three patients with established muscle disease, but without cardiac symptoms, showing conduction defects.

A, Left anterior hemiblock, indicating conduction disorder of the left Purkinje tissue.

B, Gross QRS widening, left bundle branch block and prolonged P–R interval, indicating trifascicular involvement.

C, Right bundle branch block with prolonged P–R interval.

Table 5–2. SUDDEN DEATH IN MYOTONIC DYSTROPHY

Source	Age at Death	Sex	Previous Clinical Data	Cause of Death
Spillane (1951)	51	M	Muscle symptoms for 15 years; heart clinically normal; ECG: left axis deviation	Ventricular dilatation; left heart failure; no other abnormality
Fisch and Evans (1954)	41	M	Heart clinically normal; ECG: atrial flutter with varying block	Fatty infiltration and fibrosis of myocardium; scattered hypertrophied muscle fibres
Holt and Lambert (1964)	65	F	Previous cerebral embolus; ECG: frequent ectopic beats with T-wave changes suggesting cardiomyopathy	Died unexpectedly during sleep; autopsy: diffuse enlargement of heart (450G); fatty infiltration of myocardium but no abnormality of conducting tissue noted
Rausing (1972)	32	M	Moderate muscle disease; atrial flutter; no cardiac symptoms	Ventricular fibrillation; focal myocarditis on autopsy
Parvu (1973)	49	M	No clinical cardiac abnormality; ECG: abnormal AV and IV conduction	No autopsy
Uemura et al (1975)	?	F	Younger sister of patient under study; no clinical details given	Died during sleep five days after cataract surgery; no autopsy details

bundle-branch and intraventricular block. Atrial arrhythmias were common, in particular atrial flutter, but ventricular arrhythmias less so, and complete heart block, surprisingly, was noted in only one instance. Figure 5-1 shows ECG abnormalities in patients studied personally.

Although ECG abnormalities are asymptomatic in most patients with myotonic dystrophy, some show severe symptoms as a result of arrhythmia; persistent atrial flutter is the commonest cause, and episodes lasting up to three years have been recorded (Spurney and Woolf, 1962; Salomon and Easley, 1973). Stokes-Adams attacks requiring insertion of a cardiac pacemaker have also been described (Thomson, 1968; Petkovich et al, 1964; Bulloch et al, 1967). The attacks were related to quinidine therapy for atrial flutter in the case of Cannon (1962).

Sudden death is well recognised to occur in myotonic dystrophy, and is not confined to those with advanced muscle disease. In a family studied personally a 12 year old boy, previously diagnosed as having myotonic dystrophy, collapsed and died suddenly in the school playground. Although not known to have had cardiac abnormality before his death, it is of interest that his younger brother, also affected with onset at birth, showed partial AV block on ECG. Rausing (1972) described sudden death associated with ventricular fibrillation in a man of 32, and Spillane (1951) reported a 35 year old man who died suddenly in the hospital during investigations. The existing reported data on sudden deaths are summarised in Table 5-2 along with the underlying factors where known. Although these cases are not common, they argue strongly for the avoidance of unnecessary investigations and surgery that could place the patient at risk, and support the use of ECG monitoring during anaesthesia and surgery. Other anaesthetic problems are discussed later in this chapter.

The Underlying Basis of Conduction Disorders
in Myotonic Dystrophy

The ECG abnormalities listed in Table 5-1 suggest an extensive involvement of the cardiac conducting tissue in myotonic dystrophy. This has received more precise documentation by vectorcardiography and from the more recently developed His bundle electrogram. Fearrington et al (1964) studied 17 established cases of myotonic dystrophy by vectorcardiography, and in 10 showed abnormal ventricular activation. Six patients showed records similar to that seen in myocardial infarction, despite complete lack of clinical evidence of coronary artery disease. Fearington et al suggested that the conduction abnormalities might be part of more extensive myocardial damage.

The exact localisation of conduction defects has been considerably advanced by development of the His bundle electrogram, a technique whereby various portions of the conducting bundles can be studied directly by endocardial recording from the pacing electrodes. Josephson et al (1973) examined a father and son with myotonic dystrophy by this technique. Both had shown a prolonged PR interval and intraventricular conduction defect on electrocardiography, but the His electrogram localized the defect to the His-Purkinje system in the case of the father, and the son showed prolonged conduction in the AV node, the bundle and in its branches. Subsequent studies on more extensive series of patients using this technique have confirmed that all parts of the conducting system may be affected. Griggs et al (1975) studied a further 11 patients by His bundle electrogram, and showed abnormal conduction in eight of these. In six patients conduction was prolonged between the His bundle and the ventricles, and in five it was impaired between the atria and the bundle. Similarly, only two of the eight patients examined by Schmitt et al (1974) had normal His bundle electrograms.

Pathological studies support a selective and extensive involvement of the conducting system. Thomson (1968) reported an autopsy study of the conducting tissue of a 69 year old woman with myotonic dystrophy who had repeated episodes of atrial flutter and subsequent left bundle-branch block. Serial sections through the conducting system showed severe degeneration of all parts. The myocardium of the sino-atrial node had shrunk to a few isolated fibres embedded in dense fibrous tissue; similar changes were present in the AV bundle and its branches. Similar changes in the conducting tissue have been found by Théry et al (1975) in a patient with complete AV dissociation (Fig. 5–2).

Drug Treatment of Myotonia and Cardiac Conduction

The depressant effects on cardiac conduction of drugs such as procainamide and quinine, commonly used in the treatment of myotonia, raise the question whether such drugs may have adverse cardiac effects in patients with myotonic dystrophy. Munsat (1967), in a double-blind study, found prolongation of the PR interval in three patients treated with procainamide, but this did not occur with diphenylhydantoin. Griggs et al (1975) obtained similar results, showing a lengthening of the PR interval with procainamide in 12 out of 13 patients, and with quinine in six out of 13. Diphenylhydantoin, by contrast, shortened the PR interval in eight out of ten patients. The drugs appeared equally effective in control of the myotonia. Four patients were given intravenous diphenylhydantoin during His bundle studies; no effect on conduction could be detected. From these studies it would seem wise to avoid procainamide and quinine in patients showing prolonged conduction, and to use diphenylhydantoin

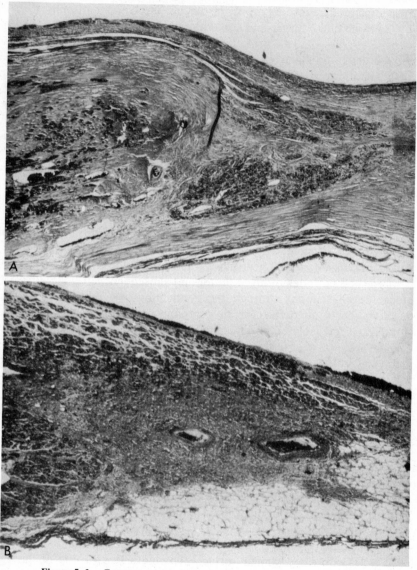

Figure 5-2. CARDIAC CONDUCTING TISSUE IN MYOTONIC DYSTROPHY.

Sections through (A) sino-atrial node and (B) bundle of His to show fibrotic and sclerotic changes. The patient died in complete heart block and His bundle electrocardiography had located the block within and below the bundle. (Photomicrographs by courtesy of Dr. C. Théry, Lille. Patient reported by Théry et al, 1975.)

where myotonia is troublesome enough to warrant drug treatment. The physiological basis of drug treatment is discussed in Chapters 13 and 15.

Mitral Valve Prolapse

Winters et al (1977) have recently documented a previously unsuspected cardiac problem in a large family with myotonic dystrophy. A 30 year old man underwent cardiological investigation for a heart murmur that was shown to be due to mitral valve prolapse, and he was also discovered to have myotonic dystrophy. The association might have been fortuitous in this patient, but 25 of his relatives were also studied. Ten had myotonic dystrophy, of whom eight had evidence of mitral valve prolapse on echocardiography. In contrast, none of the 15 relatives unaffected by myotonic dystrophy showed the cardiac defect. It seems unlikely that this family is unique, and increasing use of the echocardiogram may show at least minor degrees of mitral valve prolapse to be frequent. Since histological valve abnormalities have not been noted in autopsy studies it is unlikely that serious and progressive valve lesions occur, but the possibility of mitral valve prolapse being a factor in those patients developing significant cardiomyopathy will have to be borne in mind in future studies. Echocardiographic studies have not yet been reported in infants with congenital myotonic dystrophy; it is distinctly possible that transient valvular dysfunction might be responsible for heart murmurs that at present are attributed to congenital structural defects.

The Pathological Basis of the Cardiac Abnormality

In addition to the reports of Thomson (1968) and Théry et al (1975) on the conducting tissue, a number of more general autopsy reports have provided histological details of the cardiac abnormalities in myotonic dystrophy. Of the 29 cases reviewed by Berthold (1958) in which the heart had been examined histologically, 14 were reportedly normal, and in the remainder atrophy of myocardial muscle and increased fibrosis were the principal features. Both Holt and Lambert (1964) and Thomson (1968) found fatty infiltration, but three of the four cases studied by Orndahl et al (1964) were normal. In a number of cases histological changes were slight in comparison with the clinical or electrocardiographic abnormalities, supporting the view that selective involvement of the conducting tissue, rather than a generalised cardiomyopathy, accounts for most of the clinical cardiac problems seen in myotonic dystrophy.

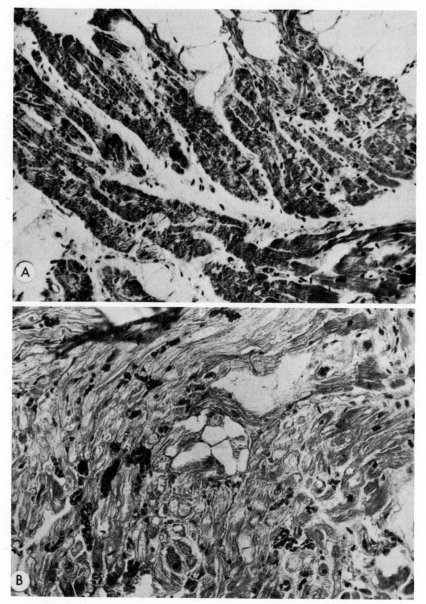

Figure 5-3. CARDIAC BIOPSY CHANGES IN MYOTONIC DYSTROPHY.*

A, Light micrograph of myocardium of right ventricle. Patient with heart block and Stokes-Adams attacks.

B, Light micrograph of right ventricle of patient without cardiac symptoms but with conduction abnormality on ECG. Marked variation of fibre size is seen in both patients, with widespread fatty infiltration and vacuolar degeneration of myocardial cells. There is no significant fibrosis or inflammatory infiltrate. (Original magnification (A) × 160 (B) × 400.)

*From Uemura et al, 1973, Electrophysiological and histological abnormalities of the heart in myotonic dystrophy. Am. Heart J. 86:616–624; by courtesy of Dr. N. Uemura, Kagoshima.

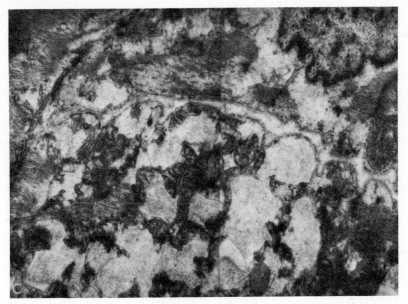

Figure 5–3. (*Continued*)

C, Electron micrograph of patient shown in (A) showing degenerating mitochondria. (Original magnification × 10,000.)

Of particular interest is the report by Rausing (1972) of autopsy studies on a mother and son who both died from myotonic dystrophy; the mother had a terminal bronchopneumonia in an advanced stage of the disease, and the son collapsed and died with ventricular fibrillation at age 32. The hearts of both patients showed patchy areas of active myocarditis with marked cellular infiltration of muscle fibres by histiocytes and leucocytes. Acute changes of this type have not been found in other autopsy studies, but Rausing suggests that some of the more chronic changes reported previously may be the result of periodic episodes of more acute myocarditis.

The value of autopsy reports is somewhat limited by the fact that the patients have mostly had advanced, longstanding disease, and biopsy material has only recently become available to allow the disorder to be studied at an earlier stage and with the use of electron microscopy.

Bulloch et al (1967) utilised the opportunity of a patient undergoing implantation of a cardiac pacemaker for heart block to study a sample of left ventricular muscle. Under the light microscope both normal areas and areas of marked destruction of fibres were seen. Fatty replacement was widespread and connective tissue was diffusely increased. The electron microscope also showed myofibrils varying from normal to marked dissolution. Numerous vacuoles, considered to be degenerating mitochondria, were seen. Biopsy material was also studied from a similar patient of Petkovich et al (1964). Uemura et al (1975) obtained myocardial biopsies from three patients with myotonic dystrophy, using an endomyocardial bioptome introduced via the femoral vein, a procedure claimed to be of low risk. Only one of the patients had cardiac symptoms (Stokes-Adams attacks), although partial ECG conduction defects were present in two of them. Both light and electron-microscopic studies showed marked myocardial changes, similar to those described by Bulloch et al (1967). Disorganised and degenerating mitochondria were the most prominent electron-microscopic features (Fig. 5–3). A patient studied by Tanaka et al (1973) showed similar features. Despite the freedom from complications claimed for this technique, one must have reservations about employing it in a patient without cardiac symptoms.

The histological changes in the heart, as in skeletal muscle, have so far contributed little to our understanding of the underlying defect in the disease, and are still essentially at a descriptive level. They are of interest in their own right, and of importance in explaining the mechanism of the observed cardiac complications, but it is possible that advances in our fundamental understanding of the disease will come more from biochemical studies on blood and on simple cultured cells than from studies of the highly specialised cardiac muscle, in which primary and secondary events are difficult to distinguish.

CORONARY ARTERY DISEASE IN MYOTONIC DYSTROPHY

The recent discovery of the relationship of myotonia and cataract with cholesterol-lowering drugs (Winer et al, 1967), and the hypothesis that a primary defect in lipid metabolism might be involved in myotonic dystrophy, makes it important to examine the question whether the cardiac involvement in this disorder is due at least in part to coronary artery disease. The evidence proves to be strongly against this possibility. Not only is the clinical evidence of angina and other clinical features of ischaemic heart disease low, but autopsy studies have shown no more coronary artery disease than expected for the age of the patient (Orndahl, 1964). Casas (1973) has provided further evidence by finding entirely normal coronary arteriograms in a patient with myotonic dystrophy presenting with cardiomyopathy.

CARDIAC ABNORMALITIES AS A PRECLINICAL TEST FOR MYOTONIC DYSTROPHY

The various approaches to detection of the individual carrying the gene for myotonic dystrophy are discussed fully in Chapter 11. Evans (1944) originally suggested that the high prevalence of ECG abnormalities might be used in preclinical detection, but opinions have been divided since that time. In general, patients showing clinical evidence of heart disease have obvious muscular abnormalities, but several interesting exceptions have been reported. Cannon (1962) described two patients presenting with paroxysmal atrial flutter who were not diagnosed as having myotonic dystrophy until several years subsequently, and the patient of Spurney and Woolf (1962), also with atrial flutter, had been noted to have an intraventricular conduction defect on routine ECG 12 years before myotonic dystrophy was diagnosed. Holt and Lambert (1964) reported a 65 year old woman, initially diagnosed as having a non-specific cardiomyopathy, in whom myotonic dystrophy was only recognised after being diagnosed in other family members. In this instance, as in many others, the diagnosis probably was missed not for lack of positive evidence but because it was not considered.

There can be no doubt that ECG abnormalities, and sometimes clinical heart disease, may be present in patients with myotonic dystrophy many years before muscle disease is complained of or recognised. However, there is no record of a patient with cardiac disease later proving to have myotonic dystrophy in whom the characteristic muscle findings were actively sought and not found. Absence of symptoms is not a dependable criterion in these notoriously uncomplaining patients.

Should the presence of ECG abnormality in an otherwise normal family member at risk be considered as evidence that he or she possesses the abnormal gene? No prospective evidence exists on this point, but the author's personal opinion is that it should not, provided that other investigations, including slit-lamp examination and EMG, are negative.

CONGENITAL HEART DISEASE IN CHILDHOOD MYOTONIC DYSTROPHY

Caughey and Myrianthopoulos (1963) have claimed that congenital heart defects are associated with the childhood form of myotonic dystrophy. Their evidence is not convincing, for only one of the children in question had both myotonic dystrophy and a congenital heart defect (pulmonary stenosis); the other three family members with heart defects were offspring of healthy sibs of a patient with myotonic dystrophy and had no signs of the disorder. The only other documented case is that of

Bell and Smith (1972), in which the affected mother of a neonate with congenital myotonic dystrophy had undergone surgery in childhood for patent ductus arteriosus. During personal studies of childhood myotonic dystrophy in America and Britain the author has encountered only two affected children with congenital heart disease; both were mentally retarded, with congenital onset of myotonic dystrophy and the mother being the affected parent. In each case atrial septal defect was the heart lesion. A third patient was considered to have a possible ventricular septal defect, not investigated cardiologically, and a fourth, thought at birth to have coarctation of the aorta, was shown on later investigation to have no heart lesion at all. Taking the evidence together, it does not seem that a true association has been proved between myotonic dystrophy and any form of congenital heart disease. Systematic autopsy studies of fatal neonatal cases should resolve the question.

Cardiomyopathy can certainly occur in childhood myotonic dystrophy. Not only are electrocardiographic abnormalities seen, but car-

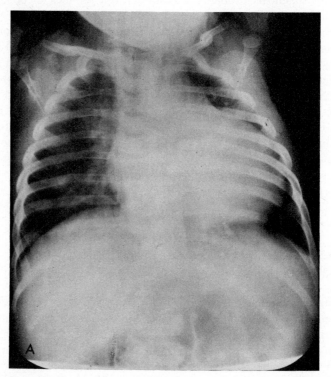

Figure 5–4.   Cardiac involvement in infantile myotonic dystrophy (see text for clinical details).

A, Chest x-ray at age 7 months showing gross cardiac enlargement.

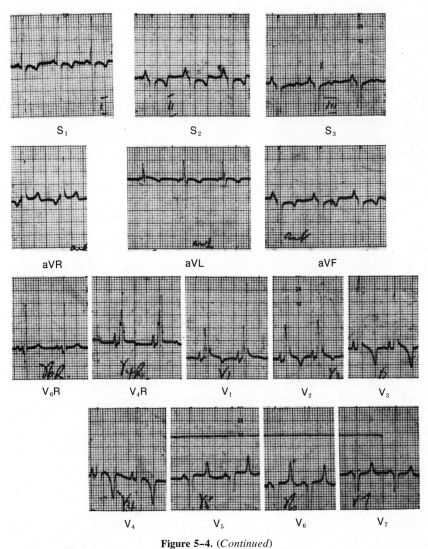

Figure 5–4. (*Continued*)

B, ECG at same age showing widespread T-wave inversion.

diomegaly and other clinical features may occur, although most of the neonatal deaths from the disease would seem to be more respiratory than cardiac. Figure 5–4 illustrates an infant with cardiac involvement and fatal outcome.*

This male infant (family 2 in Harper, 1975) was admitted to the hospital at age 7 months with increasing respiratory distress. He had been born following a normal pregnancy at 38 weeks' gestation, weighing 7 lb 12 oz at birth. Initially he was slow to feed, but subsequently was well until 1 month old when choking during feeds began. He was noted by his parents to be hypotonic but no investigation was undertaken until the onset of respiratory distress at age 7 months. Examination showed signs of bilateral basal pneumonia, with poor respiratory movements, generalised hypotonia and muscle weakness, but no muscle wasting or myotonia. Chest x-ray (Fig. 5–4*A*) showed marked cardiac enlargement in addition to bilateral lower lobe consolidation. The ECG (Fig. 5–4*B*) showed right atrial hypertrophy with incomplete right bundle-branch block as well as left ventricular hypertrophy, suggesting a generalised cardiomyopathy. Electromyography showed definite myotonic potentials. SCK was 260 mu/ml (normal 5 to 50). The infant continued to deteriorate and died. Subsequent investigation of the family revealed not only that a maternal aunt was a known case of myotonic dystrophy, but also that the mother herself showed slight but definite clinical and electromyographic myotonia, despite complete lack of symptoms.

PERIPHERAL VASCULAR DISEASE

Although there is no evidence that occlusive disease of major blood vessels is increased in myotonic dystrophy (coronary artery disease and angina pectoris have already been mentioned), peripheral vascular symptoms are frequent. In particular, vasomotor symptoms such as coldness and episodic pallor of hands and feet have been noted. These features are given more prominence in the early literature than subsequently. Steinert (1909) noted two of his original patients to have episodic coldness and numbness of the hands, and Thomasen (1948) found some degree of vasomotor symptoms in two-thirds of his patients. It is possible that improvements in home heating in recent years have reduced the prominence of these symptoms, which in any case are frequent in most wasting neuromuscular disorders. It is also of note that the patient in Thomasen's series with the most severe vasomotor disturbance, showing features of classical Raynaud's disease, had a number of relatives without myotonic dystrophy but with equally severe vasomotor symptoms.

---

*Reported by courtesy of Dr. J. R. Harper, Northampton, U.K.

RESPIRATORY COMPLICATIONS IN MYOTONIC DYSTROPHY

No evidence exists for direct involvement of pulmonary or bronchial tissue in myotonic dystrophy, but indirect involvement nonetheless may be of great importance. There are three distinct though related mechanisms for such effects:(1) aspiration of material as a result of failure in function of the pharyngo-oesophageal musculature; (2) weakness and myotonia of the respiratory muscles; and (3) less well understood, a probable cerebral abnormality of the control of respiration. Respiratory problems have long been recognised to be a major feature of patients with advanced muscle disease, but it has become clear that more mildly affected cases also may be at risk, in particular when exposed to general anaesthesia. Evidence has also been obtained recently to show that respiratory involvement is a feature of congenital myotonic dystrophy, and may be a major cause of mortality in affected infants.

Bronchial Aspiration

The abnormalities in pharyngeal and oesophageal contraction that so frequently result in aspiration of material into the bronchial tree have been discussed in Chapter 4. Although the cause is gastrointestinal, the resulting symptoms are mostly respiratory, and may have lethal results, particularly in those patients with significant weakness, because of the possibility of aspiration.

Common presenting symptoms resulting from aspiration are recurrent chest infections, unexplained fever and pleuritic chest pain. Chest x-ray may show patchy consolidation or collapse, and small areas of atelectasis are frequent in the absence of symptoms. The role of bronchial aspiration in causing these problems has already been illustrated by the patient shown in Figure 4–2, and the chest radiographs are shown in Figure 5–5. Of the 19 patients studied by Lee and Hughes (1964), ten had recurrent chest infections, and eight of these showed linear basal opacities on x-ray examination. Pruzanski (1962) reported two patients with bronchiectasis, and this was also present in one of the patients of Hughes et al (1965). The association of bronchiectasis with severe reflux has been shown by patient A. N. (Fig. 4–3), in whom swallowed contrast medium was aspirated and outlined the bronchiectatic area. This case also emphasises the fact that a near-fatal aspiration pneumonia can occur in an active patient with little muscular disability, and is not merely a terminal event in those with advanced muscle disease.

The complete prevention of bronchial aspiration is not always feasible, but it may be reduced considerably by common-sense measures such as

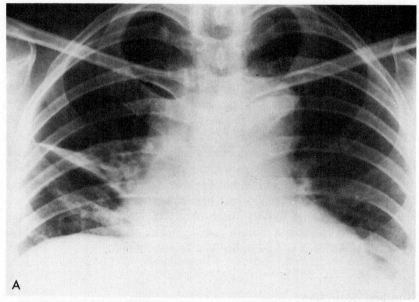

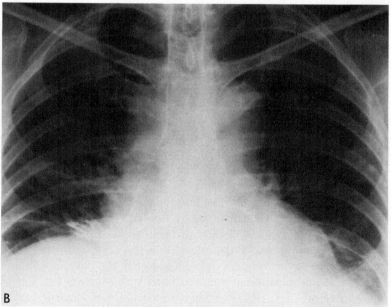

Figure 5–5. ASPIRATION PNEUMONIA IN MYOTONIC DYSTROPHY.

Chest x-rays of patient W. R. (see also Figs. 4–1 and 4–2.)

A, Initial chest x-ray on admission with acute pneumonia, showing changes of consolidation in right mid zone.

B, Persisting contrast medium in segments of right main bronchus after swallowing small amount of Dionosil contrast medium.

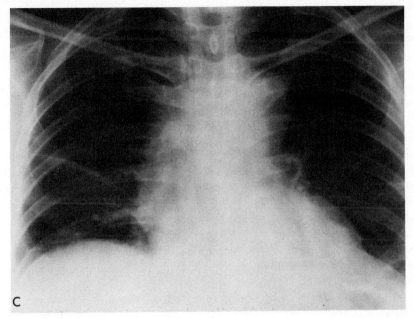

Figure 5–5. (*Continued*)

C, Repeat chest x-ray three months subsequently. The lung changes have largely cleared but the right hemidiaphragm remains elevated.

avoidance of hurried meals, thickening the consistency of liquid foods such as soups, avoiding large meals late at night, and sleeping with the head of the bed elevated. Prompt treatment of chest infections with antibiotics and physiotherapy, and a high index of suspicion that aspiration may be occurring, will also help to reduce the respiratory complications.

Diaphragmatic Involvement

As long ago as 1931 Rouquès reported that one of his cases of myotonic dystrophy showed an elevated right hemidiaphragm on x-ray examination, and that movements of both sides were reduced. Autopsy evidence of changes in the diaphragm similar to those seen in other muscles was found by Londrès (1935), although Black and Ravin (1947) encountered no diaphragmatic abnormalities in their five autopsied cases. A succession of further studies, particularly those by Caughey (Caughey and Gray, 1954; Caughey and Pachomov, 1959; Caughey and Myrianthopoulos, 1963), has confirmed that diaphragmatic function during life may be abnormal.

These authors studied seven patients, all showing unilateral elevation of the diaphragm, and of the two examined histologically (one at autopsy, one from a biopsy at cholecystectomy) both showed degenerative changes in the diaphragmatic muscle.

Radiological studies of diaphragmatic movement have suggested that the diaphragmatic abnormality is not simply the result of weakness and atrophy, but also of myotonia. Benaim and Worster-Drought (1954) and Kilburn et al (1959) reported jerky diaphragmatic movements with delayed return of the diaphragm to its normal position. The patient in the former study showed myotonia of the intercostal muscles; inaccessibility of the diaphragm until more recently has prevented attempts to record myotonia in it directly by electromyography, but Smorto et al (1972) were able to record from the diaphragmatic leaflet arising from the 12th rib in a severely affected woman, and showed myotonic potentials during inspiration.

Attention has recently been focussed on the function of the diaphragm in infants with myotonic dystrophy. Elevation of the diaphragm has been noted in a number of instances (Bell and Smith, 1972; Harper, 1975) and in some has been confused with eventration of the diaphragm (Harper, 1975; Aicardi et al, 1975). Autopsy has shown severely atrophic diaphragmatic musculature (Bossen et al, 1974; Harper, 1975), and there seems little doubt that this may be an important factor in the high mortality seen in the neonatal period in these infants. Intercostal muscle involvement has also been documented (Bossen et al, 1974) and may be responsible for the characteristically thin ribs that are seen (Fried et al, 1975). These aspects are fully discussed along with the other complications of congenital myotonic dystrophy in Chapter 9, but it is of interest to note that Caughey and Pachomov (1959) considered the possibility that the diaphragmatic elevation seen in adults was the result of a congenital defect rather than of progressive atrophy.

Alveolar Hypoventilation

One of the most intriguing aspects of respiratory function in myotonic dystrophy has been the discovery of alveolar hypoventilation in some affected individuals, and its possible relationship with the tendency to hypersomnia that is so characteristic a feature of many patients. Benaim and Worster-Drought (1954) were the first to document this, and subsequent patients were reported by Kilburn et al (1959), Bashour et al (1955), Caughey and Myrianthopoulos (1963) and others.

In all these cases there was marked hypercapnia and diminished oxygen tension, with a reduced respiratory response to inspired CO_2 and a secondary polycythaemia. Although lung function tests showed a restrictive pattern with diminished vital capacity, the abnormality of blood gases was out of proportion to that expected from the results of voluntary respiratory effort, and obesity was not more than moderate. In the early reports the possibility was raised that diaphragmatic myotonia, as evidenced by the abnormal jerky movements already mentioned, was the cause; a recent detailed study by Coccagna et al (1975) has provided interesting evidence on this point.

The patient of these authors was a 50 year old man who from adolescence had a tendency to hypersomnia, and who showed marked alveolar hypoventilation when investigated. Twenty-four-hour studies of respiratory rhythm were performed and it was shown that during sleep a marked deterioration in the blood gases occurred, along with a rise in pulmonary artery pressure, and the breathing became increasingly irregular and inadequate. The EEG showed abnormalities that were corrected by voluntary hyperventilation, and after a week on an intermittent positive-pressure breathing apparatus the blood gases were considerably improved while the patient was awake, although not during sleep. The tendency to hypersomnia persisted despite the return towards normal of blood gases.

Further evidence of an abnormal ventilatory response has come from a study of Carroll et al (1977) on seven patients with mild muscle disease, which showed a marked reduction of response to both CO_2 and oxygen in the absence of significant lung disease.

These studies raise the question whether alveolar hypoventilation may explain the more general tendency to hypersomnia and other abnormalities of the central nervous system, or whether the hypoventilation is itself a manifestation of a more general abnormality of cerebral function. Several points seem clear regarding this.

1. Weakness of the respiratory muscles cannot be the sole factor since some patients have had only mild general muscle weakness and adequate function on voluntary respiration.

2. Obesity has been only slight in most reported cases.

3. The tendency to hypersomnia has often preceded known respiratory abnormality by many years.

4. Some patients with hypersomnia do not show obvious hypoventilation, and correction of the blood gases does not abolish the hypersomnia.

5. The diminished respiratory response to CO_2 indicates an abnormality of cerebral control of respiration.

From this it seems inescapable that there is both a cerebral and a respiratory component to the problem; the question is, which is the primary abnormality? It can be argued that a longstanding immobility of the diaphragm from myotonia might produce a tendency to hypoventilation that could result in decreased CO_2 sensitivity of the brain stem and further hypoventilation, as seen in the hypoventilation syndromes associated with chronic obstructive lung disease and with obesity. Against this is the fact that hypoventilation and somnolence are not features of myotonia congenita and other non-progressive myotonias, in which the degree of myotonia is commonly much more severe than in myotonic dystrophy. The argument in favor of a primary cerebral defect is given support by the associated cerebral features of mild progressive dementia, the occurrence of histological thalamic abnormalities (Chapter 7) and by the frequency of mental retardation in congenital myotonic dystrophy, as well as by the existence of cerebral involvement in related disorders such as Duchenne dystrophy (Dubowitz, 1965). However, it could equally be argued that some of these cerebral changes themselves could be at least partly due to chronic anoxia from hypoventilation.

To resolve these questions requires the detailed study of those patients with mild muscle disease in whom somnolence is prominent without overt alveolar hypoventilation. If the respiratory abnormality should prove to be the major one it may have important implications for early treatment of the myotonic state. Meanwhile, taking into account the numerous systems that appear to be directly affected by the disease, the author suspects that both the central nervous system and the respiratory muscles will prove to be involved as primary factors.

ANAESTHETIC RISKS IN MYOTONIC DYSTROPHY

The established cases of myotonic dystrophy, with muscle wasting and respiratory impairment, clearly represent a considerable anaesthetic hazard, and as such should be treated with particular caution by anaesthetist, surgeon and physician alike. Paradoxically, such patients are not those at greatest risk, but rather the mild or undiagnosed individuals who may present with one of the systemic problems needing surgery, such as cataract, or who may require anaesthesia during childbirth or for a coincidental disorder. These patients may fail to mention or may be unaware of their muscle symptoms, and may only be recognised as having a neuromuscular problem as a result of failure to establish adequate respiration postoperatively.

Numerous individual instances of anaesthetic complications, including death, are recorded. Two patients studied by the author had postoperative respiratory failure following Caesarian section, and are discussed in Chapter 6. In one of these the cause was first considered to be cholinesterase deficiency, and then myasthenia gravis. A middle-aged man died following cholecystectomy, having been considered to have hypoparathyroidism because of cataracts and "tetany"; another patient, diagnosed as part of a family study in the absence of specific muscular symptoms, had suffered severe postoperative respiratory difficulties following cholecystectomy the previous year, which had led her physician to question whether there might not be an underlying neurological cause.

The relationship of complications to the type of anaesthetic agent used has been the subject of considerable discussion. Dundee (1952) considered that thiopentone was particularly responsible and that affected patients showed a specific sensitivity to this drug. Bourke and Zuck (1957) also reported a patient with complications related to thiopentone anaesthesia. Their patient recovered, and was subsequently given a test dose of 50 mg thiopentone which resulted in prolonged apnoea. They reasonably concluded from this that a hypersensitivity to this drug existed, and that it should be avoided. Another fatal anaesthetic disaster was reported by Caughey and Myrianthopoulos (1963), which shows that death under anaesthesia is not confined to the elderly or severely incapacitated. The patient was a 12 year old girl undergoing correction of ptosis; previous investigation had confirmed the diagnosis of myotonic dystrophy but had not shown cardiac or respiratory abnormalities.

A valuable review of the subject was provided by Kaufman (1960), who searched the records of patients previously studied by Maas in London and obtained details on 25 operations, not selected because they had given rise to problems. Fifteen were uneventful, but five produced respiratory difficulties and four others ended in death. The fatal cases all had severe muscle disease; in three of them ventilatory failure was the main trouble. A fourth died suddenly following cholecystectomy, and no specific cause could be found. Two of the fatal cases had not received thiopentone, and Kaufman concluded that the problems resulted more from the general depressant effects of the drugs used on respiration than from a specific effect of thiopentone or other agents. A further fatal case was described by Tsueda et al (1975), in which a 49 year old woman, with a previous history of periodic somnolence, died in ventilatory failure following cholecystectomy. The diagnosis of myotonic dystrophy was not firmly made until after her death when her brother was found to be affected.

Several authors subsequently have described other aspects of anaesthesia in myotonic dystrophy. Ravin et al (1975) reported two patients undergoing oral surgery, one of whom had severe airway obstruction postoperatively, and Hook et al (1975) discussed the management during Caesarian section; their patient's problems resulted more from haemorrhage than from anaesthesia. The possible role of arrhythmias in anaesthetic and postoperative deaths has not been fully explored, and deserves more attention in view of the frequency of their occurrence, and the instances of sudden death independent of anaesthesia (see Table 5–2). Most of the reported difficulties appear to be respiratory in nature, but a careful check for clinical and electrocardiographic evidence of irregularity and conduction defects is a wise precaution.

Recent interest in the association of malignant hyperpyrexia in response to anaesthetics and muscle relaxants with a specific subclinical myopathy (Denborough et al, 1970) has raised the question whether such a reaction could also occur in the myotonic disorders. Myotonia is not a feature of hyperpyrexic myopathy but muscle hypertrophy may be marked. There are isolated reports of hyperpyrexia in myotonia congenita (Saidman et al, 1964; Morley et al, 1973), but in the former case the diagnosis was doubtful, and a muscle biopsy from the latter patient did not show the characteristic pharmacological response of malignant hyperpyrexia (Moulds and Denborough, 1974); the response of muscle from patients with myotonic dystrophy and hypokalaemic periodic paralysis was also normal. A single report exists of malignant hyperpyrexia in a patient with myotonic dystrophy (Schellnack et al, 1976), but in the light of the close attention paid to anaesthetic problems in myotonic dystrophy it would not seem that malignant hyperpyrexia is a high risk for patients with this condition or related myotonic disorders.

The sensible precautions for anaesthesia in patients with myotonic dystrophy are summarised, from a physician's viewpoint, below.

1. Awareness of the diagnosis prior to anaesthesia and surgery, and avoidance of unnecessary procedures.

2. Careful preoperative clinical assessment of cardiac and respiratory function.

3. ECG, with special attention to defects of rhythm and prolonged conduction.

4. Chest x-ray, with emphasis on possible elevation of the diaphragm and atelectasis due to silent aspiration.

5. Pulmonary function tests, to assess the adequacy of the respiratory muscles and to exclude alveolar hypoventilation.

6. Careful postoperative nursing and medical care, with special attention to adequate ventilatory function and to ensuring that muscle weakness of jaw or neck does not result in obstruction of the airway.

The observation of these relatively simple procedures should considerably reduce the hazards of general anaesthesia in myotonic dystrophy.

REFERENCES

Aicardi J., Conti D. and Goutières F. (1975): Clinical and genetic aspects of the neonatal form of Steinert myotonic dystrophy. J. Genet. Hum. (Suppl.) *23*:146–157.

Bashour F., Winchell P. and Reddington J. (1955): Myotonia atrophica and cyanosis. N. Engl. J. Med. *252*:768–770.

Bell D. B. and Smith D. W. (1972): Myotonic dystrophy in the neonate. J. Pediatr. *81*:83–86.

Benaim S. and Worster-Drought C. (1954): Dystrophia myotonica with myotonia of the diaphragm causing pulmonary hypoventilation with anoxaemia and secondary polycythaemia. Med. Illus. *8*:221–226.

Berthold H. (1958): Zur pathologischen Anatomie der Dystrophia myotonica (Curschmann-Steinert). Dtsch. Z. Nervenheilkd. *178*:394–412.

Black W. C. and Ravin A. (1947): Studies in dystrophia myotonica. VII. Autopsy observations in five cases. Arch. Pathol. *44*:176–191.

Bossen E. H., Shelburne J. D. and Verkauf B. S. (1974): Respiratory muscle involvement in infantile myotonic dystrophy. Arch. Pathol. *97*:250–252.

Bourke T. D. and Zuck D. (1957): Thiopentone in dystrophia myotonica. Br. J. Anaesth. *29*:35–38.

Bulloch R. T., Davis J. L. and Hara M. (1967): Dystrophia myotonica with heart block: a light and electron microscopic study. Arch. Pathol. *84*:130–140.

Cannon P. J. (1962): The heart and lungs in myotonic muscular dystrophy. Am. J. Med. *32*:765–775.

Carroll J. E., Zwillich C. W. and Weil J. V. (1977): Ventilatory response in myotonic dystrophy. Neurology *27*:1125–1128.

Casas J. C. L. (1973): Cardiovascular changes in Steinert's disease. Arch. Inst. Cardiol. Mex. *43*:779–786.

Caughey J. E. and Gray W. G. (1954): Unilateral elevation of the diaphragm in dystrophia myotonica. Thorax *9*:67–70.

Caughey J. E. and Myrianthopoulos N. E. (1963): Dystrophia Myotonica and Related Disorders. Charles C Thomas, Springfield, Ill.

Caughey J. E. and Pachomov N. (1959): The diaphragm in dystrophia myotonica. J. Neurol. Neurosurg. Psychiatry *22*:311–313.

Church S. C. (1967): The heart in myotonia atrophica. Arch. Intern. Med. *119*:176–181.

Coccagna G., Mantovani M., Parch C., Miron F., and Lugares E. (1975): Alveolar hypoventilation and hypersomnia in myotonic dystrophy. J. Neurol. Neurosurg. Psychiatry *38*:977–984.

Denborough M. A., Ebeling P., King J. O. and Zapf P. (1970): Myopathy and malignant hyperpyrexia. Lancet *1*:1138–1140.

Dubowitz V. (1965): Intellectual impairment in muscular dystrophy. Arch. Dis. Child. *40*:296–301.

Dundee J. (1952): Thiopentone in dystrophia myotonica. Anesth. Analg. (Cleve.) *31*:257–260.

Evans W. (1944): The heart in myotonia atrophica. Br. Heart J. *4*:41–47.

Fearrington E. L., Gibson T. C. and Churchill R. E. (1964): Vectorcardiographic and electrocardiographic findings in myotonia atrophica: a study employing the Frank lead system. Am. Heart J. *67*:559–609.

Fisch C. and Evans P. V. (1954): The heart in dystrophia myotonica; report of autopsied case. N. Engl. J. Med. *251*:527–529.

Griffith T. W. (1911): On myotonia. Q. J. Med. *5*:229–247.

Griggs R. C., Davies R. J., Anderson D. C. and Dove J. T. (1975): Cardiac conduction in myotonic dystrophy. Am. J. Med. *59*:37–42.

Guillain G., Bertrand I. and Rouquès L. (1932): Les lésions de la myotonie atrophique. Ann. Med. *31*:180–197.

Harper P. S. (1975): Congenital myotonic dystrophy in Britain. 1. Clinical aspects. Arch. Dis. Child. *50*:505–513.

Harper P. S. (1975): Congenital myotonic dystrophy in Britain. II. Genetic basis. Arch Dis. Child. *50*:514–521.

Holt J. M. and Lambert E. H. (1964): Heart disease as the presenting feature in myotonia atrophica. Br. Heart J. *26*:433–436.

Hook R., Anderson E. F. and Noto P. (1975): Anaesthetic management of a patient with myotonia dystrophica. Anaesthesiology *43*:689–692.

Hughes D. T., Swann J. C., Gleeson J. E. and Lee F. I. (1965): Abnormalities in swallowing associated with dystrophia myotonica. Brain *88*:1037–1042.

Josephson M. E., Caracta A. R., Gallagher J. J. and Damato A. N. (1973): Site of conduction disturbances in a family with myotonic dystrophy. Am. J. Cardiol. *32*:114–118.

Kaufman L. (1960): Anaesthesia in dystrophia myotonica. A review of the hazards of anaesthesia. Proc. R. Soc. Med. *53*:183–188.

Kilburn K. H., Eagen J. T. and Heyman A. (1959): Cardiopulmonary insufficiency associated with myotonic dystrophy. Am. J. Med. *26*:929–935.

Lee F. I. and Hughes D. T. (1964): Systemic effects in dystrophia myotonia. Brain 87:521–536.

Londrès G. (1935): Sur l'étiologie de la myotonie atrophique. Rev. Neurol. 63:556–665.

Maas O. and Zondek H. (1920): Untersuchungsbefund an einem Fall von Dystrophia Myotonica. Z. Gesamte Neurol. Psychiatr. 59:322–331.

Morley J. B., Lambert T. F. and Kakulas B. A. (1973): Excerpta Medica International Congress Series 295, 543.

Moulds R. F. W. and Denborough M. A. (1974): Myopathies and malignant hyperpyrexia. Br. Med. J. (1974) 3:520.

Munsat T. L. (1967): Therapy of myotonia. A double-blind evaluation of diphenylhydantoin, procainamide and placebo. Neurology 17:359–367.

Orndahl G., Thulesius O., Enestrom S. and Dehlin O. (1964): The heart in myotonic disease. Acta Med. Scand. 176:479–491.

Parvu V. (1973): Inima in distrofia miotonica. Med. Interna. (Bucur) 25:71–86.

Petkovich N. J., Dunn M. and Reed W. (1964): Myotonia dystrophica with A-V dissociation and Stokes-Adams attacks. A case report and review of the literature. Am. Heart J. 68:391–396.

Pruzanski W. (1962): Respiratory tract infections and silent aspiration in myotonic dystrophy. Dis. Chest 42:608–610.

Rausing A. (1972): Focal myocarditis in familial dystrophia myotonica. Br. Heart J. 34:1292–1294.

Ravin M., Newmak Z. and Saviello G. (1975): Myotonia dystrophica — an anaesthetic hazard: two case reports. Anesth. Analg. 54:216–218.

Rouquès L. (1931): La myotonie atrophique. Thesis, Paris.

Saidman L. J., Havard E. S. and Eger E. I. (1964): Hyperthermia during anesthesia. J.A.M.A. 190:1029–1032.

Salomon J. and Easley R. M. (1973): Cardiovascular abnormalities in myotonic dystrophy. Chest 64:135–137.

Schellnack K., Regling G., Hofmann J., Buntrock P., Martin H. and Hecht H. (1976): Maligne Hyperthermie bei subklinischer myotonischer Dystrophie. Beitr. Orthop. Traumatol. 23:537–544.

Schmitt J. and Schmidt C. (1975): Steinert disease and heart. Complete expression of the gene on heart muscle tissue. J. Genet. Hum. 23:59–64.

Schmitt J., Schmidt C., Clerget M. and Luporsi D. (1974): Les troubles cardiaques de la maladie de Steinert. Ann Méd. Intern. 125:195–199.

Smorto M. P., Vignieri M. R. and Fierro B. (1972): The diaphragm in dystrophia myotonica. Riv. Neurobiol. 18:48–54.

Spillane J. D. (1951): The heart in myotonia atrophica. Br. Heart J. 13:343–347.

Spurney O. M. and Woolf J. W. (1962): Prolonged atrial flutter in myotonic dystrophy. Am. J. Cardiol. 10:886–889.

Tanaka N., Tanaka H., Takada M., Niimura T., Kanehisa T. and Terashi S. (1973): Cardiomyopathy in myotonic dystrophy. A light and electron microscopic study of the myocardium. Jap. Heart J. 14:202–212.

Théry C., Ketelers J. Y., Gosseun B., Lekieffre J., Béthouart M. and Warembourgh (1975): Le block auriculo-ventriculaire de la maladie de Steinert. Etude électrophysiologique et histologique des voies de conduction. Arch. Mal. Coeur 68:1087–1093.

Thomasen E. (1948): Myotonia. Universitetsforlaget Aarhus.

Thomson A. M. P. (1968): Dystrophia cordis myotonica studied by serial histology of the pacemaker and conducting system. J. Pathol. Bacteriol. 96:285–295.

Tsueda K., Shibutani K. and Lefkowitz M. (1975): Postoperative ventilatory failure in an obese, myopathic woman with periodic somnolence: a case report. Anesth. Analg. (Cleve.) 54: 523–526.

Uemura N., Tanaka H., Niimura T., Hashiguchi N., Yoshimura M., Terashi S. and Kanesisa T. (1973): Electrophysiological and histological abnormalities of the heart in myotonic dystrophy. Am. Heart J. 86:616–624.

Waring J. J., Ravin A. and Walker C. E. (1940): Studies in dystrophia myotonica: clinical features and treatment. Arch. Intern. Med. 65:763–799.

Winters S. J., Schreiner B., Griggs R. C., Rowley P. and Nanda N. C. (1977): Familial mitral valve prolapse and myotonic dystrophy.

CHAPTER SIX

Endocrine Abnormalities in Myotonic Dystrophy

From the time of the earliest descriptions of myotonic dystrophy (Steinert, 1909; Curschmann, 1912) testicular atrophy has been recognised to be a feature of myotonic dystrophy, and subsequently it has come to be realised that a more widespread disturbance of endocrine function is frequently seen, particularly of insulin metabolism, but also possibly of the pituitary. There is still inadequate documentation of the extent of these abnormalities, and less information still on their underlying basis, let alone how they relate to each other and to the muscle abnormalities. Much of the early work was limited by the available techniques of investigation; the advent of radioimmunoassays has enabled more precise data to be collected on some aspects of endocrine function, but others remain unexplored by modern techniques. Table 6–1 summarises the overall state of our knowledge.

THE GONADAL DEFECT

Testicular atrophy was recognised early to be a feature of adult males with myotonic dystrophy, and there now exists satisfactory evidence as to the type of lesion and its endocrine consequences, although why it should occur and its relation to the muscle abnormality is completely unknown.

The early reports of Steinert (1909) and Curschmann (1912) documented the occurrence of testicular atrophy. In the survey of Thomasen (1948), 37 out of 43 adult males (86 per cent) had testicular atrophy, and Klein (1958) found it in 71 of 113 examined (62.8 per cent). Both autopsy and biopsy studies have confirmed this high incidence of abnormality, and

115

Table 6–1.   ENDOCRINE ABNORMALITIES IN MYOTONIC DYSTROPHY

Organ	Frequent Abnormalities	Rare or Inconsistent Abnormalities
Testis	Testicular atrophy (60 to 80% clinically); degeneration of tubular cells; hyperplasia of Leydig cells; serum testosterone slightly reduced	
Ovary	No consistent evidence of abnormality; high fetal loss	
Pituitary	Increased FSH levels; slightly increased LH levels; increased LRH response	Hyperresponsiveness to exogenous growth hormone; pituitary adenoma
Pancreas	Increased insulin response to glucose load and other stimuli	Clinical diabetes; abnormal glucose tolerance test
Thyroid	No evidence of abnormality, but myotonia sometimes found in hypothyroidism	
Adrenal Parathyroid	No consistent abnormality found	

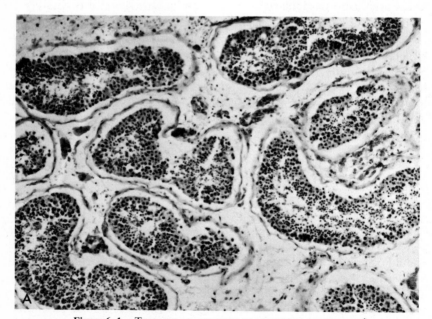

Figure 6–1.   Testicular atrophy in myotonic dystrophy*

A, Normal testis of 52 year old man (× 135).
*Preparations by courtesy of Dr. Windsor Fortt.

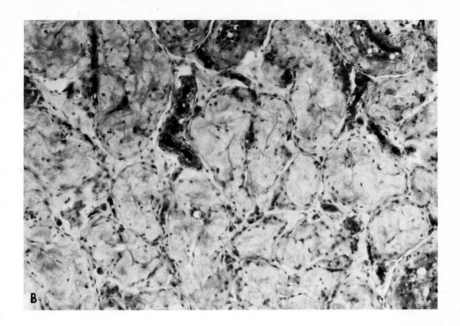

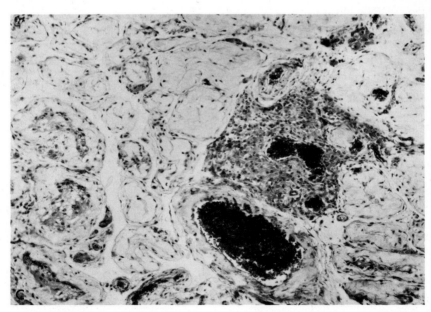

Figure 6–1. (*Continued*)

B, Testis from patient W.R. (age 60) showing severe atrophy and hyalinisation of tubular cells (× 135).

C, Patient W.R. showing area of focal hyperplasia of Leydig cells, contrasting with tubular atrophy (× 135).

have shown that the principal changes are atrophy, hyalinisation and fibrosis of the seminiferous tubules, with reduced spermatogenesis (Thomasen, 1948; Caughey and Brown, 1950; Marshall, 1959; Caughey and Myrianthopoulos, 1963). The interstitial cells, by contrast, have been shown to increase in number and size, with crystalline deposits between them. Similarity to the changes in the Klinefelter (XXY) syndrome has been noted by several authors. The changes in the testis are illustrated in Figure 6–1.

The observed structural changes correlate well with the endocrine findings. Early studies on urinary gonadotrophin excretion were conflicting (Marshall, 1959; Drucker et al, 1961; Caughey and Myrianthopoulos, 1963), but studies of plasma gonadotrophins measured by radioimmunoassay (Harper et al, 1972) showed a marked elevation of follicle stimulating hormone (FSH) levels in adult males, even in those who were mildly affected with few or no symptoms (Fig. 6–2A). Levels of luteinising hormone (LH), by contrast, were mostly normal or only moderately elevated (Fig. 6–2B), and testosterone levels were mainly moderately reduced or in the low normal range. Study by Sagel et al (1975) of the response of eight affected males to luteinising hormone–releasing hormone (LRH), the hypothalamic releasing factor considered to be responsible for control of both LH and FSH, showed a similar pattern of response. The basal level of FSH was high with an increased response to LRH in all patients except one without testicular atrophy. Basal levels of LH were normal, but the response to LRH was slightly increased. These results leave no doubt that the primary defect is gonadal, with a secondary overproduction of pituitary gonadotrophins. In addition they strongly support the histological evidence of a selective involvement of the seminiferous tubules with relative sparing of interstitial cells until a later stage; the regulation of FSH secretion is considered to be controlled by a tubular factor, so far unidentified, whereas LH secretion is primarily controlled by levels of testosterone, itself directly produced by the interstitial cells. These endocrine findings also explain the relative normality of the secondary sex characteristics in myotonic dystrophy, even when marked testicular atrophy is present.

The studies discussed above give no evidence to suggest an abnormality in the hypothalamic-gonadal axis, but one of three males studied by Febres et al (1975) showed reduced FSH and LH levels with normal pituitary responsiveness, suggesting a hypothalamic cause. The exceptional nature of this patient is shown by the total absence of gonadal tissue in two biopsies, and it cannot be excluded that a coincidental disorder was present.

Information on the prepubertal testis in myotonic dystrophy is limited, but Hamilton (1974) studied testicular material from six patients with childhood onset of the disease, most of whom had congenital onset.

Histology of the testis was essentially normal in all cases, but analysis of enzymes involved in testosterone metabolism showed a reduction in 17,20-desmolase and of 17-reductase in three and two patients respectively. Meiotic chromosome studies on the testis of a child with congenital myotonic dystrophy (family 1 in Dyken and Harper, 1973) showed no abnormality.

The high frequency of testicular tubular changes, even in mildly affected individuals, might lead one to expect a high degree of male

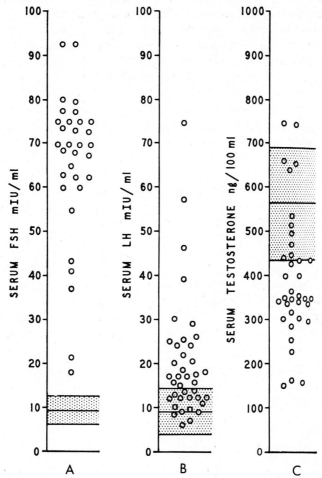

Figure 6-2. CHANGES IN SERUM GONADOTROPHINS AND TESTOSTERONE IN A SERIES OF ADULT MALES WITH MYOTONIC DYSTROPHY.*

A, FSH: the level in all patients is raised considerably above the normal adult range.

B, LH: although some patients have elevated levels there is considerable overlap with the normal range.

C, Testosterone: most patients show moderately reduced or low normal levels.

*From Harper et al, 1972.

infertility in myotonic dystrophy, but this is only partially the case. Caughey and Myrianthopoulos (1963) have recorded a man who fathered a child when already documented as having testicular tubular atrophy. On the other hand some patients complain of impotence, and others remain unmarried. Thomasen (1948) found almost half his patients aged over 25 to be unmarried, although the fertility of those who were married was no different from their healthy sibs. Klein (1958) found 55 per cent of 148 affected Swiss men over 30 years to be unmarried. The fertility data are discussed fully in relation to inheritance in Chapter 10. All series agree in showing a moderate reduction in both sexes, male fertility being more reduced than female except in the series of Bell (1948).

The possibility of gonadal abnormality in females with myotonic dystrophy has received little attention, and the cyclical nature of female gonadal hormone secretion makes study difficult except under carefully controlled conditions. Marshall (1959) found no abnormality of oestrogen excretion in two affected women studied over a three-week period, and the four women observed by Sagel et al (1975) showed no abnormality of gonadotrophin and testosterone levels, nor of response to LRH, although all complained of oligomenorrhoea. Likewise, the single amenorrhoeic woman reported by Febres et al (1975) showed normal gonadotrophins and normal response to clomiphene. Since the primary gonadal lesion in the male appears to be in the tubular cells of the testis, which have no functional homologous counterpart in the female, it is not surprising that women do not appear to show the secondary gonadotrophin changes present in men.

At a clinical level, affected women show little evidence of hypogonadism or other gonadal dysfunction. Information collected by the author on 44 affected adult females and 25 unaffected sibs and spouses in the same families is given in Table 6–2. The high incidence of gynaecological symptoms in the controls illustrates the need for caution in interpreting the results from the affected members.

Table 6–2.   REPRODUCTIVE DATA ON WOMEN WITH
MYOTONIC DYSTROPHY

	Affected	Controls
Total Studied	44	25
Age at Study (Years)	38.62 ± 12.79	38.52 ± 13.78
Liveborn Children	81	53
Live Births per Individual	1.84	2.12
Hysterectomy	13/44 (29.5%)	2/25 (8.0%)
	4/44 (9.1%)	0/25 (0%)
Menstruation: Excessively heavy	17/40 (43.5%)	11/24 (46.0%)
Excessively painful	22/40 (57.5%)	6/22 (27.3%)
Excessively irregular	14/40 (35.0%)	5/21 (23.8%)
Age at Menarche (Years)	13.13 ± 1.49	12.60 ± 0.89
Age at Menopause (Years)	40.0 ± 9.42	48.1 ± 4.19

Table 6–3.   MATERNAL COMPLICATIONS OF PREGNANCY
IN MYOTONIC DYSTROPHY

Increased muscle weakness (not common)
Increased spontaneous abortion rate
Reduced fetal movements
Hydramnios
Prolonged first stage of labour
Reduced voluntary muscle power in second stage
Retained placenta
Postpartum haemorrhage
Anaesthetic sensitivity
Increased neonatal mortality*

*See Chapter 9.

PREGNANCY

The intrauterine and neonatal problems of the infant born to the mother with myotonic dystrophy are discussed fully in the section on the disorder in childhood (Chapter 9). There is much less information available as to the effects of pregnancy on the affected mother, and no prospective study of the subject has been undertaken; the existing case reports are likely to reflect a bias towards describing the abnormal, although Shore (1975), Sarnat et al (1976) and Donaldson (1978) have provided useful reviews of the subject. The major obstetrical problems are summarised in Table 6–3.

Davis (1958) and Hopkins and Wray (1967) reported cases in which the infant was normal but in which muscle weakness in the mother was temporarily worsened during a pregnancy. The author has not encountered objective increase in weakness, although pregnancy is a time when increased medical supervision is likely to bring existing weakness to attention. Sciarra and Steer (1961) were the first to document manometrically abnormal uterine contraction during labour. The patient had inadequate uterine contractions with a delayed relaxation phase which was shortened by administration of oxytocin. The same patient had earlier suffered a cardiac arrest at 15 weeks' gestation when quinidine conversion of atrial flutter was attempted — an unwise procedure for both mother and fetus. Despite these problems the infant was apparently normal at birth.

Shore and MacLachan (1971) studied electromyographically the myometrium of a non-pregnant woman with myotonic dystrophy, and found incoordinated contraction but no relaxation delay after electrical stimulation. They observed two pregnancies and collected data on six others. Three of the eight infants had features suggestive of congenital myotonic dystrophy (see Chapter 9). Poor uterine contractions were observed in five out of the eight pregnancies. Retention of the placenta and postpartum haemorrhage due to poor uterine contraction were other complications; the first stage of labour was prolonged (over 24 hours in three cases). Shore (1975) also mentions premature delivery as a complication, but this was not a feature of the author's series (Harper, 1975a).

The significance for the fetus of hydramnios during pregnancy is discussed in Chapter 9; for the obstetrician it is a clear indication that neonatal problems are to be expected. The study of Harper (1975a) showed a high incidence of hydramnios (30 per cent) as well as a reduction in fetal movements in those pregnancies leading to an affected child, but since the mothers were ascertained through having at least one congenitally affected child, these data cannot be considered representative of pregnancy as a whole in the disorder. Hydramnios should also serve as a warning not to induce labour without good reason, as the following personal case illustrates.

A 20 year old unmarried girl with myotonic dystrophy (UHW 46772), a member of an extensive and rather uncooperative family with the disorder, became pregnant. She declined termination of pregnancy, and the obstetrician was warned of the possible maternal and fetal complications of the disease. Hydramnios was noted, and it was decided to deliver her at what was considered to be full term. The baby proved to be premature (wt 2.3 kg), was hypotonic and developed fulminating respiratory distress, dying aged 48 hours. Whether prematurity alone was the cause of death or whether the infant also had myotonic dystrophy is debatable, but it is likely that the hydramnios contributed to an inaccurate assessment of fetal maturity.

The cause of the hydramnios has now been documented as inadequate fetal swallowing. Dunn and Dierker (1973) demonstrated delayed swallowing of intra-amniotic Hypaque in the second pregnancy of a woman who had hydramnios in both her pregnancies and who was only subsequently realised to have myotonic dystrophy. It is important to recognise that the incidence of hydramnios is not increased in those pregnancies resulting in a genetically normal infant, nor when the disorder is paternally transmitted — i.e., both mother and fetus must be abnormal for the hydramnios to occur (Harper, 1975a).

The author has observed two almost fatal episodes following Caesarian section in mothers of congenitally affected children (families 16 and 22 in Harper, 1975b). Both mothers were mildly affected, and were not known to have muscle disease at the time. In both cases prolonged artificial ventilation was required, acute tubular necrosis developing in one case, but fortunately with complete recovery in both instances. Gardy (1963) reported a milder case of prolonged hypoventilation after spontaneous delivery. Details of one of these cases are given below.*

---

*Courtesy of Dr. Nigel Royston, Taunton, Somerset, U.K.

A 23 year old, symptomless primagravida was admitted for induction of pregnancy because of post-maturity. Poor progress resulted from an oxytocin drip, and following the appearance of meconium-stained liquor Caesarian section was undertaken. One half-minute after induction of anaesthesia with nitrous oxide, Fluothane and Scoline she became cyanosed, but improved with additional oxygen; tubocurarine was also given. A healthy boy was delivered, but immediately postoperatively cyanosis and inadequate respiration occurred, with hypotonia and dilated pupils. Reintubation was required and the patient was maintained on an artificial respirator for 24 hours; temporary renal shutdown occurred. Spontaneous respiration was re-established after 24 hours and she recovered rapidly with no residual renal damage. No cause was found at this time for her anaesthetic sensitivity, cholinesterase deficiency being excluded. One year later she again became pregnant and Caesarian section was required because of placenta praevia. Special care was taken during anaesthesia owing to the previous episode, and there were no complications. The infant, however, was born severely hypotonic, with facial diplegia and talipes, and subsequent mental retardation (case 16 in Harper, 1975b). Examination of the mother at this stage showed obvious myotonia of grip and slight facial weakness, leading to the diagnosis of myotonic dystrophy in both mother and child; subsequently both the mother's brother and the maternal grandmother were shown to be affected.

REPRODUCTIVE LOSS

Individual case reports on pregnancies of women with myotonic dystrophy do not give an accurate picture of the overall pregnancy pattern of those affected, nor of the rate of fetal and perinatal mortality. It is important to know this in order to predict the prospective degree of risk to mother and fetus, but no published data exist; Table 6–4 gives information based on two series of patients studied by the author. The first series (Harper, 1975a) is of women ascertained through their affected children, and therefore likely to be biased towards a high incidence of neonatal

Table 6–4. REPRODUCTIVE LOSS IN WOMEN WITH MYOTONIC DYSTROPHY

	Harper (1975) AFFECTED	*Harper (1972)* AFFECTED	CONTROL
Total Live Births	149	80	53
Abortions	28	26	5
Rate per 100 live births	18.8	32.5	9.45
Stillbirths	2	3	1
Rate per 100 live births	1.34	3.75	1.89
Neonatal Deaths	24	8	0
Rate per 100 live births	16.2	10.0	0
Total Reproductive Loss	54	37	6
Rate per 100 pregnancies	30.2	34.0	10.2

problems; the second series is more representative, consisting of adult American women examined personally as part of the study of genetic linkage (Harper, 1972). The controls in this series were spouses and unaffected sibs (all examined personally); they were comparable in age distribution and social background but the use of spouses as controls inevitably meant that some of the pregnancies in the "control" series were genetically affected.

It is clear from Table 6–4 that both the rate of abortion and the neonatal death rate are sharply increased in the pregnancies of women with myotonic dystrophy; the control series by contrast shows rates comparable to those recorded for many general populations, suggesting that the poor social conditions of many affected families are unlikely to be responsible.

Figure 6–3 shows clearly that the mortality is bimodal in distribution, and that true stillbirths are not common. Most instances recorded as stillbirths proved to be liveborn infants with inadequate respiration, surviving only a few hours. The bimodal distribution suggests that different factors are likely to be operating in early pregnancy from those in the perinatal period.

Details of the neonatal deaths are given in connection with the discussion of congenital myotonic dystrophy in Chapter 9; there is strong evidence that many, probably the majority, represent severe undiagnosed instances of the congenital form of the disease, with respiratory muscle involvement and pulmonary immaturity as the immediate fatal factors. Since the first series of patients was selected through a patient being congenitally affected, a high neonatal death rate among sibs is not surprising; it is thus important that the neonatal death rate is still high (10 per cent) in the unselected series, suggesting that the risk of a child with

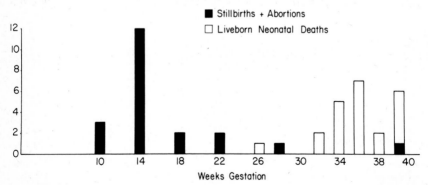

Figure 6–3. REPRODUCTIVE LOSS IN MYOTONIC DYSTROPHY IN RELATION TO GESTATIONAL AGE.

Data from Harper, 1975, including only those cases of known gestational age. Grouped by four-week periods before 26 weeks; by two-week periods after 26 weeks.

congenital myotonic dystrophy is not confined to a small subgroup of affected women.

Both series of affected women show a high rate of spontaneous abortion, raised two or three times above that in the control series and the general population rate of around 10 per cent. The peak of incidence at around three months' gestation makes it improbable that fetal neuromuscular abnormality is responsible, nor is there evidence suggesting that chromosomal or other major developmental abnormality in the fetus is a likely cause, although these abortuses have not been specifically studied. Possible maternal causes are abnormality of uterine muscular activity, as has been documented in labour, or abnormal levels of gonadal hormones. Although both are plausible, there is total lack of evidence on these matters at present.

PITUITARY

The secondary elevation of pituitary gonadotrophic hormones in males with myotonic dystrophy, resulting from the primary hypogonadism, is now well-documented (Harper et al, 1972), but the occurrence of clinically important abnormalities in other pituitary hormones, in particular growth hormone, remains doubtful, and clinical impressions have not yet been confirmed adequately by detailed endocrine study. Initial suggestions of an abnormality in growth hormone production were prompted by the superficial similarity of some of the radiographic changes to those seen in acromegaly, in particular the tendency to prognathism, the frequent occurrence of hyperostosis frontalis interna and the enlargement of the frontal air sinuses. The pituitary fossa is generally small (Caughey, 1952; Caughey and Myrianthopoulos, 1963). Autopsy studies of the pituitary gland collected by Caughey showed hyperplasia of the basophil cells in eight out of 30 cases, but in only two was there evidence of eosinophilic cell hyperplasia.

Two instances of pituitary tumour occurring in men with myotonic dystrophy have been noted, one an eosinophilic adenoma with acromegaly (Caughey, 1958), the other a massive chromophobe adenoma (Banna et al, 1973). A third instance, of a small chromophobe adenoma and without clinical abnormalities, was discovered at autopsy by Benda and Bixby (1947). The occurrence could be coincidental, but longstanding hypogonadism and secondary pituitary overaction from various causes have been recognised to be associated with the development of pituitary tumours, as discussed by Caughey, and this seems a reasonable explanation in the cases associated with myotonic dystrophy.

Endocrinological evidence of growth hormone disturbance is sparse and unconvincing. Chyatte et al (1972, 1974) found a hyperresponsiveness to exogenous human growth hormone, measured by nitrogen retention, even though these patients showed no evidence of growth hormone deficiency. The authors' claim that this might be used as therapy to arrest muscular wasting seems improbable, and no objective change was seen in the muscle status of their patients.

Caughey and Koochek (1974) found high basal growth hormone levels in two patients with myotonic dystrophy, one of whom showed a steep rise of growth hormone in response to insulin. Yamamoto et al (1974) noted a variable serum growth hormone response to intravenous insulin and to arginine infusion, which was elevated in some patients and depressed in others. In view of the abnormality in insulin metabolism documented below, and the intimate relationship between growth hormone and insulin, it would indeed be surprising if no disturbance of growth hormone were to be found in myotonic dystrophy. Nevertheless, it would appear likely that the pituitary is not primarily involved in the disorder, any disturbances being secondary to the well-established gonadal changes and the alterations in insulin metabolism.

DIABETES MELLITUS

An association between myotonic dystrophy and diabetes mellitus was first noted in the reports of Caughey and Brown (1950), Stanbury et al (1954) and Jacobson et al (1958); numerous studies have since been carried out in an attempt to document the precise nature of the abnormality in carbohydrate metabolism seen in myotonic dystrophy, and to relate it to other aspects of the disease. Surprisingly, the question of the frequency of clinical diabetes in this disorder has received little attention, and this will be considered before the detailed metabolic studies are discussed.

The individual case reports and small series on which the association was initially proposed are not sufficiently representative to enable the frequency in the general population to be inferred. Information is available, however, from several large population series that are unlikely to have missed overt clinical diabetes, and the data are summarised in Table 6–5. The author's control series consisted of spouses and unaffected

Table 6–5. CLINICAL DIABETES IN MYOTONIC DYSTROPHY

	Diabetic	Non-diabetic	Total	% Diabetic
Thomasen (1948)	0	101	101	0
Klein (1958)	7	234	241	2.90
Harper (unpublished data):				
Myotonic dystrophy	11	158	169	6.50
Controls	2	120	122	1.64

Table 6–6.   CLINICAL DIABETES IN MYOTONIC DYSTROPHY

Case Number	Sex	Age at Study	Degree of Muscle Involvement	Age at Diagnosis of Diabetes	Treatment	Known Diabetic Relatives
AFFECTED						
1	M	49	severe	40	oral hypo-glycaemic drugs	none
2	F	50	moderate	46	oral	none
3	M	53	severe	45	oral	mother, sister, first cousin
4	M	55	moderate	52	oral	first cousin (case 3)
5	F	18	severe	12	insulin	none
6	M	40	mild	36	oral	mother (case 7)
7	F	62	minimal	?	nil	son (case 6)
8	M	78	minimal	52	insulin	none
9	F	50	mild	39	oral	brother (case 10)
10	M	43	moderate	40		sister (case 9)
11	M	45	severe	41	oral	none
CONTROLS						
1	F	70		57	insulin	none
2	F	81		75	oral	none

relatives, all examined personally, but with a slightly reduced mean age (29.6 years, compared with 36.7 years for the affected group). Table 6–6 summarises the type of diabetes. It should be emphasised that these population studies give prevalence rates and underestimate the risk of diabetes developing during the lifetime of an individual; nevertheless, they suggest that the incidence of clinical diabetes is not as high as early reports suggested. The author's results suggest a fourfold increase in risk, but the difference is only significant at the 5 per cent level ($0.05 > P > 0.02$).

Information on asymptomatic glucose intolerance is not available from population studies, but combining the data of those detailed metabolic studies in which carbohydrate intolerance was not the basis of selection gives a frequency of 20 out of 123 patients (16 per cent) with a glucose tolerance curve graded as definitely diabetic. Only two out of 123 (1.6 per cent) were clinically diabetic (Table 6–7).

Considering the relative infrequency of clinical and chemical diabetes in myotonic dystrophy, it is perhaps surprising that more detailed studies have shown a consistent and specific abnormality to exist, but there is now no doubt that such is the case. Huff, Horton and Lebowitz (1967) were the first to report an increased insulin response to a glucose load. All of their six patients showed an elevated fasting plasma insulin, and the insulin response to both oral and intravenous glucose was both abnor-

Table 6–7.   ABNORMAL GLUCOSE TOLERANCE IN
MYOTONIC DYSTROPHY

	Total	Clinical Diabetes	Diabetic GTT	Insulin Hyperresponsive
Walsh et al (1970)	20	0	2	19
Huff et al (1967)	6	0	0	6
Barbosa et al (1974)	29	2	9	21 (out of 26)
Poffenbarger et al (1976)	8	0	3	5
Bird and Tzagournis (1970)	10	0	2	4
Bjorntorp et al (1973)	17	0		
Cudworth and Walker (1975)	10	0	1	6
Gorden et al (1969)	12	0	0	7
Mendelsohn et al (1969)	11	0	3	1
Total	123	2	20	69 (110 studied)

mally rapid and prolonged, with an increased peak value. Despite the high insulin levels there was relatively little change in blood glucose, although there was a normal response to exogenous insulin.

Subsequent investigators have confirmed this abnormality. Gorden et al (1969) studied 12 patients, all with a normal glucose tolerance test; seven showed an abnormal insulin response to glucose, and these authors found no correlation with severity of the dystrophy. Walsh et al (1970) found an increased insulin response in 17 out of 20 patients, and although Mendelsohn et al (1969) found only one of 11 patients with an abnormal insulin response, the total data of the eight major reports (Table 6–7) show an abnormally raised insulin response to glucose in 69 out of 110 patients studied (63 per cent). The response has also been shown to be increased to stimuli other than glucose, including glucagon, tolbutamide and arginine (Gorden et al, 1969), whereas it is inhibited in the normal manner by fasting and by epinephrine (adrenaline) (Huff and Lebowitz, 1968).

A number of hypotheses, not all mutually exclusive, have been proposed to explain these observations (Table 6–8); insensitivity to circulating insulin was ruled out early by the finding by Huff et al (1967) and

Table 6–8.   ABNORMALITY OF INSULIN RESPONSE IN
MYOTONIC DYSTROPHY: HYPOTHESES

Insensitivity to circulating insulin
Biologically ineffective form of insulin produced
Abnormal sensitivity of pancreatic insulin secretion
Excessive growth hormone production
Abnormal receptor site in β cell or peripheral tissues
Abnormality only in those already predisposed to diabetes for other reasons

subsequent workers of a normal response to exogenous insulin. The production of a biologically ineffective form of insulin was initially suggested by Huff et al, but they could find no discrepancy in the insulin produced by their patients when tested by bioassay on rat adipose tissue and muscle as well as by immunoassay. Poffenbarger et al (1976) have confirmed this and have shown no increase in the proinsulin fraction of insulin in patients with myotonic dystrophy, so that a biologically ineffective insulin molecule seems improbable. A growth hormone-mediated effect seems similarly unlikely in view of the essentially normal growth hormone studies found by most investigators in myotonic dystrophy.

At present an abnormal sensitivity of the pancreatic β cell in response to a variety of stimuli seems the most likely explanation of the facts, if only by exclusion, but no evidence exists as to the underlying basis for such a response. The increasing evidence for a widespread cell membrane abnormality in myotonic dystrophy (discussed in Chapter 14) makes it intriguing to speculate that this might also be involved in the abnormality of the insulin response. Abnormality of insulin binding sites in peripheral tissues would be expected to cause insulin insensitivity, which is not the case; such binding sites have recently been studied in white blood cells (Kohbayashi et al, 1977) and have proved to be normal. Involvement of receptor sites on the pancreatic β cell could affect the normal control of insulin production, but evidence on this point is totally lacking.

Finally, consideration must be given to the possibility that the association between diabetes and myotonic dystrophy is essentially indirect, with only individuals environmentally or genetically predisposed to diabetes for other reasons showing the abnormality. This may be valid for the relatively infrequent occurrence of clinical diabetes, but it does not explain adequately the increased insulin response in most patients, which seems likely to be causally related to the biochemical basis of the disease.

Several investigators have attempted to use the abnormality of insulin response as a preclinical test to detect the disorder in asymptomatic relatives. Walsh et al (1970) whose patients were drawn mainly from one large family, found nine out of 23 clinically unaffected relatives to show an abnormal insulin response, and Barbosa et al (1974) discovered 11 of 32 relatives, many of them children, to be abnormal. The authors suggested that insulin response to a glucose load might prove to be a useful predictive test, but there are a number of reasons for caution in this approach at present. The results show no clear bimodal distribution between normal and abnormal values, and even in definitely affected individuals the proportion showing the abnormality is only 60 to 80 per cent. Barbosa et al showed marked variation in the same individuals on retesting at intervals of more than one year; several members would have been considered normal on one occasion but not on another. Finally, no prospective evidence exists as to whether family members showing an abnormal insulin response will in fact develop signs of the disorder at a later stage, nor is the proportion of false positives known. Until there is more information on some of these questions it would seem unwise to use the insulin response as more than supportive evidence as to whether or not an individual is carrying the myotonic dystrophy gene.

THYROID

The slowness and apathy of many patients with myotonic dystrophy may give a superficial similarity to that of the myxoedematous patient, an impression that may be reinforced by the presence of bradycardia and of hair loss. The basal metabolic rate may also be depressed (Thomasen, 1948; Caughey and Brown, 1950), but nevertheless specific tests of thyroid function are entirely normal in the great majority of patients (Drucker et al, 1961; Caughey and Myrianthopoulos, 1963), and no benefit results from thyroid hormone.

A few patients have been reported in whom myotonic dystrophy and thyroid disease have coexisted, probably as a coincidence. Stanbury et al (1954) described one patient presenting with hypothyroidism who later developed myotonic dystrophy and diabetes, and a second patient had recurrent thyroid adenocarcinoma.

A larger number of patients have been recorded with colloid goitre (Benda et al, 1954; Caughey and Myrianthopoulos, 1963), but in the absence of clear evidence of thyroid dysfunction it is difficult to accept a true association. No studies of thyroid (or other organ-specific) antibodies appear to have been reported.

The delayed relaxation of tendon reflexes characteristic of hypothyroidism should not be confused with myotonia, which is not a reflex phenomenon, but occasional hypothyroid patients may show muscle stiffness clinically, although the EMG is not similar to that seen in true myotonia. This association, often termed Hoffmann's syndrome, has already been mentioned in Chapter 3.

OTHER ENDOCRINE FUNCTIONS

Adrenocortical activity in myotonic dystrophy was the subject of much early study, notably by Marshall (1959), Drucker et al (1961) and Caughey (Caughey and Brown, 1950; Caughey and Myrianthopoulos, 1963). No clinical features of adrenal insufficiency are seen, and although autopsy reports have shown varying degrees of atrophy (Berthold, 1958) this is difficult to interpret in a chronic disease of this type. Similarly, while some patients have shown low excretion of 17-ketosteroids, more specific studies of plasma cortisol, ACTH response and the metyrapone test have all failed to show evidence of hypoadrenalism, nor has the hypothalamo-pituitary-adrenal axis been shown to be abnormal (Bernard-Weil, 1972).

The reports quoted above have also shown essentially normal blood levels and urinary excretion of calcium and phosphate, with no evidence of parathyroid abnormalities, a point of some relevance in view of the possibility of confusion between myotonia and tetany (see Chapter 3) and the common occurrence of cataract in both myotonic dystrophy and hypoparathyroidism. Bernard-Weil (1972) found a failure of phosphate response to calcium infusion and a number of other equivocal abnormalities, but it seems unlikely that any major defect of parathyroid function exists. No radioimmunoassays of parathyroid hormone have been reported.

EARLY BALDING

This common but little studied abnormality is seen in most males with myotonic dystrophy (Fig. 6–4). Walsh et al (1964) noted it in 24 out of 28 males studied. The hair loss may be both frontal and temporal, and shows no obvious differences from ordinary familial balding. In general there is a correlation with the severity of muscle disease. The author has seen moderate balding in two severely affected women, but never in children of either sex.

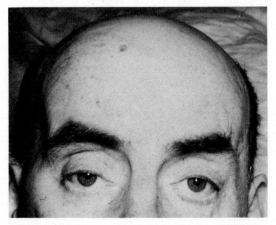

Figure 6–4. Balding in myotonic dystrophy (ptosis also present).

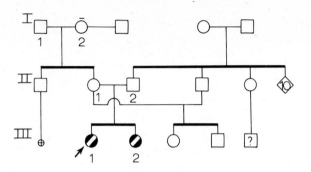

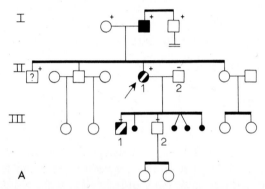

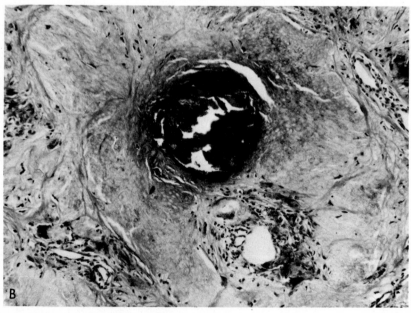

A

B

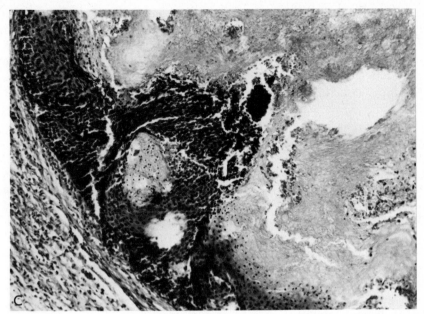

Figure 6–5. Calcifying epithelioma of Malherbe and myotonic dystrophy.

A, Pedigree (family 41 of Harper, 1972a). Myotonic dystrophy (*solid square*); myotonic dystrophy (*solid square + flash*). Examined personally (−); deceased (+).

Patient III-1. Born 1938; mentally retarded. Progressive muscle weakness since puberty; also paralytic poliomyelitis of right leg at age 18 months. Myotonia of grip and percussion present, weakness of jaw and facial muscles, early cataract. Thirteen scalp tumours present, 0.5- to 4-cm diameter, containing yellowish calcified material. Marked balding. Histology of tumour removed from left temporal region in 1966 is shown in *B* (magnification × 160). Basophilic cells, giant cells and "shadow cells" are shown.

Patient II-1. Born 1918. Mother of III-1. Severely disabled by myotonic dystrophy with generalised muscle weakness and heart block. Died from pulmonary oedema after examination in 1970. An infected scalp swelling, 5.5- × 7-cm diameter, was removed at age 46 years (Indiana University Medical Center), several smaller lesions being present. Microscopy was typical of calcifying epithelioma, with multinucleate giant cells, areas of necrosis and plasma cell and lymphocyte infiltrate of the dermis.

C, Histology of tumour removed from an unrelated patient (case 12 of Harper, 1972a) (magnification × 160). Focal calcification and giant cells can be seen.

The basis of the hair loss is unknown; the testicular atrophy frequently observed in males might be expected to delay balding, although it should be noted that the testicular changes primarily involve the tubules; hypertrophy of the normally active Leydig cells is seen, but no elevation of plasma testosterone (Fig. 6–2). An alternative explanation is that expression of the gene or genes for common male baldness is enhanced, but the family members without muscle disease do not appear to have an increased incidence of early balding.

Early balding has been used to an unjustified extent in the early diagnosis of myotonic dystrophy, and in the author's view it is far too common and non-specific a feature to use as a diagnostic criterion. Lynas (1957) classed balding along with weakness, myotonia, and cataract as one of the main modes of presentation in her analysis of the disease. Until some specific histological or other method is developed of differentiating the balding of myotonic dystrophy from that occurring in otherwise healthy males, this seems unjustified.

CALCIFYING EPITHELIOMA OF MALHERBE

Calcifying epithelioma of Malherbe, also known as pilomatrixoma, is a well-recognised benign neoplasm believed to originate from primitive cells of the hair matrix (Forbis and Helwig, 1961). In 1965 Cantwell and Reed reported a patient with myotonic dystrophy who had multiple calcifying epitheliomas. This could have been a coincidental occurrence, but during the course of the author's genetic study of American families with myotonic dystrophy a further seven patients were unexpectedly found to have histologically documented tumours of this type, tumours being multiple in four patients (Harper, 1972b). In no case were such tumours found in unaffected relatives, who were also closely examined in this study (Harper, 1973). The histological appearance and pedigree of one family in which both mother and son had the tumours are shown in Figure 6–5. Since the lesions may be confused clinically with simple sebaceous cysts they may well be commoner than is realised at present. The underlying basis for the association is entirely unknown; no other diseases are known to occur with calcifying epithelioma (Forbis and Helwig, 1961).

SKELETAL ABNORMALITIES

A variety of skeletal changes has been noted in myotonic dystrophy, both clinically and radiologically, some of which may be related to endocrine disturbances; these are summarised in Table 6–9 and illustrated in Figure 6–6. The skull changes have received most attention and have been thoroughly documented by Walton and Warrick (1954) as well

Table 6–9. SKELETAL CHANGES IN MYOTONIC DYSTROPHY

Cranial hyperostosis
Air sinus enlargement
Small pituitary fossa
Temporo-mandibular dislocation
Talipes }
Arthrogryposis } childhood cases

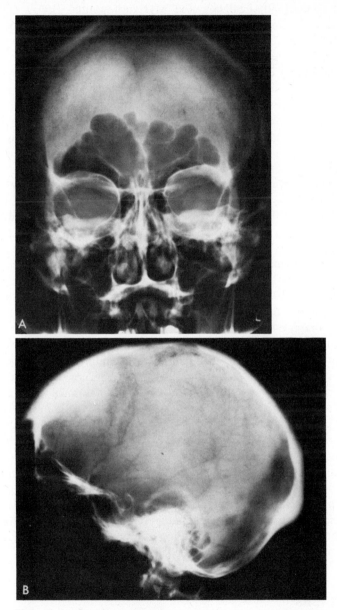

Figure 6-6. SKELETAL ABNORMALITIES IN MYOTONIC DYSTROPHY.

Patient K.A., aged 52 years (seen in Fig. 2–5), with moderately severe muscle involvement.

A, Enlargement of frontal air sinuses.

B, Hyperostosis cranii.

as in a series of studies by Caughey (Caughey and Brown, 1950; Di Chiro and Caughey, 1960; Caughey and Myrianthopoulos, 1963). The most frequent change in the series of Di Chiro and Caughey was hyperostosis frontalis interna (23 out of 52 patients studied), together with more diffuse hyperostosis of the calvarium. Hyperostosis frontalis interna is a common incidental finding in normal females but is rarely seen in healthy males. The pituitary fossa was abnormal in 24 patients, being reduced in size in 22, and enlarged in two. One of these patients had acromegaly, the other "acromegaloid" features. Enlarged air sinuses and prognathism were other frequent findings, and Caughey concluded that the changes were likely to have an endocrine basis; he postulated an increased growth hormone secretion resulting from longstanding hypogonadism, which in some cases might result in true acromegaly, but more frequently in lesser skeletal changes. Di Chiro and Caughey found a correlation between severity of skeletal changes and degree of hypogonadism, but subsequent endocrine studies, as already discussed, have not confirmed a consistent abnormality of growth hormone secretion, nor is it clear why the pituitary fossa should be small in most cases. Nevertheless, it does seem likely that the skull changes are in some way related to endocrine disturbances.

Lee et al (1972) have reported a variety of detailed radiological measurements, confirming the increased thickness of the calvarium (mean 11.5 mm compared with a normal series of 5 to 8 mm), and also providing volumetric measurements on the sella turcica (mean 425.5 cu mm compared with normal mean of 594 cu mm). Other findings included decreased orbital distance, pectus excavatum, loss of normal cervicothoracic spinal contour, and in two cases scoliosis. The combination of skeletal abnormalities seen in myotonic dystrophy contributes to the generally asthenic and lanky physical build which these patients commonly show and which is reinforced by the pattern of muscle wasting. This appearance on occasion may cause diagnostic confusion, and the author has seen patients with myotonic dystrophy diagnosed as the Marfan syndrome and Klinefelter syndrome on this account. The resemblance is increased by the fact that many Marfan patients show true muscle hypoplasia (McKusick, 1972), and the presence of hypogonadism in the Klinefelter syndrome is a further point of confusion. The finding of myotonia firmly excludes these and other superficially similar disorders.

REFERENCES

Banna M., Bradley W. G. and Pearce G. W. (1973): Massive pituitary adenoma in a patient with dystrophia myotonica. J. Neurol. Sci. 20:1–6.
Barbosa J., Nuttall F. Q., Kennedy W. and Geotz F. (1974): Plasma insulin in patients with myotonic dystrophy and their relatives. Medicine 53:307–323.
Bell J. (1948): The Treasury of Human Inheritance. 4. Nervous Diseases and Muscular Dystrophies, Part V. Dystrophia Myotonica and Allied Diseases. Cambridge University Press.

Benda C. E. and Bixby E. M. (1947): Urinary excretion of 17-ketosteroids in various conditions of oligophrenia correlated with some autopsy observations. J. Clin. Endocrinol. Metab. 7:503–518.

Benda C. E., Maletskos C. J., Hutchinson J. C. and Thomas E. B. (1954): Studies of thyroid function in myotonia dystrophica. Am. J. Med. Sci. 228:668–672.

Bernard-Weil E. (1972): Données neuro-endocriniennes nouvelles sur la maladie de Steinert, particulièrement en ce qui concerne l'axe hypothalamo-hypophyso-surrénalien et la régulation du métabolism phospho-calcique. Ann. Endocrinol. (Paris) 33:251–266.

Berthold H. (1958): Zur pathologischen Anatomie der Dystrophia Myotonica (Curschmann, Steinert). Dtsch. Z. Nervenheilkd. 178:394–412.

Bird M. and Tzagournis M. (1970): Insulin secretion in myotonic dystrophy. Am. J. Med. Sci. 260:351–358.

Bjorntorp P., Schroder G. and Orndahl G. (1973): Carbohydrate and lipid metabolism in relation to body composition in myotonic dystrophy. Diabetes 22:238–242.

Caughey J. E. (1952): Radiological changes in the skull in dystrophia myotonica. Br. Med. J. 1:137.

Caughey J. E. (1958): Hypogonadism and pituitary tumours. Report of a case of dystrophia myotonica with hypogonadism and acromegaly. N. Z. Med. J. 57:482–486.

Caughey J. E. and Brown J. (1950): Dystrophia myotonica: endocrine study. Q. J. Med. 19:303.

Caughey J. E. and Koochek M. H. (1974): Growth hormone in dystrophia myotonica. N. Z. Med. J. 79:685–687.

Caughey J. E. and Myrianthopoulos N. C. (1963): Dystrophia Myotonica and Related Disorders. Charles C Thomas, Springfield, Ill.

Chyatte S. B., Rudman D., Patterson J. H., Ahmann P. and Jordon A. (1974): Human growth hormone in myopathy: myotonic dystrophy, Duchenne muscular dystrophy, and limb-girdle muscular dystrophy. South. Med. J. 67:170–172.

Chyatte S. B., Rudman D., Patterson J. H., Gerron G. G., O'Beirne I. F., Barlow J. A., Ahmann P., Jordon A. and Mosteller R. C. (1972): Myotonic dystrophy in men: hyper-responsiveness to human growth hormone. Arch. Phys. Med. Rehabil. 53:470–475.

Cudworth A. G. and Walker B. A. (1975): Carbohydrate metabolism in dystrophia myotonica. J. Med. Genet. 12:157–161.

Culebras A., Podolsky S. and Leopold N. A. (1977): Absence of sleep-related growth hormone elevations in myotonic dystrophy. Neurology 27:165–167.

Curschmann H. (1912): Über familiare atrophische Myotonie. Dtsch. Z. Nervenheilkd. 45:161–202.

Davis H. (1958): Pregnancy in myotonica dystrophia. J. Obstet. Gynaecol. Br. Emp. 65:479–480.

Di Chiro G., and Caughey J. E. (1960): Skull changes in eighteen cases of dystrophia myotonica. Acta Radiol. (Stockh.) 54:22–28.

Donaldson J. O. (1978): Neurology of Pregnancy. W. B. Saunders Co., London, Philadelphia.

Drucker W. D., Rowland L. P., Sterling K. and Christy N. P. (1961): On the function of the endocrine glands in myotonic muscular dystrophy. Am. J. Med. 31:941–950.

Dunn L. J. and Dierker L. J. (1973): Recurrent hydramnios in association with myotonia dystrophica. Obstet. Gynecol. 42:104–106.

Dyken P. R. and Harper P. S. (1973): Congenital dystrophia myotonica. Neurology (Minneap.) 23:465–473.

Febres F., Scaglia H., Lisker R., Epinosa J., Morato T., Shlurovich M. and Perex-Palacios G. (1975): Hypothalamic-pituitary-gonadal function in patients with myotonic dystrophy. J. Clin. Endocrinol. Metab. 41:833–840.

Forbis R. and Helwig E. B. (1961): Pilomatrixoma (calcifying epithelioma). Arch. Dermatol. 83:606–618.

Gardy H. H. (1963): Dystrophia myotonica in pregnancy. Report of a case. Obstet. Gynecol. 21:441–445.

Gorden P., Griggs R. C., Nissley S. P., Roth J. and Engel W. K. (1969): Studies of plasma insulin in myotonic dystrophy. J. Clin. Endocrinol. Metab. 29:684.

Hamilton W. (1974): Testicular function in myotonic dystrophy of childhood. Clin. Endocrinol. 3:215–222.

Harper P. S. (1972a): Genetic studies in myotonic dystrophy. Thesis for degree of D.M., University of Oxford, U.K.

Harper P. S. (1972b): Calcifying epithelioma of Malherbe. Association with myotonic muscular dystrophy. Arch. Dermatol. 106:41–44.

Harper P. S. (1973): Presymptomatic detection and genetic counselling in myotonic dystrophy. Clin. Genet. 4:134–140.

Harper P. S. (1975a): Congenital myotonic dystrophy in Britain. 1. Clinical aspects. Arch. Dis. Child. 50:505–513.

Harper P. S. (1975b): Congenital myotonic dystrophy in Britain. 2. Genetic basis. Arch. Dis. Child. 50:514–521.

Harper P. S., Penny R., Foley T., Jr., Migeon C. J. and Blizzard R. M. (1972): Gonadal function in males with myotonic dystrophy. J. Clin. Endocrinol. Metab. 35:852–856.

Hopkins A. and Wray S. (1967): The effect of pregnancy on dystrophia myotonica. Neurology 17:166–168.

Huff T. A., Horton E. S. and Lebowitz H. E. (1967): Abnormal insulin secretion in myotonic dystrophy. N. Engl. J. Med. 277:837–841.

Huff T. A. and Lebowitz H. E. (1968): Dynamics of insulin secretion in myotonic dystrophy. J. Clin. Endocrinol. Metab. 28:992–998.

Jacobson W. E., Schultz A. L. and Anderson J. (1955): Endocrine studies in eight patients with dystrophia myotonica. J. Clin. Endocrinol. Metab. 15:801–810.

Klein D. (1958): La dystrophie myotonique (Steinert) et la myotonie congénitale (Thomsen) en Suisse. J. Genet. Hum. (Suppl.) 7:1–328.

Kobayashi M., Meek J. C. and Streib E. (1977): The insulin receptor in myotonic dystrophy. J. Clin. Endocrinol. Metab. 45:821–824.

Lee K. F., Lin S. R. and Hodes P. J. (1972): New roentgenologic findings in myotonic dystrophy. An analysis of 18 patients. Am. J. Roentgenol. 115:179–185.

Lynas M. A. (1957): Dystrophia myotonica, with special reference to Northern Ireland. Ann. Hum Genet. 21:318–351.

Marshall J. (1959): Observations on endocrine function in dystrophia myotonica. Brain 82:221–231.

McKusick V. A. (1972): Heritable Disorders of Connective Tissue, 4th ed. C. V. Mosby Co., St. Louis.

Mendelsohn L. V. Friedman L. M., Corredor D. G, Sieracki J. C., Sabeh G., Vester J. W. and Danowski T. S. (1969): Insulin responses in myotonia dystrophica. Metabolism 18:764–769.

Poffenbarger P. L., Bozefsky T. and Soeldner J. S. (1976): Direct relationship of proinsulin-insulin hypersecretion to basal serum levels of cholesterol and triglyceride in myotonic dystrophy. J. Lab. Clin. Med. 87:384–396.

Sagel J., Distiller L. A., Morley J. E. and Issacs H. (1975): Myotonia dystrophica: studies on gonadal function using luteinizing hormone-releasing hormone (LRH) J. Clin. Endocrinol. Metab. 40:1110–1113.

Sarnat H. B., O'Connor T. and Byrne P. A., (1976): Clinical effects of myotonic dystrophy on pregnancy and the neonate. Arch. Neurol. 33:459–465.

Sciarra J. J. and Steer C. M. (1961): Uterine contractions during labor in myotonic muscular dystrophy. Am. J. Obstet. Gynecol. 82:612–615.

Shore R. N. (1975): Myotonic dystrophy: hazards of pregnancy and infancy. Dev. Med. Child Neurol. 17:356–361.

Shore R. N. and MacLachlan T. B. (1971): Pregnancy with myotonic dystrophy. Course, complications and management. Obstet. Gynecol. 38:448–454.

Stanbury J. B., Goldsmith R. R. and Gillis M. (1954): Myotonic dystrophy associated with thyroid disease. J. Clin. Endocrinol. Metab. 14:1437–1443.

Steinert H. (1909): Myopathologische Beitrage. 1. Über des klinische und anatomische Bild des Muskelschwunds der Myotoniker. Dtsch. Z. Nervenheilkd. 37:58–104.

Thomasen E. (1948): Myotonia. Universitetsforlaget Aarhus.

Walsh J. C., Turtle J. R. Miller S. and McLeod J. G. (1970): Abnormalities of insulin secretion in dystrophia myotonica. Brain 93:731–742.

Walton J. N. and Warrick C. K. (1954): Osseous changes in myopathy. Br. J. Radiol. 27: 1–15.

Yamamoto M., Kito S., Fujimori N. and Kosaka K. (1974): Endocrinological studies on myotonic dystrophy. Clin. Neurol. (Tokyo) 14:406–414.

CHAPTER SEVEN

Peripheral and Central Nervous Involvement in Myotonic Dystrophy

The concept of the muscular dystrophies as primary degenerative disorders of muscle has been challenged by a series of studies over the past decade, some based on electrophysiological techniques (McComas et al, 1971), others on the use of transplantation and tissue culture of nerve and muscle (Salafsky, 1971; Gallup and Dubowitz, 1973), which have proposed the alternative hypothesis that a primary neural defect is responsible for the observed changes in muscle. This subject is discussed fully in Chapter 14; most of the controversy has revolved around Duchenne dystrophy, but the discovery of abnormalities in the peripheral nerves of patients with myotonic dystrophy, as well as in the central nervous system, has raised the question whether these abnormalities are secondary to the muscular defect or whether they represent a primary denervating process.

PERIPHERAL NERVE

Clinical abnormalities suggesting involvement of peripheral nerves or spinal cord are scanty; most patients have relatively well-preserved reflexes, although in some cases they are lost early (Caughey and Myrianthopoulos, 1963). Minor sensory disturbance has been found in some series but not by others (Caughey and Myrianthopoulos, 1963). Occasional patients with more marked sensory changes have been reported (Pilz et al, 1974; Kalyanarran et al, 1973) but may have had coincidental disorders. Similarly, the family "L" described by Caughey and Myrianthopoulos (1963) as suffering from both myotonic dystrophy and Charcot-Marie-Tooth disease proved on further study to have inherited the disorders separately from different parents (Harper, 1972).

Early autopsy studies found no obvious changes in the peripheral nerves, but Coers (1955) and Coers and Woolf (1959), using intravital methylene blue staining on biopsies, found abnormalities in the terminal nerve fibres, and similar changes were also found in ten patients by MacDermot (1961) using the same technique. Changes were observed in the distal nerve fibres and intramuscular bundles, and consisted of globular swellings alternating with abnormally narrowed areas, increased tortuosity of fibres, elongation and variation in size of the motor end-plates, and a striking increase in terminal branching of nerve fibres, in some cases forming a network on the muscle fibre surface. The changes were similar to those seen in myasthenia gravis (Coers and Woolf, 1959). Woolf and Coers (1974) have produced a quantitative measure of the number of terminal arborisations arising from a given number of motor neurons, the "terminal innervation ratio", and they showed this to be significantly increased in myotonic dystrophy in contrast to muscle from Duchenne and other dystrophies, in which it was normal.

Electron-microscopic studies have not been as helpful as was hoped in elucidating the changes seen with methylene blue staining. The studies of Klinkerfuss (1967) and Johnson (1969) showed no abnormalities of nerve endings, but Allen et al (1969) found elongations and abnormal shape of the motor end-plates. The other electron-microscopic changes seen in muscle are discussed in Chapter 12.

Engel et al (1975) made a special study of the neuromuscular junction in myotonic dystrophy and other myopathies, using quantitative techniques; although they found a slight increase in mitochondria and decrease in density of synaptic vesicles, there was no visible abnormality of intramuscular nerves, nor of the postsynaptic region. They particularly commented on finding atrophic muscle fibres with normal innervation, strong evidence against the atrophic process being dependent on a neural abnormality. Studies on the main nerve trunks (superficial peroneal) by Pollock and Dyck (1976) were also entirely normal, including the fibre density and the morphology of teased fibres from four patients.

Functional evidence of peripheral nerve involvement has come from electrophysiological studies. McComas et al (1971) studied 17 patients, and estimated the number of motor units in the extensor digitorum brevis muscle. They found a mean reduction in number of motor units but normal function of those units that were surviving, suggesting a primary disorder of motor innervation. Nerve conduction velocities were normal.

Similar abnormalities have been found by Panayiotopoulos and Scarpalezos (1976) and by Ballantyne and Hansen (1974), using a different technique. Both noted a reduced number of motor units when recording from the extensor digitorum brevis in patients with myotonic dystrophy; this agreement is particularly significant since Ballantyne and Hansen did not encounter such changes in other forms of dystrophy, disagreeing strongly with McComas et al on the findings in Duchenne dystrophy. Panayiotopoulos and Scarpalezos also found slowed conduction in the main trunk of the deep peroneal nerve, and Caccia et al (1974) noted reduction in conduction velocity of both motor and sensory nerves in a mildly affected patient.

Taking the evidence as a whole there seems little doubt that involvement of peripheral nerve does occur in myotonic dystrophy and that it cannot satisfactorily be explained as secondary to changes in muscle. Although patients who are disabled with muscle disease are subject to entrapment neuropathies, many of those showing neural abnormalities were not severely affected, and the changes have not been found by most investigators in other more severely disabling forms of dystrophy.

If primary abnormalities of nerve function are accepted as existing in myotonic dystrophy, is it possible that they could be responsible for the myotonia and progressive degeneration seen in the muscles? Although McComas et al (1971) propose this for myotonic dystrophy, along with a neural origin for other dystrophies, the evidence is greatly against this hypothesis. Not only have some patients with severe muscle disease shown minimal or absent changes in peripheral nerve structure or function, but there is no general correlation of severity of the neural and muscle changes; the basic phenomenon of myotonia is likewise remarkably independent of innervation, in contrast to the syndromes characterised by continuous fibre activity. The conclusion seems to be in little doubt: primary involvement of peripheral nerve exists but is not a constant finding and is largely independent of primary muscle involvement. Taking into account the numerous systems that appear to be independently involved in the disorder, this is hardly a surprising conclusion to reach; it is possible that it will be found to apply to other human dystrophies also, and thus to resolve the continuing controversy regarding "neurogenic" and "myogenic" origins of these diseases.

SPINAL CORD

Apart from the original report of Steinert (1909), whose patient with spinal cord abnormalities probably also had tabes dorsalis, most investigators have found few abnormalities (Berthold, 1958). The suggestions of reduced motor unit number and abnormal peripheral nerve function discussed above have given relevance to a reassessment of the spinal cord, and this has been provided by Walton et al (1977) who made careful quantitative studies of the cell numbers in five autopsied cases of myotonic dystrophy. The numbers of motor neurons were entirely normal and the only consistent change seen was an increase in the glial cell count. This would certainly appear to rule out a significant role for the spinal cord in the production of any of the major features of myotonic dystrophy.

THE BRAIN

Abnormalities in mental function in adults with myotonic dystrophy have been recognised since the earliest studies (Adie and Greenfield, 1923), and these contrast with the lack of such defects in a number of other equally disabling neuromuscular disorders such as the limb-girdle and facio-scapulo-humeral dystrophies and the spinal muscular atrophies. Most of the authors of large regional surveys, including Thomasen (1948), De Jong (1955) and Klein (1958), have reported a high frequency of abnormalities and have regarded them as an integral part of the condition. In addition to reduced intelligence, the main characteristics noted have been "reduced initiative", "inactivity" and "apathetic temperament", and social deterioration of the families through the generations has been particularly stressed by Caughey and Myrianthopoulos (1963). Documentation of these features for the most part has been imprecise, being noted by investigators who were concentrating on other features; however, the fact that they have been observed in family or population studies rather than by neurologists or psychiatrists suggests that they are not being overestimated in importance. The author's own impressions from family studies based principally on home visits bear out Caughey's assessment of the situation:

"While in the country in search of a certain "myotonic's" home, it was often possible to identify a residence by its neglected appearance, the obvious need of repairs, the unkempt yard and garden choked with overgrown grass and weeds, which provided a vivid contrast with the surrounding well-kept homes." (Caughey and Myriathopoulos, 1963.)

Thomasen (1948) considered 36 of his 99 patients to be of reduced intelligence, and 63 showed diminished initiative or other emotional change. In general he found the degree of these changes to correlate with the severity of muscle disease. Klein (1958), on the basis of 100 personal cases and 158 reviewed from previous publications, found mental abnormalities in 86 patients (35 percent), of whom 54 showed reduced intelligence. Various authors pass comment on the temperament of their patients, although from the lack of consistency one suspects that the observations may reflect on the investigator as much as on the patients! Adie and Greenfield (1923) found hostility and unreliability, whereas Thomasen (1948) and Caughey and Myrianthopoulos (1963) found most patients to be cooperative and cheerful, in spite of poor living conditions and considerable disability. The author's own experience agrees with this, he having been received hospitably by patients in their own homes despite inconvenience of timing and sometimes lack of prior warning. All authors agree in finding a high proportion of patients with a general apathy and inertia, not readily explicable by the degree of muscular disability. Caughey may again be quoted:

"We have found that affected individuals, when just mildly incapacitated, were often content to sit or lie idly for hours."

Hypersomnia is a prominent feature of many patients with myotonic dystrophy, although it is more often remarked on by relatives than by the patient himself. This is discussed in relation to alveolar hyperventilation in Chapter 5; respiratory abnormalities may be a factor in its production, but they do not satisfactorily explain its occurrence as a longstanding feature in individuals who otherwise are affected in a relatively mild way. One 18 year old boy seen by the author had no muscular symptoms. Inappropriate somnolence was the presenting complaint, and narcolepsy had been diagnosed by a neurologist unaware of the family history of myotonic dystrophy. The EEG was normal, but classical early signs of myotonic dystrophy were present, including myotonia and lens opacities. One of the four patients with hypersomnia reported by Phemister and Small (1961) was likewise a previously unrecognised case of myotonic dystrophy. Hypoventilation was not an obvious feature of these patients, and they also noted increased restlessness during nocturnal sleep. Phemister and Small considered whether the hypersomnia represented true narcolepsy, and decided it was not, since the tendency to sleep did not occur in episodic fashion, nor during activity, but only when attention was not being held.

Severe psychotic changes are uncommon; Thomasen found none in his series, neither did Klein (1958), although Maas and Paterson (1937) reported two patients with such changes; their findings of a high frequency of mental changes and minor physical abnormalities among the otherwise unaffected relatives have not been supported by other studies. It may be noted in passing that when Dr. Julius Thomsen described myotonia congenita in his own family he also considered a tendency to psychosis to be part of the disorder, a finding not confirmed by subsequent workers.

A thorough neuropsychiatric study of myotonic dystrophy using standardised assessment of intelligence and personality in a representative series of patient seems never to have been performed, suprisingly; such an endeavour might throw valuable light on the likely nature and distribution of the underlying presumed cerebral defect, and is badly needed to supplement the incomplete and largely anecdotal information on which we have to rely at present.

Evidence from pathological and other investigations that bears on the involvement of the brain is as fragmentary as the clinical data. Most autopsy studies have found no obvious cerebral abnormality but have given little detail on fine microscopy of the brain. Rosman and Kakulas (1966), however, provided details of three autopsied patients who had clinical evidence of mental retardation as well as of one who did not. The three retarded patients, one of whom had also had alveolar hypoventilation, all showed reduced brain weight, minor abnormalities in gyral architecture, and microscopically a disordered cortical cellular arrangement with neurons present in the subcortical white matter, suggesting a disturbed migration of neurons during fetal life. The brain stem was considered to be normal. These changes were not seen in the single patient without clinical cerebral abnormality, but comparable findings were present in the brains of three retarded patients with Duchenne dystrophy. More recently, Culebras et al (1973) and Wisniewski et al (1975) have found microscopic evidence of inclusion bodies in thalamic neurons. Culebras et al studied material from six patients, two of whom had been included in the report of Rosman and Kakulas (1966). All patients showed numerous eosinophilic inclusion bodies in neurons of the thalamus; the inclusions were also visible on electron microscopy, and their staining properties suggested that they were composed of protein. Although occasional inclusions (less than 1 percent) were found in the thalamus of ageing normal people, 10 to 30 percent of thalamic cells were affected in those with myotonic dystrophy. Two of the patients in the series had no mental changes clinically, and Culebras et al suggested that the abnormalities reflected a progressive degeneration, whereas those noted by Rosman and Kakulas were the result of an intrauterine influence.

Wisniewski et al (1975) have also noted thalamic inclusion bodies in a patient with myotonic dystrophy. Their case was complicated by a fatal coexistent posterior fossa meningioma, but it seems improbable that the thalamic changes could be attributed to this. Electron-microscopic study of the inclusions showed an appearance different from that found by Culebras et al, not being membrane-bound, and with an internal structure of alternating dark and light bands. Under the light microscope the bodies were eosinophilic and stained densely purple with toluidine blue.

Electroencephalographic studies have been performed by Barwick et al (1965), who reported results from 18 patients whose mean age was 45 years and from those affected with other dystrophies and normal controls. Abnormalities were found in 11 patients with myotonic dystrophy (61 percent), although the fact that 20 percent of controls also showed abnormalities is disturbing. The main abnormalities were excessive theta or delta wave activity, and focal sharp wave discharges. Unfortunately no clinical details were given and no attempt was made to correlate the EEG findings with other neurological data.

Refsum (1961) and Refsum et al (1967) have shown diffuse enlarge-

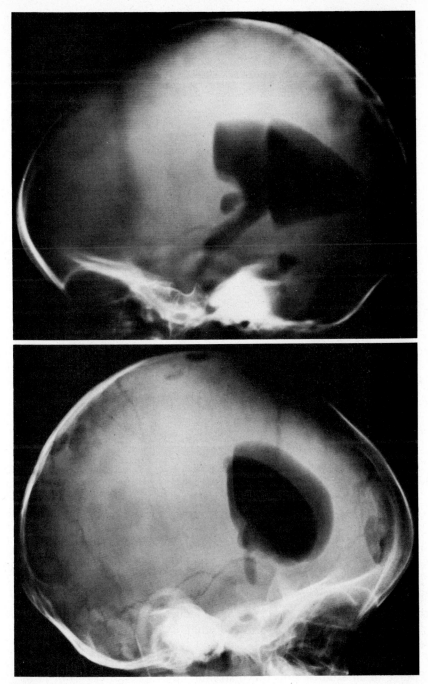

Figures 7–1 and 7–2. CEREBRAL INVOLVEMENT IN CHILDHOOD MYOTONIC DYSTROPHY.

7–1, Air study of patient G.H., aged 2 years, showing generalised ventricular dilatation. Full clinical details of this child with congenital myotonic dystrophy are given in Chapter 9.

Illustration continued on following page

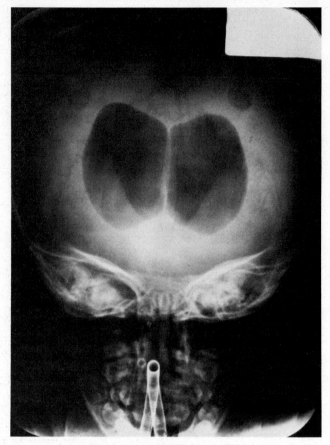

Figures 7-1 and 7-2 *Continued*

ment of the cerebral ventricles to occur in myotonic dystrophy, and serial air encephalograms showed a progression of the changes in five of ten patients, including all three with an interval of more than five years between the studies. This is further evidence that a progressive atrophic process may take place in affected adults as well as a static abnormality.

A raised CSF protein level was noted by Refsum et al (1959) in the course of air studies, and was also found by Pilz et al (1974) in 15 of 36 patients, with levels of 50 to 190 mg percent. Three of these had other neurological disorders that might have been responsible for the elevation, but this did not apply to the remainder. Pilz et al performed electrophysiological studies and found evidence of lower motor neuron abnormalities

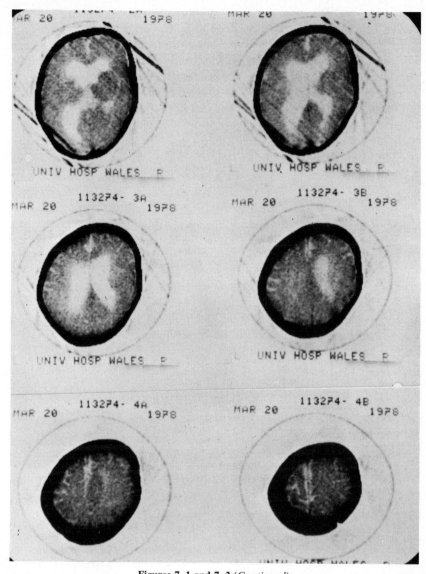

Figures 7–1 and 7–2 (*Continued*)

7–2, CAT scan of same patient aged 6 years. The ventricular dilatation persists and increased space can be seen over the cerebral cortex.

in ten of the patients with raised CSF protein; interestingly, all ten were male, a finding difficult to explain on genetic or other grounds.

The greater severity of mental changes in patients with childhood onset of disease has long been recognised, and the high incidence of mental retardation in congenital cases is discussed fully in Chapter 9.

Figures 7–1 and 7–2 show the ventricular dilatation of one congenital case studied by the author, as demonstrated by air studies and computerised axial tomography. Although most of the author's cases did not show evidence of progressive mental deterioration (Harper, 1975), there has not been any series as yet in which the cerebral changes have been followed radiologically. The advent of computerised tomography provides a harmless method whereby serial studies can be performed, and should give valuable information on the frequency and degree of cerebral involvement by the disease in childhood.

REFERENCES

Adie W. J. and Greenfield J. G. (1923): Dystrophia myotonica (myotonia atrophica). Brain 46:73–127.

Allen D. E., Johnson A. G. and Woolf A. L. (1969): The intramuscular nerve endings in dystrophia myotonica — a biopsy study by vital staining and electron microscopy. J. Anat. 105:1–26.

Ballantyne J. P. and Hansen S. (1974): New methods for the estimation of the number of motor units in a muscle. 2. Duchenne, limb-girdle and myotonic muscular dystrophies. J. Neurol. Neurosurg. Psychiatry 37:1195–1201.

Barwick D. D., Osselton J. W. M. and Walton J. N. (1965): Electroencephalographic studies in hereditary myopathy. J. Neurol. Neurosurg. Psychiatry 28:109–114.

Berthold H. (1958): Sur pathologischen Anatomie der Dystrophia myotonica (Curschmann-Steinert). Dtsch. Z. Nervenheilkd. 178:394–412.

Caccia M. R., Negri S. and Parvis V. P. (1974): Myotonic dystrophy with neural involvement. J. Neurol. Sci. 16:253–269.

Caughey J. E. and Myrianthopoulos N. C. (1963): Dystrophia Myotonica and Related Disorders. Charles C Thomas, Springfield, Ill.

Coers C. (1955): Etude histologique et histochimique de la jonction neuromusculaire dans les syndromes myotoniques. Acta Neurol. Psychiat. Belg. 55:18–22.

Coers C. (1955): Les variations structurelles normales et pathologiques de la jonction neuromusculaire. Acta Neurol. Psychiat. Belg. 55:741–746.

Coers C. and Woolf A. L. (1959): The Innervation of Muscle. Oxford.

Culebras A., Feldman R. G. and Merk F. B. (1973): Cytoplasmic inclusion bodies within neurons of the thalamus in myotonic dystrophy. J. Neurol. Sci. 19:319–329.

Culebras A., Podolsky S. and Leopold N. A. (1977): Absence of sleep-related growth hormone elevations in myotonic dystrophy. Neurology 27:165–167.

De Jong J. G. Y. (1955): Dystrophia myotonica, paramyotonia and myotonia congenita. Acta Genet. (Basel) 7:310.

Engel A. E., Jerusalem F., Tsojihata M. and Gomez M. R. (1975): The neuromuscular junction in myopathies. A quantitative ultrastructural study. In Recent Advances in Myology (Eds.: W. G. Bradley, D. Gardner-Medwin and J. N. Walton). Excerpta Medica, Amsterdam.

Gallup B. and Dubowitz V. (1973): Failure of 'dystrophic' neurones to support functional regeneration of normal or dystrophic muscle in culture. Nature 243:287–289.

Harper P. S. (1972): Genetic studies in myotonic dystrophy. Thesis for degree of D. M., University of Oxford, U. K.

Harper P. S. (1975): Congenital myotonic dystrophy in Britain. I. Clinical aspects. Arch. Dis. Child. 50:505–513.

Johnson A. G. (1969): Alteration of the Z lines and I band myofilaments in human skeletal muscle. Arch. Neuropathol. (Berlin) 12:218–226.

Kalyanarran K., Smith B. H. and Chadha Z. L. (1973): Evidence for neuropathy in myotonic muscular dystrophy. Bull. Los Angeles Neurol. Soc. 38:188–196.

Klein D. (1958): La dystrophie myotonique (Steinert) et la myotonie congénitale (Thomsen) en Suisse. J. Gen. Hum. (Suppl.) *1* 1–328.

Klinkerfuss G. H. (1967): An electron microscopic study of myotonic dystrophy. Arch. Neurol. *16*:181–193.

Maas O. and Paterson A. S. (1937): Mental changes in families affected by dystrophia myotonica. Lancet *1*:21–23.

MacDermot V. (1961): The histology of the neuromuscular junction in dystrophia myotonica. Brain *84*:75–84.

McComas A. J., Sica R. E. P. and Campbell M. J. (1971): "Sick" motoneurons. A unifying concept of muscle disease. Lancet *1*:321–326.

Panayiotopoulos C. P. and Scarpalezos S. (1976): Dystrophia myotonica. Peripheral nerve involvement and pathogenetic implications. J. Neurol. Sci. *27*:1–16.

Phemister J. C. and Small J. M. (1961): Hypersomnia in dystrophia myotonica. J. Neurol. Neurosurg. Psychiatry *24*:173–175.

Pilz H., Prill A. and Volles E. (1974): Kombination von myotonischer Dystrophie mit "idiopathischer" Neuropathie. Z. Neurol. *206*:253–265.

Pollock M. and Dyck P. J. (1976): Peripheral nerve morphometry in myotonic dystrophy. Arch. Neurol. *33*:33–39.

Refsum S. (1961): Luftencephalographi wed dystrophia myotonica. Nord. Med. *65*:822–824.

Refsum S., Engeset A. and Lonnum A. (1959): Pneumoencephalographic changes in dystrophia myotonica. Acta Psychiatr. Scand. *34*:98–99.

Refsum S., Lonnum A., Sjaastad O. and Engeset A. (1967): Dystrophia myotonica. Repeated pneumoencephalographic studies in ten patients. Neurology (Minneap.) *17*:345–348.

Rosman N. P. and Kakulas B. A. (1966): Mental deficiency associated with muscular dystrophy. A neuropathological study. Brain *89*:769–787.

Salafsky B. (1971): Functional studies of regenerated muscles from normal and dystrophic mice. Nature *229*:270–272.

Steinert H. (1909): Über das klinische und anatomische Bild des Muskelschwunds der Myotoniker. Dtsch. Z. Nervenheilkd. *37*:38–104.

Thomasen E. (1948): Myotonia. Universitetsforlaget Aarhus.

Walton J. N., Irving D. and Tomlinson B. E. (1977): Spinal cord limb motor neurons in dystrophia myotonica. J. Neurol. Sci. *34*:199–211.

Wisniewski H. M., Berry K. and Spiro A. J. (1975): Ultrastructure of thalamic neuronal inclusions in myotonic dystrophy. J. Neurol. Sci. *24*:321–329.

Woolf A. L. and Coers C. (1974): Pathological anatomy of the intramuscular nerve endings. *In* Disorders of Voluntary Muscle (Ed.: J. N. Walton). Churchill Livingstone, Edinburgh, pp. 274–309.

CHAPTER EIGHT

The Eye in Myotonic Dystrophy

The involvement of the eye in myotonic dystrophy provides some of the most helpful diagnostic information and is the reason why many patients seek medical attention. The long tradition of interest in genetic disorders shown by ophthalmologists not only has given particularly thorough documentation of this aspect of the condition, but has meant that the ocular involvement has been considered in close association with other clinical and genetic problems of the disease. Indeed, some of the major genetic studies, such as that of Klein (1958), have been undertaken by ophthalmologists; good general reviews of the ocular complications of the disease and of other features from the ophthalmologist's viewpoint are to be found in the books by Waardenburg et al (1961) and Walsh and Hoyt (1969). These works are also valuable sources of references to the early literature on the subject, particularly from Continental Europe.

Cataract was first established as an integral feature of myotonic dystrophy by Greenfield (1911), although previous workers, notably Bartels (1906), had noted an association between lens opacities and myotonia. The full significance of cataract as an indicator of the abnormal gene was documented by Fleischer (1918), who clearly showed that cataract in previous generations without obvious muscle disease could link apparently unrelated patients with myotonic dystrophy. At the same time the studies of Curschmann (1912) demonstrated the variability of cataract in relation to muscle disease within individual families. The early workers fully realised the significance of lens opacities in the early diagnosis of myotonic dystrophy, and the slit-lamp rapidly became and has remained one of the major diagnostic aids. The genetic studies of Thomasen (1948), Klein (1958) and others have explored the use of lens opacities as a presymptomatic test for the disease, and this is fully discussed in Chapter 11.

150

The character of the cataract was early realised to be unusual and distinctive; Vogt (1921) was the first to emphasise the specific character of the early lens changes as seen through the slit-lamp, and to document the remarkable multi-coloured, iridescent nature of the early dust-like opacities, as well as their distribution in the subcapsular layers of the lens (see Figs. 8–1 and 8–2). The specificity of these changes has been upheld by subsequent studies, and provided the lenses can be examined at an early stage there is rarely cause for confusion with other forms of cataract.

Considering the detailed study of cataract in myotonic dystrophy over many years it is surprising that the existence of retinal abnormalities was not appreciated until quite recently. In fact, as with almost every other aspect of myotonic dystrophy, it has become apparent that there is generalised involvement of the eye, and when the muscular component is also taken into consideration it is plain that ocular symptoms should not be attributed to cataract without careful investigations of other aspects. Table 8–1 summarises the principal ways in which the eye may be involved, and before detailed discussion of the different abnormalities the following case history may be appropriate to emphasise how widespread the ocular problems can be.

J. G., a 54 year old train driver, was seen with a primary complaint of visual deterioration over the preceding five years, in addition to general tiredness and slight weight loss. Two sisters and a nephew were already known to have myotonic dystrophy, but the patient denied specific muscle symptoms. General examination showed obvious myotonia of grip and thenar percussion, with muscle weakness and wasting of the characteristic distribution. Ophthalmic examination showed marked bilateral ptosis, and extensive external ocular muscle weakness, with a left divergent squint and bilateral weakness of the medial rectus muscles. Early cataract was observed with the ophthalmoscope, and slit-lamp examination showed typical multi-coloured opacities in the posterior subcapsular regions of both lenses. The visual acuity was 6/36 in both eyes, correctible to 6/18. The lens changes were not considered to account adequately for the loss of acuity, but retinoscopy showed abnormalities of both macular regions, with a pigmentary disturbance more marked in the right eye. The periphery of the retina was normal.

**Table 8–1. OCULAR ABNORMALITIES IN
MYOTONIC DYSTROPHY**

Cataract
Retinal degeneration
Low intraocular pressure, enophthalmos
Ptosis
Corneal lesions
Extraocular myotonia
Extraocular muscle weakness

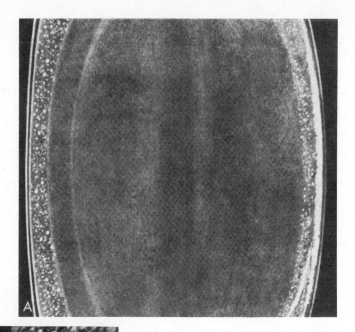

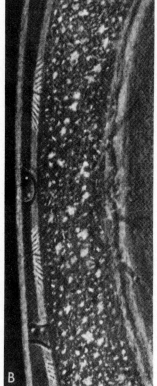

Figures 8–1 and 8–2. CATARACT IN
MYOTONIC DYSTROPHY.

These drawings, reproduced from the
classical "Atlas" of Vogt (1931) by permission of the publishers, are still probably the
clearest illustrations of the lens changes in
myotonic dystrophy and are much superior
to modern photographs. The originals are in
colour and give a vivid impression of the
iridescent opacites seen with the slit-lamp.

1*A*, Slit-lamp microscope view of lens
opacities in a 30 year old male with myotonic dystrophy. Note the distribution of the
punctate opacities in the anterior and posterior subcapsular regions of the lens and
the relative lack of central changes.

1*B*, Higher-powered slit-lamp microscope view of lens opacities in a 56 year old
woman with myotonic dystrophy. The punctate opacities vary in size; some are whitish,
others coloured.

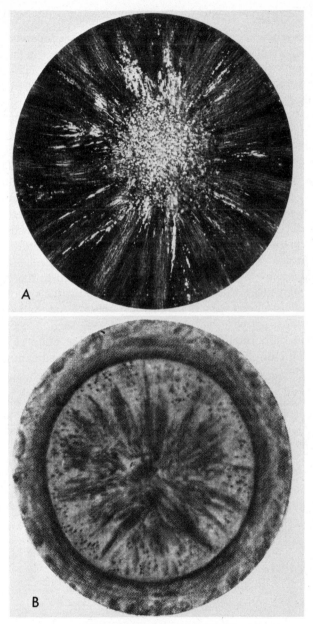

Figures 8–1 and 8–2 *Continued*

2*A*, Rosette-type cataract in myotonic dystrophy seen under direct illumination (same patient as in Fig. 8–1).

2*B*, Cataract from the patient shown in Figure 8–2, seen under direct illumination. Note peripheral opacities in addition to central rosette.

CATARACT

The incidence of cataract in myotonic dystrophy depends on the age range of the patients studied and the thoroughness with which abnormalities are sought. Studies of adults have shown the great majority of patients to have abnormalities, but not necessarily of a degree or specificity to allow myotonic dystrophy to be diagnosed had other signs of the disease not been present. Klein (1958) found lens opacities in 237 of 242 patients studied (97.9 percent), although it is clear from his data that few of his patients were examined during childhood. The author's own data are shown in Table 8–2 and Figure 8–3, and may well be an underestimate since most examinations were carried out using a portable slit-lamp instrument in the patient's own home. This allowed the examination of many family members who would not otherwise have attended the hospital for the slit-lamp procedure, but it is likely that minor changes may have been missed on occasion owing to the conditions under which the examination was performed.

The data show a number of points relevant both to the ophthalmic and genetic aspects of the disease. First, many individuals with abnormal lenses would have been passed as normal if only the ophthalmoscope had been used; most of these had no eye symptoms. Second, most patients show obvious abnormalities only in old age, and in children the lenses frequently are entirely normal (*see below*). Third, a significant proportion

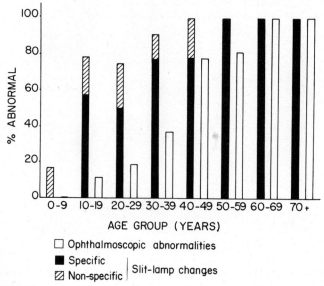

Figure 8–3. INCIDENCE OF LENS OPACITIES IN MYOTONIC DYSTROPHY.*

*From Harper, 1973.

Table 8–2.   LENS CHANGES IN INDIVIDUALS WITH
MYOTONIC DYSTROPHY

Age Group (years)	Slit-lamp Changes				Ophthalmoscopic Changes		
	DIAG-NOSTIC	ABSENT	NON-SPECIFIC	TOTAL	PRESENT	ABSENT	TOTAL
0–9	0	5	1	6	0	6	6
10–19	12	4	3	19	3	22	25
20–29	12	6	6	24	5	21	26
30–39	17	2	3	22	10	17	27
40–49	18	0	5	23	21	6	27
50–59	14	0	0	14	17	4	21
60–69	11	0	0	11	13	0	13
70+	5	0	0	5	5	0	5
Total	89	17	18	124	74	76	150

of the opacities seen with the slit-lamp are not of the classical iridescent type but non-specific, whitish opacities of a varying degree of abundance. In a patient with definite muscle disease there is little doubt that these are related, but in otherwise normal relatives their significance is much less certain, as discussed in the section on presymptomatic detection (Chapter 11).

The frequency of cataract as the mode of presentation in myotonic dystrophy also varies according to the nature of the study. In the author's series of 170 patients only nine presented with cataract, but other series have shown a higher frequency. Thus, 17 out of 55 patients of Lynas (1957) presented in this way.

Cataract surgery was required in 21 out of 164 patients in the author's series, and (as mentioned below) was more common in those with diabetes. Ophthalmic studies have naturally shown a much higher proportion of patients requiring operation, but they form a selected group from which general conclusions cannot be drawn.

The Relationship of Cataract and Muscle Disease

Although lens changes are one of the most consistent extramuscular features of myotonic dystrophy, it has long been recognised that, whereas some patients with severe muscle disease have only insignificant opacities, others have mature cataract at a stage when muscle symptoms are minimal or even absent. In particular the question has been raised whether special genetic factors that may result in cataract, as opposed to muscle disease, are predominant in certain families, or particular generations within a family.

The genetic studies of Bell (1948) and Lynas (1957) have shown that the mean age at onset of those patients presenting with cataract is higher by 15 to 20 years than those in whom myotonia or weakness are the presenting features. This in itself tells us little except that the muscular features are exceptionally variable. Lynas also found close correlation for sibs and for parents and children showing cataract as the mode of onset. The predominance of cataract in older, mildly affected individuals has been used to support the existence of "anticipation", or a tendency for progressively earlier onset and greater severity of disease in successive generations; the biases and pitfalls of interpretation of this situation are discussed in Chapter 10, as is the question of possible genetic heterogeneity.

The constancy of lens changes in myotonic dystrophy, despite the variability in development of established cataract, is one of the strongest arguments in favor of myotonic dystrophy being controlled by a single gene. No family with myotonic dystrophy has ever been reported in whom lens abnormalities were consistently absent, nor have the specific lens abnormalities ever been documented in the other inherited myotonic disorders or muscle dystrophies.

The Evolution of Cataract in Myotonic Dystrophy

Although the detailed features of the myotonic cataract are familiar to ophthalmologists, other clinicians may be less aware of the features to look for, and an approximate classification is given below as a guide to what may be expected. Further details can be found in the studies of Vos (1938) and Junge (1966), and Buschke (1943) gives a valuable comparison of myotonic and other forms of metabolic cataract.

Stage 1. No visual symptoms are produced and ophthalmoscopic examination of the lenses is normal. Slit-lamp examination of the lenses shows scattered dust-like opacities, principally in the posterior subcapsular regions. Many of the opacities are iridescent, glinting blue or red as the angle of the lamp is changed; others are whitish. In some patients only whitish opacities can be seen.

Stage 2. Cortical spokes may be seen with the ophthalmoscope, and the lens surface appears reticulated. Slit-lamp examination shows the iridescent opacities to be increased in size and number; confluent posterior subcapsular plaques may be seen.

Stage 3. Diminution of visual acuity is usually present. Star-shaped opacities and spokes may be seen with the ophthalmoscope. Slit-lamp examination shows numerous opacities throughout the lens. The iridescent opacities may be less conspicuous as the general clouding increases.

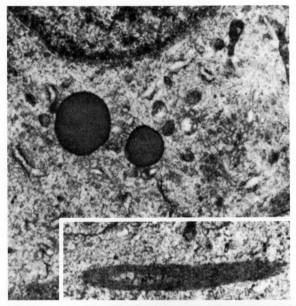

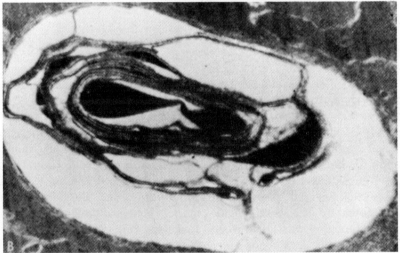

Figure 8–4. Ultrastructural changes in the lens in myotonic dystrophy*

A, Anterior lens epithelium showing lipid droplets (× 29,600). Inset illustrates a protein crystalloid (× 21,800).

B, Anterior subcapsular cortex. Larger (12 μm) vacuole containing multi-laminar whorls (× 13,300).

*From Dark and Streeten, 1977. Am. J. Ophthalmol. *84*:666–674, by permission of the authors and publishers.

Stage 4. Mature cataract. The appearances may be impossible to differentiate from cataract of other cause; the specific early changes are rarely distinguishable.

It should be clear from the above discussion that there is no substitute for a careful examination of the lenses by an experienced ophthalmologist. For the general physician or neurologist who is involved with most patients with myotonic dystrophy, however, several points should be emphasised.

1. A normal ophthalmoscopic examination is no guarantee of normal lenses; the earliest and most specific opacities are not visible with the ophthalmoscope.

2. Opacities seen with the ophthalmoscope should be confirmed with the slit-lamp. In two patients seen by the author apparent lens opacities proved to be pigment spots on the lens surface when examined with the slit-lamp.

3. Quantitative studies of lens opacities have been shown to be helpful in distinguishing myotonic dystrophy gene carriers from normal individuals (Pescia and Emery, 1976), as discussed fully in Chapter 11.

4. Mature cataract in an elderly member of a family with myotonic dystrophy is not sufficient ground for diagnosing the disease in the absence of other abnormalities, unless the specific features of myotonic cataract have been noted at an earlier stage of its development.

Cataract in Childhood

Although some authors (e.g., Klein, 1958) state that lens opacities can always be found in myotonic dystrophy, they are referring to series composed almost exclusively of adults. The author's own study (Harper, 1972, 1973) showed no diagnostic lens changes in patients under the age of 10 years, although the difficulty of making a thorough slit-lamp examination in the home may have resulted in some being missed. The relationship of lens changes to age is shown in Table 8-2 and Figure 8-3, which also reveals the inadequacy of ophthalmoscopy alone. Burian and Burns (1967) found no iridescent opacities in their youngest patients of 10 to 15 years, although whitish "snowball" opacities were present. Junge (1966) noted no specific lens changes in patients under 20 years, six patients in this age group being the only ones in his series with entirely normal lenses.

Cataract similarly is not a common feature of infants with congenital myotonic dystrophy, although it may occur later in patients with the congenital form; in one case (24-III-5 of Harper, 1972), a girl with severe congenital myotonic dystrophy developed diabetes at age 12 years and required cataract extraction at age 13 years. None of the 70 children with congenital myotonic dystrophy studied by the author (Harper, 1975) had lens opacities before 10 years of age, with the exception of one child born with congenital cataracts. Caughey and Barclay (1964) have also described a child with congenital cataract and myotonic dystrophy, as have Sarnat et al (1976), so it is possible that the association is more than fortuituous. Lens changes clearly are not usual, however, in congenital myotonic dystrophy, and congenital cataract as an isolated finding in a family with myotonic dystrophy should not be considered as grounds for diagnosing the disease. The following case, encountered by the author in his study (Harper, 1975) but not included in that series, provides a salutary example.*

A. C. (male), born to a father with diagnosed myotonic dystrophy, was noted to have a unilateral cataract at birth. The other lens was normal, and the child was otherwise healthy, with no signs of congenital myotonic dystrophy. Initially he was considered to have myotonic dystrophy on the basis of the cataract, and to be an exception to the maternal transmission of the neonatal form. Later investigation showed that the mother had been exposed to rubella, and that the father's myotonic dystrophy was likely to be unrelated. The child has remained well subsequently.

Cataract and Diabetes

Simon (1962) suggested that the occurrence of diabetes accelerated the development of cataract in patients with myotonic dystrophy. Data of the author (Table 8–3) appear to support this, showing cataract surgery required in 45 percent of those patients with diabetes and only 13 percent of those without. The age distributions of the two groups are not comparable, however, and the coexistence of the two complications may simply be a function of advancing age, although their close temporal association, as in the girl with congenital myotonic dystrophy mentioned above, would seem to be causally related.

---

*Reported by courtesy of Dr. R. Forrester.

Table 8–3. DIABETES AND CATARACT IN MYOTONIC DYSTROPHY*

	Diabetic	Non-diabetic	Total
Cataract surgery	5	16	21
No cataract surgery	6	137	143
Total	11	153	164

*Based on data of Harper, 1972.

Drug-induced Myotonia and Cataract

The drugs triparanol (MER/29) and diazacholesterol both inhibit the formation of cholesterol from its precursor desmosterol, and in consequence have been used both in man and animals as cholesterol-lowering agents. Both have been found to produce myotonia, in particular diazacholesterol (Winer et al, 1966); the mechanism for this and its possible relationship to the metabolic basis of myotonic dystrophy are discussed in Chapter 14. It is thus of considerable interest that triparanol has been reported as causing cataract in man. Kirby et al (1962) described three patients, one a child with familial hypercholesterolaemia, who developed cataract following triparanol treatment. Posterior and anterior subcapsular opacities were present. Examination of 16 other patients taking triparanol showed no lens opacities. Peter et al (1973) demonstrated that chronic diazacholesterol administration to rats resulted in cataract formation.

Biochemical and Ultrastructural Abnormalities in the Lens

Considering the number of patients with myotonic dystrophy undergoing cataract removal, the biochemical studies have been meagre in the extreme. Horvath (1973) described a single instance of myotonic cataract analysed for sodium and potassium content. A level of 10.9 mg percent potassium was found in comparison with levels of 92 to 309 mg percent in senile cataracts and 635 mg percent for normal lens. Further studies on more extensive series are needed, and might provide information regarding the general metabolic basis of myotonic dystrophy as well as on the pathogenesis of the cataract itself.

The ultrastructure of the lens in myotonic dystrophy has recently been studied by Dark and Streeten (1977) who have shown a number of unusual features, including lipid droplets, vacuoles containing whorled material, and protein crystalloid deposits. Some of these changes are shown in Figure 8–4.

RETINAL CHANGES

The occurrence of cataract as a major clinical feature in myotonic dystrophy has been recognised for many years by ophthalmologists and other clinicans alike. The existence of retinal changes, although well-documented in the ophthalmological literature, is little appreciated elsewhere and deserves greater attention. Not only are these changes yet another indication of the multi-systemic effects of the disorder, but they

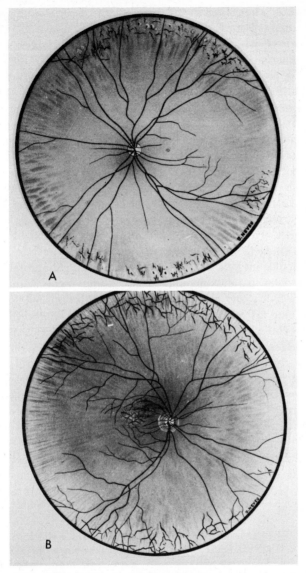

Figure 8–5. RETINAL CHANGES IN MYOTONIC DYSTROPHY.*

A, Left eye of 47 year old man with severe myotonic dystrophy showing a peripheral pigmentary degeneration. The patient showed concentric reduction of visual fields, enlarged blind spot and an abnormal and greatly reduced electroretinogram. Crystalline lens opacities were also present.

B, Right eye of a 45 year old man with severe myotonic dystrophy, showing degenerative changes and pigmentation in the macular region, together with peripheral pigmentary retinopathy.

*Fundus drawings from Babel and Tsacopoulos, 1970, Ann. Ocul. (Paris) *203*:1049–1065, by courtesy of Professor J. Babel and the publishers.

are of practical importance in the assessment of patients in whom cataracts are a minor feature or have been removed, and who nevertheless show reduced visual acuity.

Gotfredsen (1949) first described the coexistence of myotonic dystrophy and a pigmentary retinal degeneration, but it only became established that this was a genuine association after the study of a number of extensive series of patients by Junge (1966), Burian and Burns (1967) and Babel and Tsacopoulos (1970), whose findings are illustrated in Figure 8–5. The visible retinal abnormalities may be either a peripheral pigmentary degeneration similar to that seen in retinitis pigmentosa, or a central macular lesion, described as star-shaped in some patients or as a yellowish plaque in others. Marked loss of visual acuity, except where due to cataract, is seen in only a minority, but appears to be greatest in those with obvious macular degeneration rather than in patients with peripheral retinal changes. Table 8–4 summarises the main abnormalities found in the principal studies.

Of particular interest has been the finding of an abnormal electroretinogram in most patients examined, including those with no visible fundus abnormality and no ocular symptoms. Burian and Burns (1967) particularly emphasise the occurrence of this abnormality in members of their series who did not have advanced muscle disease, and found it present in patients as young as 10 years of age. These findings not only demonstrate the existence of retinal changes as an integral part of the disorder, but raise the possibility of the electroretinogram being used as a preclinical test in the same way as the occurrence of early lens opacities. So far, no study has been performed on asymptomatic first-degree relatives to test this possibility, nor are there data on retinal changes in congenital myotonic dystrophy.

Histological details of the retinal changes have now been studied in several patients; most have been examined at autopsy (Manschot, 1968; Burns, 1969; Houber and Babel, 1970), but in one case (a woman aged 44)

Table 8–4. RETINAL ABNORMALITIES IN MYOTONIC DYSTROPHY:
COMBINED RESULTS OF THREE LARGE STUDIES

	Babel and Tsacopoulos (1970)	Burian and Burns (1967)	Junge (1966)	Total
Peripheral pigmentary changes	11	4	1	16
Macular degeneration	5	6	2	13
Visual acuity reduced (apart from cataract)	2	8	–	10
Dark adaptation	3	–	43	46
Electroretinogram reduced or abolished	10	25	42	77
Colour vision abnormal (dyschromatopsia)	7	0	3	10
Total studied	12	25	52	89

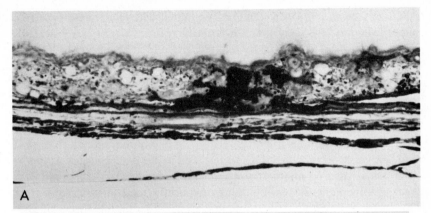

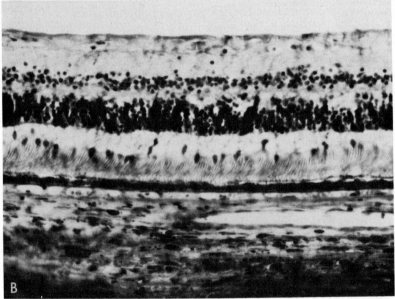

Figure 8–6. RETINAL CHANGES IN MYOTONIC DYSTROPHY.*

A, Photomicrograph of retina to show atrophy and proliferation of pigment.

B, Photomicrograph of retina from near the equator, showing rarefaction of internal nuclear layer and irregular distribution of pigment in the epithelium.

*From Houber and Babel, 1970, Ann. Ocul. *203*:1067–1076, by courtesy of Professor J. Babel and publishers.

the eye was removed for a coincidental malignant melanoma (Betten et al, 1971). The main changes found in this case were disorganisation of the peripheral retina with cystic changes, pigment increase and loss of photoreceptors; the macula was normal apart from foci of pigmented cells. In the two cases of Houber and Babel (1970) (Fig. 8–6) the loss of photoreceptors was less marked, and hyalinisation and fibrosis of small blood vessels were present; these authors suggested a vascular basis for the retinal defect, a view difficult to reconcile with the early functional changes demonstrated by the electroretinogram.

Myotonic dystrophy is by no means unique in showing a retinal defect alongside a primary neurological abnormality. A combination of peripheral neuropathy and pigmentary retinal degeneration is seen in Refsum's syndrome, together with other systemic involvement such as ichthyosis. All the abnormalities are now known to result from a single enzyme defect involving phytanic acid oxidation. Betten et al (1971) postulated that quinine might be responsible for the retinal changes in myotonic dystrophy, since this drug as well as derivatives such as chloro-quine are known to affect the retina. Mansoelf et al (1972) ruled out a direct involvement, reviewing the patients reported by Burian and Burns (1967) and noting that only three had received quinine, none of these showing visible retinal lesions. However, a common factor between the two processes cannot be discounted; it is of interest that quinine, a drug relieving myotonia, should cause retinopathy, and that triparanol and dia-zacholesterol, both producing myotonia, should result in cataract. When the metabolic basis of myotonic dystrophy is better understood such relationships may prove to be more than coincidental.

OTHER OPHTHALMIC DEFECTS

Ptosis

This has already been discussed as one of the major diagnostic signs of myotonic dystrophy, and its presence frequently alerts the clinician to the diagnosis in an uncomplaining family member before formal examina-tion is made. Old family photographs may reveal its existence many years before the patient presents (see Figs. 2–1 and 2–2). Other individuals with marked myotonia by contrast may show no ptosis, although Burian and Burns (1967) recorded it as absent in only four of their 25 patients. The ptosis is rarely as marked as in some with isolated congenital ptosis or with an acquired oculomotor palsy, and in general is little complained of by the patient. The train driver described at the beginning of this chapter was reported by his relatives to use matchsticks to hold his eyes open while watching television; whether this measure was required at work could not be ascertained!

Blepharospasm

Prolonged contraction of the orbicularis oculi muscles due to myo-tonia is frequent in myotonia congenita (Fig. 3–9), and is also a feature of the Schwartz-Jampel syndrome, but is not usually seen in myotonic dystrophy. When present it generally is associated with severe myotonia of grip and relative lack of muscle wasting, and it may be easy to misdiagnose the patient as having myotonia congenita unless a careful examination for other features of myotonic dystrophy is made in both patient and relatives. A patient studied by the author illustrates this, as well as a further occupational hazard.

A 48 year old man (7-III-1 in Harper, 1972) had developed muscle stiffness at age 7 years. He complained of involuntary spasm of the eyelids lasting several seconds after sneezing, which interfered with his occupation as a lorry driver. For a year he had also noted increasing weakness of the legs. Examination showed severe myotonia of grip and of the orbicularis oculi, but no muscle wasting or weakness. No cataract was observed ophthalmoscopically but slit-lamp examination showed numerous scattered multi-coloured opacities in both lenses. The patient had no sibs; his mother had developed difficulty with walking at age 30 years and had bilateral cataract extraction at age 57; on examination she showed both myotonia and distal muscle weakness.

Extraocular Muscles

Symptoms of extraocular muscle weakness, such as diplopia, are uncommon in myotonic dystrophy, but there is no doubt that these muscles are frequently involved. Walton and Nattrass (1954) found six out of their 15 patients with extraocular muscle abnormalities. Burian and Burns (1967) noted completely normal extraocular muscle function in only four of their 25 patients, 11 showing restriction of gaze in all directions. Electromyographic evidence of myotonia was found by Davidson (1961) in the extraocular muscles of seven patients, and histological changes were shown both by Davidson and by Houber and Babel (1970). A detailed histological description of changes in the orbicularis oculi in a surgically obtained specimen was given by Ketelsen and Schmidt (1972); Kuwabara and Lessell (1975) performed full electron-microscopic examination of the external ocular muscles in specimens taken immediately after death from two men with myotonic dystrophy and documented ophthalmoplegia. Striking changes were found, similar to those seen in skeletal muscle elsewhere and discussed in Chapter 12.

Dyken (1967) emphasised the importance of extraocular myotonia as an early diagnostic sign in myotonic dystrophy, finding a persistent involuntary elevation of the eyeballs in five members of two large families after forceful voluntary closure of the eyes. Incoordination of eye movements has also been recorded by the electro-oculogram (von Noorden et al, 1964), and appears to be due to a central defect rather than purely the result of muscle weakness. The author does not consider these findings sufficiently specific for use in preclinical diagnosis, but it should be noted that in Huntington's chorea incoordinate eye movements have been found to occur at a stage earlier than other clinical features, and may prove to be of use in preclinical diagnosis in this disorder (Went, 1975).

Iris Abnormalities

Since the iris is composed largely of smooth muscle, it is not surprising that morphological abnormalities might be found in myotonic dystrophy. Two reports have suggested that an abnormal vascular pattern of the iris exists, and that this may be specific for myotonic dystrophy. Cobb et al (1970) using anterior segment fluorescein angiography found abnormal "vascular tufts" in five of ten patients, and Stern et al (1978) noted more extensive abnormalities, with irregularity and increased tortuosity of vessels and increased leakage of fluorescein from vessels, as well as the tufting seen by Cobb et al. They found the changes in all nine patients satisfactorily examined, but no abnormalities were seen in Duchenne or other dystrophies. Whether these changes indicate a more general microvascular defect is uncertain; Stern et al excluded patients with diabetes and respiratory failure, both of which have been associated with iris changes, but a connection with the preclinical abnormality of carbohydrate tolerance usual in myotonic dystrophy (see Chapter 6) cannot be ruled out.

Pupillary Reactions

It should be noted that the "myotonic" or "Adie" pupil seen in some other neurological disorders has nothing to do with myotonia, and is not a clinical feature of myotonic dystrophy or other myotonic disorders. There is some disagreement as to whether minor abnormalities of the pupillary reactions occur (Thompson et al, 1964), but Walsh and Hoyt (1969) conclude that if so they are not detectable clinically.

Intraocular Pressure

This is consistently low in myotonic dystrophy, resulting in enophthalmos, but without harmful effects recorded. Since the low tension presumably protects against glaucoma, it can perhaps be considered as one of the few advantages of myotonic dystrophy. Junge (1966), using unaffected family members as controls, found significant reduction in intraocular pressure in 84 per cent of 51 patients, and Burian and Burns (1967) noted a reduction in all 23 patients examined, with a tendency to decrease in tension with increasing age. Degeneration of the ciliary muscle would seem the likely cause of this phenomenon, and has been documented histologically by Houber and Babel (1970).

Corneal Lesions

Keratoconjunctivitis sicca was found by Burian and Burns (1967) in several of their patients, and one had old healed corneal ulcers. More dramatic corneal lesions requiring corneal grafting have been reported by Eustace (1969) in one patient; the histology of the cornea was not specific, and it is not clear at present whether a primary corneal change occurs or whether the lesions are secondary to failure to blink and other neurological problems. A high incidence of epiphora together with a greatly reduced frequency of blinking has been found by Webb et al (1978) in an isolated kindred from Labrador.

The widespread nature of the ophthalmic abnormalities in myotonic dystrophy may surprise those clinicians who have considered cataract to be the only major eye defect in this disease. All patients with myotonic dystrophy deserve a thorough examination by an ophthalmologist, whether or not they have visual symptoms, and those with decreasing visual acuity require a careful assessment of retinal appearance and function before and after cataract surgery. A particular plea should be made to ophthalmologists to search for signs of myotonic dystrophy among their otherwise uncomplaining patients with presenile cataract; recognition of the muscle abnormality may avoid preventable anaesthetic and postoperative problems and also provide the clue to apparently unrelated symptoms. Whenever possible the lens should be studied histologically, and part kept deep-frozen (*not* in formalin) for biochemical study. If no facilities are available for this, arrangements can usually be made with a suitable laboratory from a distance provided advance notice is given. In the author's opinion a closer study of the ocular defects is likely to give valuable information on the fundamental metabolic abnormality in myotonic dystrophy.

REFERENCES

Babel J. and Tsacopoulos M. (1970): Les lésions rétiniennes de la dystrophie myotonique. Ann. Ocul. (Paris) *203*:1049–1065.

Bartels R. (1906): Ein Beitrag zur Tetaniekatarakt. Klin. Monatsbl. Augenheilkd. *44*:374–381.

Bell J. (1948): Dystrophia myotonica and allied diseases. *In* Treasury of Human Inheritance. Cambridge University Press, U.K.

Betten M. G., Bilchik R. C. and Smith M. E. (1971): Pigmentary retinopathy of myotonic dystrophy. Am. J. Ophthalmol. *72*:720–723.

Burian H. M. and Burns C. A. (1967): Ocular changes in myotonic dystrophy. Am. J. Opthalmol. *63*:22–34.

Burns C. A. (1969): Ocular histopathology of myotonic dystrophy. Am. J. Ophthalmol. *68*: 416–422.

Buschke W. (1943): Dystrophic cataracts and their relation to other "metabolic" cataracts. Arch. Ophthalmol. *30*:751–762.

Caughey J. E. and Barclay J. (1954): Dystrophia myotonica and the occurrence of congenital physical defects in affected families. Australas. Ann. Med. *3*:165–170.

Cobb B., Shilling J. S. and Chisholm I. H. (1970): Vascular tufts at the pupillary margin in myotonic dystrophy. Am. J. Ophthalmol. *69*:573–582.

Curschmann H. (1912): Über familiäre atrophische Myotonie. Dtsch. Z. Nervenheilkd, *45*:161–202.

Dark A. J. and Streeten B. W. (1977): Ultrastructural study of cataract in myotonia dystrophica. Am. J. Ophthalmol. *84*:666–674.

Davidson S. I. (1961): The eye in dystrophia myotonica. Br. J. Ophthalmol. *45*:183–196.

Dyken P. R. (1967): Extraocular myotonia in families with dystrophia myotonica. Neurology (Minneap.) *16*:738–740.

Eustace P. (1969): Corneal lesions in myotonic dystrophy. Br. J. Ophthalmol. *53*:633–637.

Fleischer B. (1918): Über myotonische Dystrophie mit Katarakt. Albrecht von Graefes Arch. Klin. Ophthalmol. *96*:91–133.

Gotfredsen E. (1949): Concurrence of dystrophia myotonica and dystrophia pigmentosa retinae. Acta Psychiatr. Neurol. Scand. *24*:435–441.

Greenfield J. (1911): Notes on a family with myotonia atrophica and early cataract with report of an additional case of myotonia atrophica. Rev. Neurol. Psychiatr. *9*:169–181

Harper P. S. (1972): Genetic studies in myotonic dystrophy. Thesis for degree of D. M., University of Oxford, U.K.

Harper P. S. (1973): Pre-symptomatic detection and genetic counselling in myotonic dystrophy. Clin. Genet. *4*:134–140.

Harper P. S. (1975): Congenital myotonic dystrophy in Britain. 1. Clinical aspects. Arch. Dis. Child. *50*:505–513.

Horvath A. (1973): Untersuchungen and Ergebnisse ueber Cataracta Myotonica. Klin. Monatsbl. Augenheilkd. *163*:86–91.

Houber J. P. and Babel J. (1970): Les lésions uvéo-rétiniennes de la dystrophie myotonique. Étude histologique. Ann Ocul. (Paris) *203*:1067–1076.

Junge J. (1966): Ocular changes in dystrophia myotonica, paramyotonia and myotonia congenita. Doc. Ophthalmol. *21*:1–115.

Ketelsen U. P. and Schmidt D. (1972): Augensymptome und elektronenmikroskopische Befinde des M. orbicularis oculi bei dystrophischer Myotonie (Curschmann-Steinert). Albrecht von Graefes Arch. Klin. Ophthalmol. *185*:245–268.

Kirby T. J., Achor R. W., Perry H. O. and Winkelmann R. K. (1962): Cataract formation after triparanol therapy. Arch. Ophthalmol. *68*:486–489.

Klein D. (1958): La dystrophie myotonique (Steinert) et la myotonie congénitale (Thomsen) en Suisse. J Genet. Hum. (Suppl). *7*:1–328.

Kuwabara T. and Lessell S. (1975): Electron microscopic study of extraocular muscles in myotonic dystrophy. Am. J. Ophthalmol. *82*:303–309.

Lynas M. A. (1957): Dystrophia myotonica, with special reference to Northern Ireland. Ann. Hum Genet. *21*:318–351.

Manschot W. A. (1968): Histological findings in a case of dystrophia myotonica. Ophthalmologica (Basel) *155*:294–296.

Mansoelf F. A., Burns C. A. and Burian H. M. (1972): Morphologic and functional retinal changes in myotonic dystrophy unrelated to quinine therapy. Am. J. Ophthalmol. *74*: 1141–1143.

Pescia G. and Emery A. E. H. (1976): The importance of biomicroscopic examination of the lens in the detection of heterozygotes for certain hereditary diseases, in particular myotonic dystrophy. J. Genet. Hum. *24*:227–234.

Peter J. B., Andiman R. M., and Bowman R. L. (1973): Myotonia induced by diazacholesterol: increased (Na + K$^+$)-ATPase activity of erythrocyte ghosts and development of cataracts. Exp. Neurol *41*:738–744.

Sarnat H. B., O'Connor T. and Byrne P. A. (1976): Clinical effects of myotonic dystrophy on pregnancy and the neonate. Arch. Neurol. *33*:459–465.

Simon K. A. (1962): Diabetes and lens changes in myotonic dystrophy. Arch. Ophthalmol. 67:312–315.
Stern L. Z., Cross H. E. and Crebo A. R. (1978): Abnormal iris vasculature in myotonic dystrophy: an anterior segment angiographic study. Arch. Neurol. 35:224–227.
Thomasen E. (1948): Myotonia. Universitetsforlaget Aarhus.
Thompson H. S., van Allen M. W. and von Noorden G. K. (1964): The pupil in myotonic dystrophy. Invest. Ophthalmol. 3:325–328.
Vogt A. (1921): Die Cataract bei myotonische Dystrophie. Schweiz. Med. Wochenschr. 29:669–674.
Vogt A. (1931): Spaltlampenmikroskopie des lebenden Augnes. 2 Linse und zonula.
von Noorden G. K., Thompson H. S. and van Allen M. W. (1964): Eye movements in myotonic dystrophy. An electro-oculographic study. Invest. Ophthalmol. 3:314–324.
Vos T. A. (1938): La cataracte de la dystrophie myotonique. Ann Ocul. (Paris) 175:641–666.
Waardenburgh P. J., Franceschetti A. and Klein A. (1961): Genetics and Ophthalmology, Vol. 1. Royal van Gorcum, Assen.
Walsh F. B. and Hoyt W. F. (1969): Clinical Neurophthalmology, Vol. 2. Williams and Wilkins Co., Baltimore.
Walton J. N. and Nattrass F. J. (1954): On the classification, natural history and treatment of the myopathies. Brain 77:169–231.
Webb D., Mathews A., Harris M., Muir I., Hostetter J., Marshall W., Salimonu L., Gray J., Faulkner J. and Johnson G. (1978): Myotonia dystrophica: unusual features in a Labrador family. Can. Med. Assoc. J. 118:497–500.
Went L. N., Vegter-van der Vlis M., Volkers W. and Collewijn H. (1975): Huntington's chorea. In Early Diagnosis and Prevention of Genetic Diseases (Eds.: L. N. Went, Chr. Vermeij-Keers and A. G. J. M. van der Linden). Leiden University Press, Leiden, pp. 13–25.
Winer N., Klachko D. M., Saer R. D., Langley P. L. and Burns T. W. (1966): Myotonic response induced by inhibitors of cholesterol biosynthesis.

CHAPTER NINE

Myotonic Dystrophy in Infancy and Childhood

Myotonic dystrophy until recently has been considered a disorder that is largely if not completely confined to adult life. The older studies mentioned its occurrence in childhood rarely or not at all, and even the extensive family studies such as those of Bell (1948) and Klein (1958) largely disregarded young children in their data. There were some exceptions to this neglect: Thomasen (1948) noted myotonia in affected individuals' children as young as 3 years of age, and stressed that many cases could be diagnosed by careful clinical examination in adolescence, even though asymptomatic at this time. Other authors, in particular Maas (1937) and Bell (1948), were impressed by the high frequency of spontaneous abortions, stillbirths and infant deaths in affected families, and by the apparent increased frequency of other congenital stigmata, a feature studied in more detail by Caughey and Barclay (1954). These authors were inclined to attribute these problems to obstetrical difficulties encountered by affected women and to general social and genetic deterioration occurring in families with this disease, and it was only later realised that myotonic dystrophy might itself present in infancy or early childhood, with clinical features very different from those seen in adult life.

The first clear description of myotonic dystrophy in young children came from Vanier (1960) who studied a series of six children seen at the Hospital for Sick Children, London, by Sandifer and other paediatricians. Although some patients were in late childhood when seen, they gave a history of symptoms dating back to around the time of birth, with hypotonia, difficulty in sucking and swallowing, facial weakness, and congenital talipes in three cases. Vanier noted that some of these features suggested onset of the disease in utero and that the course was not rapidly

170

progressive. Her youngest patient was aged 9 months when studied and was still fully active when seen 15 years later by the author as part of his survey of the condition in Britain (Harper, 1975a).

Following Vanier's report a steady flow of case studies and larger series appeared, giving a fuller picture of the characteristic features and the range of variation of the disease in early childhood.

Dodge et al (1966) emphasised the distinctness of the disorder in infancy, and related the difficulties of sucking and swallowing in some of their cases to the facial weakness; they also found severe hypotonia and respiratory problems to be an important feature, as did Watters and Williams (1967). The diagnostic value of the facial appearance produced by the bilateral facial weakness was recognised by these authors, and the illustrations accompanying their cases underline this and provide a visual image that is probably of more practical help than a detailed description. Both Vanier and Dodge et al stressed the importance of distinguishing the condition from the central type of facial diplegia seen in the Möbius syndrome (*see below*).

Mental retardation had already been recognised to be a common accompaniment of myotonic dystrophy starting early in life, but it was the paper of Calderon (1966) which showed that many of these retarded patients also had the features of congenital onset, and that mental retardation was an integral though not invariable part of congenital myotonic dystrophy. It was also clear from his report and that of Dodge et al that, although patients might present soon after birth with hypotonia and facial diplegia, others might not come to attention until mental retardation was recognised at a later stage, and that patients with congenital onset gradually developed the more classical features of myotonic dystrophy, such as myotonia, progressive weakness and cataract, as they grew older.

By this stage the appearance of case reports from a variety of centres in Continental Europe and America had shown that congenital onset of myotonic dystrophy was by no means as rare as originally had been thought. Reports of fatal cases with respiratory involvement (Bell and Smith, 1972; Aicardi et al, 1974) also showed that some patients died within hours or days of birth, and that many of the unexplained neonatal deaths in families with myotonic dystrophy could be attributed to the congenital form of the disease. The absence of clinical myotonia in the neonatal period and the mildness of disease in the affected parent were also recognised, both factors that had contributed to the condition being overlooked in neonatal life. The occurrence of various congenital abnormalities, already noted and termed "myotonic dysembryoplasia" by Pruzanski (1965), were also realised to be part of the syndrome of congenital myotonic dystrophy, and to represent for the most part in utero onset of muscle dysfunction.

Histological changes in muscle are discussed fully in Chapter 12; initially, few specific changes were noted, but fuller studies using histochemistry and electron microscopy have shown a rather characteristic appearance (Karpati et al, 1973; Farkas et al, 1974). Many of the histological changes can be regarded as a failure of maturation of the muscle fibres (Sarnat and Silbert, 1976).

Alongside the evolution of the clinical entity came the discovery that the pattern of inheritance was strikingly, indeed disconcertingly, different from that to be expected in the disease as a whole. Vanier (1960) commented that the mother was usually the affected parent, but the full implications of this were not realised until the larger series of Harper and Dyken (1972) and Dyken and Harper (1973) were analysed, together with the numerous scattered reports that by this time had appeared in the literature. The author's subsequent study (Harper, 1975b) confirmed that the inheritance of congenital myotonic dystrophy was indeed overwhelmingly maternal, and that this could not be explained by biases of ascertainment. The possible reasons underlying this situation are discussed later and in Chapter 10.

Some confusion has arisen over the nomenclature of myotonic dystrophy in childhood, such terms as "congenital myotonic dystrophy", "early onset myotonic dystrophy" and "infantile myotonic dystrophy" being used interchangeably by authors without clear definition of their meaning or with wide differences of usage. The author prefers the term "congenital myotonic dystrophy" since in his view the abnormalities dating from birth are the unique feature of the syndrome. This term obviously needs to be distinguished carefully from the entirely separate entity of myotonia congenita.

The clinical picture of myotonic dystrophy in the newborn period and early childhood is now sufficiently well established to allow an accurate comparison with the disease in adult life. Nevertheless, although most paediatricians are familiar with the syndrome, many neurologists and other clinicians are not, and an attempt will be made here to give a clear picture of the essential features and the differences from the more generally recognised adult disease. The description is based on a series of 70 cases with onset at birth studied personally by the author, together with a further 56 cases reported in the literature. Table 9–1 summarises the main

Table 9–1. CONGENITAL MYOTONIC DYSTROPHY:
MAJOR CLINICAL FEATURES

Bilateral facial weakness
Hypotonia
Delayed motor development
Mental retardation
Neonatal respiratory distress
Feeding difficulties
Talipes
Hydramnios in later pregnancy
Reduced fetal movements

**Table 9-2. CONGENITAL MYOTONIC DYSTROPHY:
RELATIVE FREQUENCY OF MAJOR FEATURES**

	Harper (1975a)		Combined Other Sources*		Total	
	Number	%	Number	%	Number	%
TOTAL STUDIED	70	100	56	100	126	100
Facial weakness	61	87.1	47	83.9	108	85.7
Hypotonia	47	67.1	41	73.2	88	69.8
Delayed motor development	60	85.7	21	37.5	81	64.3
Mental retardation	48	68.5	31	55.4	79	62.7
Talipes	33	47.1	33	58.9	66	52.4
Neonatal respiratory distress	33	47.1	27	48.2	60	47.6
Neonatal feeding difficulties	38	54.3	35	62.5	73	57.1
Hydramnios	25	35.7	7	12.5	32	25.4
Reduced fetal movements	24	34.3	4	7.1	28	22.2

*Cases of congenital onset from the following reports: Aicardi et al (1974), Bell and Smith (1972), Bossen et al (1974), Calderon (1966), Dodge et al (1966), Giovanucci et al (1967), Gordon and Hilson (1967), l'Hirondel et al (1970), Karpati et al (1973), Messer et al (1973), Mundler (1970), Parker (1963), Sarnat et al (1976), Serradell (1972), Simpson (1975), Swift et al (1975), Vanier (1960), Verger et al (1967), Watters and Williams (1967), Zellweger and Ionasescu (1973).

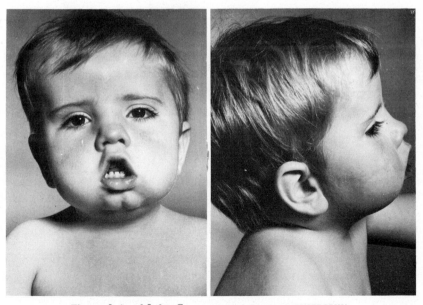

Figures 9-1 and 9-2. CONGENITAL MYOTONIC DYSTROPHY.

Patient G.H., aged 2 years, showing facial diplegia, jaw weakness and inability to stand unaided.

Illustration continued on following page

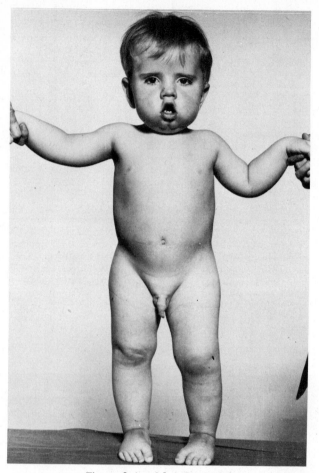

Figures 9–1 and 9–2 *Continued*

clinical features, and Table 9–2 shows their relative frequency; histological changes in muscle are considered in Chapter 12. Before the individual clinical features are discussed in detail, the following case history provides an illustration of the way in which the disorder can present (Fig. 9–1 to 9–6).

G.H. (113274), born 20 August 1970 after a full-term forceps delivery, weight 3.2 kg. He was noted at birth to be hypotonic, with an unusual facial appearance, small jaw and lack of movement in the lower limbs. Several episodes of respiratory distress occurred, with a single convulsion at 24 hours. He was reluctant to feed and while in the hospital had an episode of aspiration pneumonia. The initial diagnosis was considered to be cerebral birth trauma, and normal investigations included

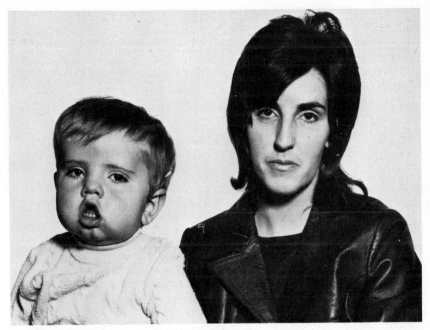

Figure 9–3. Mother of patient G.H. at time of diagnosis, showing mild facial weakness and ptosis; there were no symptoms at this time but obvious myotonia was present clinically and electromyographically.

chromosomes, EEG and SCK (35 mU/ml). Following discharge from the hospital at age 1 month his progress was slow and he was unable to sit unsupported until 18 months old, walking alone at age 3 years. Asymmetry and excessive enlargement of the cranium led to reinvestigation at 18 months, and air studies showed ventricular enlargement, more marked on the right, but no obstruction (see Fig. 7–1).

When first seen by the author shortly after these investigations the striking feature was the facial diplegia with a tented upper lip, sagging jaw but no significant ptosis. There was generalised hypotonia and muscle weakness, particularly of the lower limbs, with equinus deformities of the feet that were not present at birth. The reflexes were present; no active or percussion myotonia could be detected, nor were lens opacities seen by ophthalmoscope or subsequently with the slit-lamp. The head

Figure 9–4. Pedigree of family (see also Fig. 2–5).

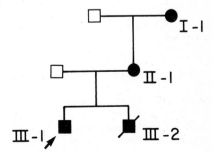

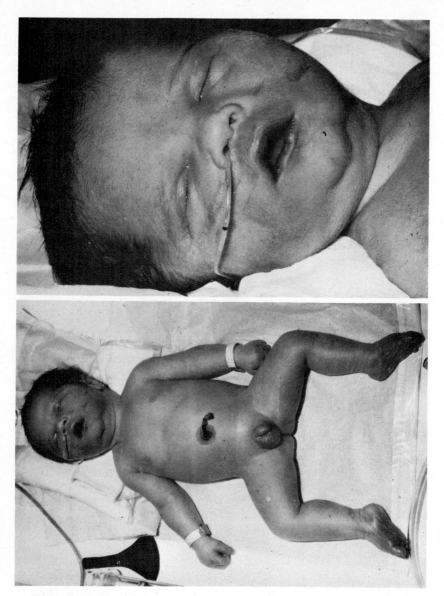

Figure 9–5. Younger sib of patient G.H., aged 24 hours, showing facial weakness and immobile posture characteristic of severe congenital myotonic dystrophy.

was still asymmetrical, with circumference at the 98th percentile. The heart and other systems were normal. He had no intelligible speech but appeared alert despite his immobile expression.

The diagnosis of myotonic dystrophy was confirmed by electromyography, which showed numerous myotonic discharges, although an earlier study at age 9 months had been considered normal. Electromyography was also performed on the

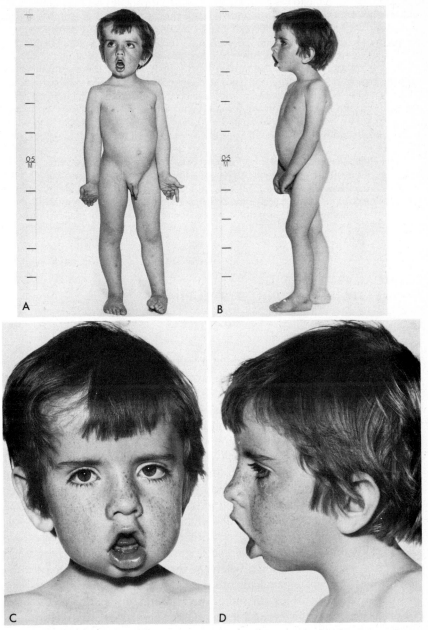

Figure 9–6. *A* to *D*. Patient G.H., aged 6 years. Motor and mental development have steadily improved, but the foot deformity persists and the facial diplegia and constantly open jaw remain striking features.

mother and showed profuse myotonic discharges. She denied symptoms but on examination had definite facial weakness, ptosis, active and percussion myotonia, and characteristic early lens opacities (Fig. 9–3). The maternal grandmother (Fig. 2–5) gave a history of cataract extractions at age 40 years but denied muscle symptoms. On examination at age 55 years she showed definite myotonia of grip and percussion but no weakness, wasting or other abnormalities.

At the time of diagnosis the mother was again 18 weeks' pregnant, and after secretor typing of the family had shown them not to be informative for linkage prediction she elected to continue with the pregnancy. Marked hydramnios was noted during the last trimester and a male infant was born at 40 weeks' gestation, weighing 2.8 kg. Marked hypotonia and respiratory distress were present from birth, with facial weakness (Fig. 9–5), and despite assisted respiration the infant died aged 48 hours.

The older sib has continued to improve over the subsequent five years; despite delay and indistinctness of speech this has steadily improved; initial assessment of IQ at age 2 years was 83 (Ruth Griffiths scale) and he is now able to attend normal school. The equinus deformities of the feet have persisted and he continues to show striking facial diplegia, with prominent weakness of jaw and sternomastoid muscles (Fig. 9–6).

CLINICAL FEATURES OF CONGENITAL MYOTONIC DYSTROPHY

Hypotonia

This is one of the most prominent features of affected neonates, and one of the main reasons for their coming to medical attention. The profound immobility and hypotonia of severe cases resembles that of the premature infant, even though most cases of congenital myotonic dystrophy have normal birth weight and gestation. In contrast to some other neuromuscular diseases presenting with hypotonia, there is a steady improvement in patients who survive, and hypotonia is rarely prominent beyond the age of 3 to 4 years. In the author's survey of congenital myotonic dystrophy in Britain, numerous children were encountered who had marked hypotonia documented in infancy, but who had lost all trace of it when examined in later childhood.

The differential diagnosis from other causes of infantile hypotonia may be difficult when the associated features such as facial diplegia and talipes are not prominent, and when the disorder is not recognised to be present in the parent. Specific disorders to be considered include a variety of congenital myopathies, including myotubular myopathy and central core disease, anterior horn cell disorders such as Werdnig-Hoffmann disease and more benign forms, type II glycogenosis (Pompe's disease), and congenital myasthenia gravis.

The principal conditons to be distinguished are discussed more fully later in this chapter and are summarised in Table 9–7. In addition there are numerous generalised metabolic causes of hypotonia, as well as generalised infections and cerebral disorders, which cannot be considered here. In both the author's series and other reported cases hypotonia frequently was attributed initially to a cerebral disorder, before it was realised that primary muscle disease was present.

Myotonia

This abnormality, the cardinal feature of adult myotonic dystrophy, is notable by its absence in the congenital form. Indeed, one can safely predict that an infant clinically showing myotonia does not have myotonic dystrophy, but one of the other myotonic disorders such as myotonia congenita. The clinical picture of extreme hypotonia that characterises myotonic dystrophy in the newborn is indeed the antithesis of myotonia, and raises the speculation whether some humoral agent in the mother might not result in the antagonistic picture in the infant.

Despite a total lack of clinical myotonia, some evidence of electrical myotonia can usually be obtained at a very early age, although it may be missed unless the diagnosis is suspected and myotonia is being actively sought. Swift et al (1975) detected electrical myotonia at 5 days of age in a severely affected infant, but other cases have shown negative or equivocal findings in the neonatal period (Sarnat et al, 1976). Studies on patient G.H. were initially negative at age 6 months, but electrical myotonia was found on re-examination one year later after the diagnosis had been made clinically. From the diagnostic point of view electromyography is more productive when performed on the mother than on the infant, and the finding of myotonia in the mother will remove any doubt as to the diagnosis.

A direct relationship exists between the occurrence of clinical myotonia and age; Table 9-3 shows that it is rarely detectable under the age of 5 years, but that it is uniformly present over the age of 10. This applies equally to those in whom no myotonia was found at an earlier age and to those not diagnosed until later, and provides strong evidence that children with the congenital form of the disease do actually possess the myotonic

Table 9-3. INCIDENCE OF CLINICAL MYOTONIA WITH AGE IN CONGENITAL MYOTONIC DYSTROPHY

Age Group (Years)	Harper (1975a)		% Present
	Present	Absent	
<1	0	4	0
1–5	2	15	12
6–10	9	3	75
11+	25	0	100

dystrophy gene and are not solely the recipients of some intrauterine environmental insult.

Facial Weakness

Bilateral facial weakness, frequently of severe degree, is perhaps the most characteristic feature of congenital myotonic dystrophy. It can be recognised in the newborn both by general appearance of the infant (Figs. 9–5 and 9–7) and by the inability to suck that results from weakness of facial, jaw and palatal muscles. Table 9–2 shows facial weakness to be the most constant abnormality noted in affected children, present in over 80 percent of cases. As the affected child grows older the facial diplegia becomes even more striking, with the immobility of expression accompanied by the shortened median part of the upper lip giving a characteristic tented or "carp-mouth" appearance (Fig. 9–2). This, along with the open jaw, is largely responsible for the characteristic facies that frequently allows an immediate diagnosis of the syndrome to be made. The remark-

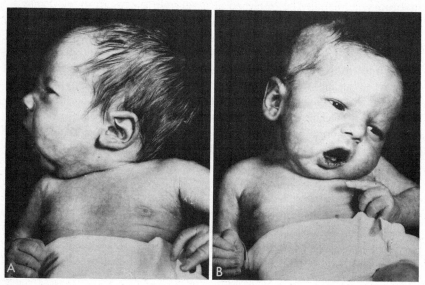

Figure 9–7. FACIAL AND JAW WEAKNESS IN NEONATE WITH CONGENITAL MYOTONIC DYSTROPHY.*

Ths infant, whose pedigree is given in Figure 10–2, was born after a 38-week pregnancy complicated by hydramnios, with a precipitate delivery. At 24 hours of age he was noted to be hypotonic, with lack of facial expression, and at 2 days poor feeding and vomiting resulted in hospital admission. When examined at age 6 days, the child showed striking facial diplegia, with a sagging jaw and a weak cry. The hypotonia and feeding problems gradually improved, but motor development was slow and facial diplegia still persisted at age 9 months. No myotonia could be detected clinically or electromyographically. The maternal grandfather was previously known to have myotonic dystrophy; the mother was symptom-free, but on examination was shown clearly to be affected. (Family studied by courtesy of Dr. G. McKhan and Dr. D. Drachman, Johns Hopkins Hospital, Baltimore.)
    *From Harper, 1972.

able similarity in facial appearance of published cases is shown in Figure 9–8. Facial weakness is also a feature of myotonic dystrophy with onset in late childhood or adult life, but these patients lack the tented upper lip which is likely to reflect intrauterine or neonatal immobility (Dyken and Harper, 1973).

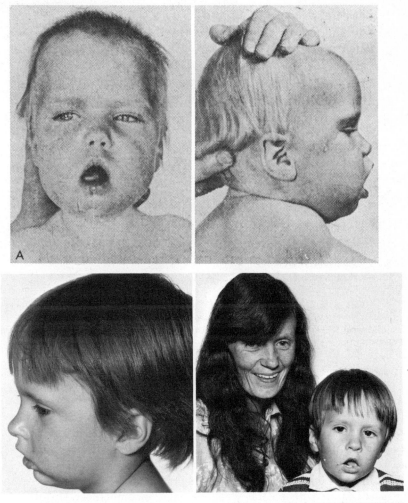

Figure 9–8. FACIAL FEATURES OF CONGENITAL MYOTONIC DYSTROPHY AT DIFFERENT AGES.

A, Patient of Vanier, 1960, aged 9 months. From Vanier, 1960, Brit. Med. J., 2:1284-8.

B, Five year old boy with congenital myotonic dystrophy, showing facial diplegia. The patient presented aged 4 years with speech problems and had shown general delay in motor and mental development. Poverty of fetal movement was the only definite abnormality during pregnancy and talipes was not present. The mother showed mild facial weakness and marked active myotonia. Although this had been present for over 20 years, she had never sought medical advice. The son showed electromyographic myotonia, but this could not be detected clinically.

Illustration continued on following page

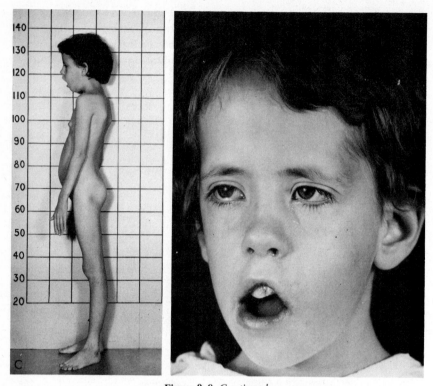

Figure 9–8. *Continued*

C, Patient R.K. (family 24 in Harper, 1972), previously studied by Calderon, 1966. Diabetes developed at age 12 years and cataract at age 13.

Despite the difference in ages the patients show a remarkable similarity in facial features.

Feeding, Swallowing and Speech Difficulties

These may be major problems in severe neonatal cases, and such a history is frequently obtained in retrospect in patients diagnosed in later childhood as a result of mental retardation or other features. Two-thirds of reported cases with onset at birth showed feeding difficulties (Table 9–2); in some instances this was mainly choking and regurgitation of feeds in association with palatal weakness and incompetence; in others, inability to suck was more related to weakness of facial and jaw muscles. Aspiration of feeds may well be one of the factors causing death in infancy, and must be guarded against in the management of these infants.

An intrauterine onset to abnormalities of swallowing is suggested by the high frequency of hydramnios (Table 9–2), which has been demonstrated radiographically to result from delayed fetal swallowing (Dunn and Dierker, 1973). So far, however, there is little detailed evidence on oesophageal function in affected neonates, although older children have been studied (Pruzanski, 1965). "Laxity" of the oesophagus was noted on barium swallow in one of the author's cases.

Children surviving infancy rarely have serious feeding problems, but the persistence of muscle weakness of the same groups is reflected in indistinct and poorly-formed speech. Although delay in speech development may also result from associated mental retardation, it is important that the mechanical component of the problem is recognised since not only may the degree of mental retardation be overestimated, but a response to speech therapy may be obtained that would not be the case if the condition were of purely cerebral origin. Patient G.H., already discussed, provides a good example of a child in whom feeding problems were succeeded by speech difficulty of muscular origin, and in whom, in spite of initial suspicions of severe retardation, improvement with speech therapy has been sufficient to allow him to attend normal school.

Colonic Involvement

Constipation and faecal soiling are of frequent occurrence in mentally retarded children and until recently there has been little definite evidence of colonic involvement in congenital myotonic dystrophy, although one of the cases of Watters and Williams (1967) had a laparotomy for colonic obstruction. A detailed report by Lenard et al (1977) of two brothers with severe colonic problems in childhood is thus of great interest. One brother presented with classical congenital disease and had severe constipation from 2 years of age, with dilatation of the colon, poor motility and abnormal haustration all seen on barium enema. The second brother had shown no evidence of muscle disease in early childhood, but had recurrent diarrhoea and abdominal distension with colonic dilatation and abnormal colonic peristalsis noted at the time of appendectomy. Despite a search for myotonia because of the family history of myotonic dystrophy, EMG was normal until the age of 8 years, when myotonic potentials were seen. This family thus provides evidence that smooth muscle involvement not only occurs in childhood myotonic dystrophy, but may be the presenting, and indeed the only feature for some years.

It thus seems clear that all abdominal symptoms in children with myotonic dystrophy must be thoroughly investigated for a possible basis of smooth muscle dysfunction. Equally important is the possibility raised by the report of Lenard et al that such features occurring in an apparently unaffected sib may be the first indication that the individual in fact has myotonic dystrophy.

Respiratory Distress

The frequency and importance of respiratory complications in adults with myotonic dystrophy has already been stressed in Chapter 5. There is growing evidence that they are of even greater importance in neonates with myotonic dystrophy and that they are largely responsible for a previously unrecognised group of neonatal deaths from the disease. Four main causes of neonatal respiratory difficulty exist:

1. Diaphragmatic and intercostal muscle involvement.
2. Pulmonary immaturity.
3. Aspiration pneumonia.
4. Failure of cerebral respiratory control.

At present there is considerable evidence that all four factors are involved, but their relative importance and their extent in any individual case is difficult to document precisely, since most of the author's data and those in the literature have been recorded retrospectively.

The clinical picture of affected infants gives a good indication of the severity of the problem, but not of its causes. The most severely affected infants may never establish effective respiration following delivery, and may expire rapidly unless resuscitated. Table 9–6 suggests that this may have been the case in a number of undiagnosed sibs in the author's series in whom associated features of the disease gave strong retrospective evidence that they were affected. With hospital delivery and active resuscitation now the rule, such infants now more frequently survive long enough for the correct diagnosis to be made, but even when the possibility is anticipated, ventilation and other measures may not ensure survival, as in the younger sib of patient G.H. described earlier (Fig. 9–5). How far active measures should be pursued in such cases is a difficult decision in view of the relatively good prognosis for life but high incidence of mental retardation when the hazards of the first days of life are successfully past. There can be little doubt that increased survival is one of the reasons for the increasing recognition of the disorder in infancy.

Less severely affected infants may have episodes of cyanosis and apnoea, or tachypnoea with rib retraction; these features may be aggravated by feeding. With few exceptions respiratory complications are rare beyond the first month of life. One of the author's 70 patients (case 2) died from pneumonia at age 6 months, but the others with respiratory problems who survived the first month showed a striking improvement.

Involvement of the respiratory muscles in the immediate postnatal period has now been well documented in a number of ways. Radiological evidence of a raised right hemidiaphragm has been noted by a number of authors, notably Aicardi et al (1974), and was present in at least eight of the 56 cases summarised in Table 9–2. Confusion with a true diaphragmatic hernia occurred in one of the author's series (Fig. 9–12), and one of the patients of Aicardi et al was actually subjected to surgery for this diagnosis, which was not confirmed. Another fatal case of Aicardi et al showed hypoplasia of the diaphragm at autopsy, and this was present in one of the sibs of the author's series (case 87, Harper 1975b). The preferential involvement of the right dome of the diaphragm has been attributed by Aicardi et al to the greater resistance from the liver on this side. Histological changes in the diaphragm have been documented by Bossen et al (1974) and by Sarnat and Silbert (1976), and have shown diminished fibre size, increased central nuclei and immaturity of differentiation.

Intercostal muscle involvement is supported by the finding of abnormally thin ribs on chest x-ray (see Fig. 9–13), and by histological changes shown at autopsy by Bossen et al (1974). Although Fried et al (1975) suggest that the radiological sign of thin ribs may be specific to myotonic dystrophy, this seems improbable, and there seems no reason why this change should not occur in any neuromuscular disease with onset in utero that involves the intercostal muscles.

Evidence of pulmonary immaturity is seen both in the clinical picture of the "respiratory distress syndrome", and from autopsy evidence of atelectasis, failure of expansion of the lungs, and hyaline membrane changes (Aicardi et al 1974; Harper, 1975). Aicardi et al considered that the reduced birth weight in their cases might contribute to pulmonary immaturity, but in many instances where severe respiratory distress has occurred birth weight and gestation have been entirely normal. In view of the clear evidence of hypoplasia of the respiratory and other muscles, and other features of intrauterine immobility such as hydramnios, talipes and reduced fetal movements, it seems reasonable to attribute the pulmonary immatury to lack of respiratory movements in utero. With improvement in techniques of fetal monitoring it may become possible to detect this before delivery and to predict which affected individuals will have severe respiratory problems.

Bronchial aspiration in severely affected infants from palatal weakness and incompetence is a constant hazard in the newborn period, although reduced by improved methods of tube feeding. Whether oesophageal involvement plays as significant a part as it does in adult life is uncertain, as already discussed. Finally, the role of cerebral factors in ventilatory failure in newborns with myotonic dystrophy is questionable. Apnoea as a result of anoxic brain damage may directly affect respiration, but it is difficult either to establish or exclude a primary abnormality of cerebral control of respiration in view of the multiple other factors usually present. The strong evidence for a cerebral respiratory abnormality in adults and the high incidence of mental retardation in affected neonates must make such a cerebral factor likely, although not yet proved.

Delayed Motor Development

This is almost invariable in cases with severe neonatal difficulties, and closely parallels the degree of hypotonia. Significant motor delay was seen in 60 of the author's 70 patients, and the lower proportion among other case reports reflects lack of information or early death rather than normal development. Although some reports refers to generalised "psychomotor retardation", there are patients in whom marked motor delay occurs with near-normal mental development; as with speech delay it is important that the relative contributions of the mental and motor aspects are accurately assessed.

Regardless of the degree of delay in passing the motor landmarks, the prognosis for being able to walk and be actively mobile is excellent, in contrast to some other congenital myopathies and anterior horn cell disorders. None of the survivors among the author's 70 cases had failed to walk, nor was any member of the series confined to a wheelchair as a result of subsequent deterioration. A number of parents had been categorically told that their child would never walk or be independent in any way, and it is important for paediatricians and others involved in the early care of these children to recognise that in those infants who survive the early weeks the prognosis is one of steady improvement throughout early childhood.

Mental Retardation

This is arguably the most important feature of congenital myotonic dystrophy in its effects on the child's development, even though it is not of diagnostic help in infancy and may be difficult to assess accurately even at a later stage. It is also a feature in which there is real doubt as to the underlying pathogenesis, and where there is no clear demarcation between the congenital form of the disease and those cases with onset in later childhood.

In the author's series 48 out of 70 patients showed definite mental retardation, and only nine showed clearly normal mental development; a further 13 were either too young for accurate assessment or were incompletely documented. The distribution of IQ in the series is shown in Figure 9–9, but it should be noted that the children were assessed by different observers and methods. The experience of other authors is similar —Table 9–2 shows that 31 of the 56 collected cases were recorded as retarded, and only four were specifically stated to be mentally normal.

Several points require emphasis regarding the type of mental retardation seen in this disease.

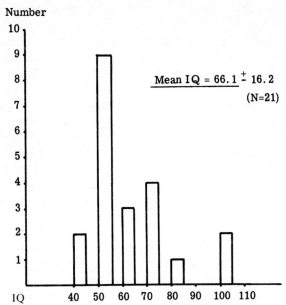

Figure 9–9. Distribution of IQ in a series of mentally retarded patients.

1. It is usually moderate to mild in degree, with an IQ level commonly between 40 and 80; even those individuals ascertained through mental subnormality hospitals have rarely been severely retarded (Jean et al, 1968), being able to speak and look after themselves to a limited degree.

2. The retardation appears to be present from birth, and in the author's series there was no evidence of deterioration in intellectual function, although this did occur in one of Vanier's (1960) patients who had repeated assessment by the same investigator.

3. It is unlikely that the mental retardation is attributable solely to perinatal anoxia, although this is undoubtedly an aggravating factor in some cases. Only a few cases have been recorded with spasticity or other generalised neurological features to suggest anoxic brain damage; although in the USA study of Dyken and Harper (1973) a higher incidence of mental retardation was seen in those infants with a history of perinatal distress, the larger British series (Harper, 1975) showed an identical level of IQ in the two groups (66 $\pm$ 15 for those with neonatal respiratory distress, 65 $\pm$ 20 for those without). It thus appears inescapable that a significant part of the mental retardation is the direct result of a primary cerebral abnormality due either to the action of the myotonic dystrophy gene itself, or to the associated maternal factor that appears to be acting in the congenital form of the disease *(see below)*.

Despite the high neonatal mortality from congenital myotonic dystrophy, information is sadly lacking on cerebral changes. Several autopsy reports state that no abnormality was noted in the brain, but detailed neuropathological evidence is lacking. In view of the microscopic abnormalities found by Rosman and Kakulas (1966) in adult patients with myotonic dystrophy and mental retardation, the origin of which was thought to be in fetal life, it is important that more detailed studies of cerebral microscopy are performed in fatal neonatal cases.

Not all cases of myotonic dystrophy associated with mental retardation are identified in the newborn period. Early studies (Maas, 1937; Thomasen, 1948) acknowledged mental retardation to be a frequent accompaniment of adult myotonic dystrophy, even though at this time the specific syndrome of congenital myotonic dystrophy was not recognised. Studies in mental subnormality hospitals have produced a number of previously undetected cases (Jean et al, 1968), and other patients are diagnosed at the time of school entry. What proportion of these represents unrecognised cases of congenital myotonic dystrophy is open to doubt. In some a clear history of neonatal problems can be obtained in retrospect: thus, one member of the author's series (case 17, Harper 1975b) denied all muscle symptoms when examined at the age of 30 years. He had attended a school for the educationally subnormal and had been born with talipes. In addition to myotonia, examination showed a striking facial diplegia which photographs showed to have been present since childhood.

In other cases no history of neonatal problems can be obtained —five of the 17 cases of Dyken and Harper (1973) with onset before the age of 5 years had mental retardation as the only feature in the first year of life. It is difficult to draw a clear demarcation between such patients and others who develop myotonia and other muscle symptoms in adolescence, and are found to have mild or moderate mental retardation at this time.

Talipes

Talipes was present at birth in half the cases reported in the literature and by the author (Table 9–2); several of the author's cases required surgical correction, and in some it was a major cause of motor delay. Most cases were bilateral, and in the equinovarus position. A smaller number of children have been born with more generalised contractures sufficient to warrant the term arthrogryposis (Dyken and Harper, 1973; Aicardi et al, 1974; Sarnat et al, 1976), and two such children are shown in Figure 9–10. It is clear that congenital myotonic dystrophy has to be considered among the numerous causes of both talipes and generalised arthrogryposis. Active surgical correction should be pursued, since the

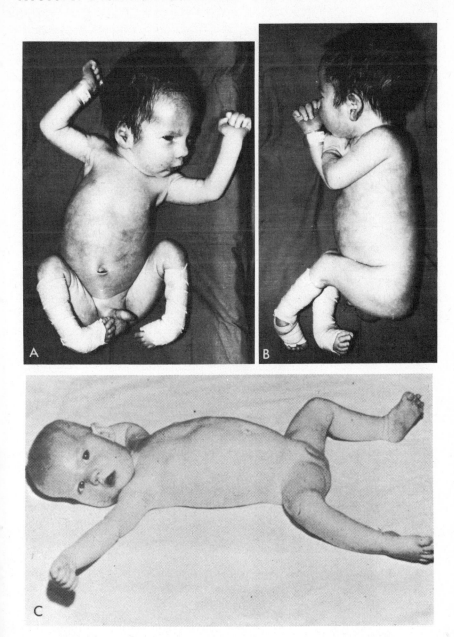

Figure 9–10. GENERALISED ARTHROGRYPOSIS IN MYOTONIC DYSTROPHY.

A, B, Affected male infant (family 22 of Harper, 1975b) (see also Fig. 9–13).

C, Female infant aged 3 months with bilateral talipes and restricted movement at hips and other joints. Note facial diplegia.*

Illustration continued on following page

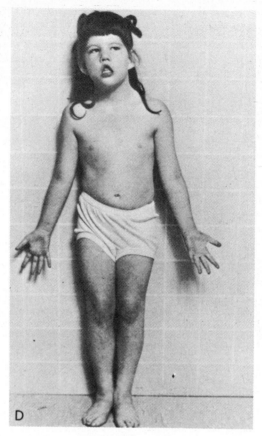

Figure 9–10. *Continued*

D, Same child as in *C* aged 5 years following surgical correction of arthrogryposis.*
*Reproduced from Dyken and Harper, 1973, by permission of the Editor.

prognosis for both life and mobility is good once the neonatal period is passed.

Strabismus

Strabismus (Fig. 9–11) is a relatively common finding in infants and young children with myotonic dystrophy, although rarely noticeable in the newborn period. Six of the children in the author's series had strabismus of varying degree, two of whom required surgery; a number of the cases in the literature were noted to have strabismus. It should be noted that affected children do not have the severe oculomotor nerve defects that may be seen in the Möbius syndrome.

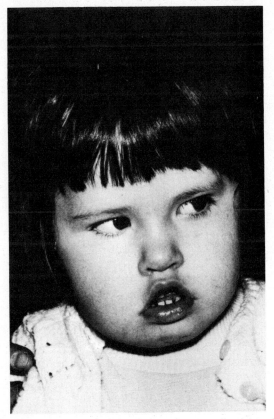

Figure 9–11. Strabismus in congenital myotonic dystrophy (see Fig. 9–12 for further clinical details).

Abnormalities in Pregnancy

The hazards of pregnancy in myotonic dystrophy have already been discussed from the maternal viewpoint in Chapter 6, but not all the problems can be blamed directly on the uterine muscle or on difficulties of delivery. Table 9–4 summarises the major problems seen in pregnancies resulting in a child with congenital myotonic dystrophy. Study of the sibships of patients show that abnormalities of pregnancy are confined to those in which the infant proves to be affected (Harper, 1975b), and that those ending in an apparently normal infant are relatively problem-free. Analysis of the pregnancies ending in infants with congenital myotonic dystrophy has shown several abnormalities, all directly attributable to failure of fetal muscle action. Reduced fetal movements were noted in

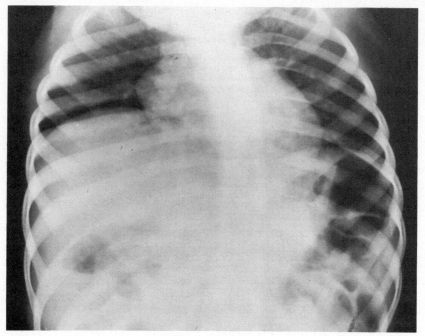

Figure 9–12. Raised diaphragm in congenital myotonic dystrophy.

This female infant was born at 39 weeks gestation weighing 1500 gm. There were severe respiratory problems shortly after birth and the radiograph was initially suspected of showing eventration of the right diaphragm. There was slow spontaneous improvement, but she showed slow motor and mental development, with facial diplegia and strabismus (Fig. 9–11). At 2 years of age the right diaphragm was only slightly elevated. (Family 23 of Harper, 1975a, studied by courtesy of Dr. Lewis Rosenbloom, Liverpool.)

Table 9–4. INTRAUTERINE INVOLVEMENT IN CONGENITAL MYOTONIC DYSTROPHY

| | *Harper (1975a)* | | |
	Present	*Absent*	*Uncertain*
Hydramnios			
Definite (18)			
Probable (7)	25	29	16
Reduced fetal movements	24	28	18
Talipes	33	36	1

Birth weight (kg) (no. = 68)	
Mean	3.22
SD	0.64
Gestation (w) (no. = 63)	
Mean	39.5
SD	2.2

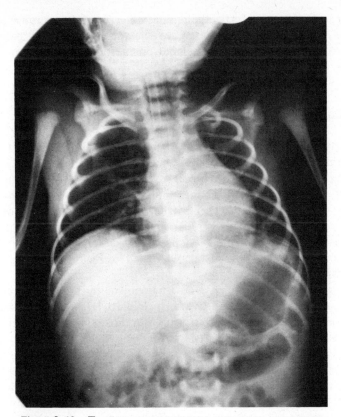

Figure 9–13. THIN RIBS IN CONGENITAL MYOTONIC DYSTROPHY.

Chest radiograph of male infant aged 2 days. The pregnancy was complicated by hydramnios, but delivery was at full term. There was no spontaneous respiration for eight minutes after delivery and intubation was required, but intermittent cyanotic attacks occurred during the first 36 hours of life requiring mechanical ventilation for five days. Generalized arthrogryposis was also present (see Fig. 9–10*A* and *B*). There have been no subsequent respiratory problems. (Family studied by courtesy of Dr. Lewis Rosenbloom, Liverpool.)

almost half (24 out of 52) the pregnancies for which information was available, and hydramnios occurred in a similar proportion (25 out of 54). Hydramnios was severe in some instances, requiring removal of liquor, and the simplest explanation — failure of fetal swallowing — has been demonstrated radiographically, as discussed earlier. A high frequency of breech presentation was also found.

Intrauterine growth, by contrast, is little disturbed. Although Aicardi et al (1974) found reduced birth weight in their patients, the birth weight and gestation in the author's series were close to normal.

If these abnormalities are considered together with the talipes, arthrogryposis, and evidence of respiratory and other muscle hypoplasia seen immediately after birth, the picture emerges of a generalised intrauterine myopathy, with the pathology well-established in many patients by the time of birth. Supporting evidence comes from a variety of apparently unrelated malformations, discussed below.

Other Congenital Abnormalities

Early studies such as those of Maas (1937), Bell (1948) and Caughey and Barclay (1954) stressed the frequency of "congenital stigmata" in the offspring of patients with myotonic dystrophy. We now recognise that most of these children had congenital myotonic dystrophy, but there remains genuine doubt whether a true increase in unrelated congenital defects actually exists. This is of some aetiological significance, for such an increase might favour the existence of a true teratological agent being responsible for what Pruzanski (1965) had termed "myotonic dysembryoplasia."

Data specifically collected on this subject by the author are summarised in Table 9–5. The results are particularly relevant if the abnormalities are divided (somewhat arbitrarily) into those that might be related to dysfunction of fetal muscle and those that would appear to require a separate pathogenesis. It is clear that most abnormalities fall into the first group, and in the future it may be more appropriate to consider them as an integral part of the general fetal muscle abnormality that characterises the disorder, along with such defects as talipes, diaphragmatic hypoplasia and hydramnios. The second group of abnormalities form a heterogeneous assortment, and cannot be related immediately to the disease or to

**Table 9–5. ASSOCIATED MALFORMATIONS IN 70 PATIENTS
WITH CONGENITAL MYOTONIC DYSTROPHY**

Harper (1975a)	
Possibly Attributable to Muscle Involvement (10)	
Inguinal hernia	2
Undescended testis	4
Congenital dislocation of hip	2
Hiatus hernia	1
Torticollis	1
Not Attributable to Muscle Involvement (10)	
Congenital heart defect (unconfirmed)	2
Hydrocephalus	2
Spasticity	1
Blocked nasolacrimal duct	1
Hydronephrosis	1
Congenital cataract	1
Transverse palm crease	1
Cleft lip	1

each other. Anoxia could be responsible for the spasticity and related neurological abnormalities, and it is arguable whether the occurrence of the other defects is more than coincidental. The data on congenital heart disease have been discussed in Chapter 5, and the subject of congenital cataract has also been argued in Chapter 8. Coexistent abnormalities in case reports from the literature are almost all directly attributable to muscle dysfunction, with the exception of patent ductus arteriosus (Zellweger and Ionasescu, 1973), hypertrichosis (Bell and Smith, 1972; Aicardi et al, 1974) and micrognathia (Mundler, 1970). The same is true for the reports in the older literature collected by Caughey and Barclay (1954). A final decision will have to await more systematic autopsy studies of fatal neonatal cases. There certainly seems to be no evidence from the author's data or elsewhere of an increased malformation rate in offspring who are not affected by congenital myotonic dystrophy.

MORTALITY AND PROGNOSIS

The potentially lethal nature of the respiratory complications in congenital myotonic dystrophy has already been stressed, and there is no doubt that the increased mortality among offspring of mothers with the disease noted by Bell (1948) and other early investigators is due at least partly to the congenital form of the disease. There is also strong evidence that many fatal cases remain undiagnosed, judging by the frequency with which case reports mention previous pregnancies ending in neonatal death, and from those fatal cases diagnosed retrospectively (Dunn and Dierker, 1973; Fried et al, 1975). The author's study of the condition in Britain, based largely on patients ascertained through paediatricians at a time when the neonatal problems were less well recognised, contained only four fatal cases, but study of the families showed 24 neonatal deaths among sibs; details are given in Table 9–6. Although not all these infants may have had congenital myotonic dystrophy, the occurrence of talipes, hydramnios and other suspicious features makes it probable that a considerable proportion were indeed affected. These deaths represent 16 per cent of all live births in the sibships, compared with a rate of 19 per 1,000 in the population as a whole over a comparable time.

By far the greatest part of the mortality in fatal cases of congenital myotonic dystrophy and in suspected cases among sibs is concentrated in the first hours and days of life, although active resuscitation is likely to prolong the period. It is noteworthy that true stillbirths are rare — although several of the neonatal deaths shown in Table 9–6 were referred to as stillbirths, closer examination of records showed that the infants in fact had lived for a short period after birth, death in most cases resulting from failure to establish adequate respiration.

Table 9-6.   NEONATAL DEATHS AMONG SIBS OF PATIENTS WITH CONGENITAL MYOTONIC DYSTROPHY*

Family No.	Sex	Age at Death	Birth Weight (kg)	Gestation (w)	Hydramnios	Talipes	Necropsy	Cause of Death	Details
4	M	2 d	1·9	36	+			Uncertain	
6	F	Few hours	1·4	36	+			Cerebral haemorrhage	
7	M	Few hours		34	+			Prematurity	
8	F	2 h	3·3	38	+	+	+	Cerebral haemorrhage	Rapid delivery; hypotonic, cyanosed, bilateral talipes; subtentorial tear with haemorrhage into posterior fossa; no note of muscle abnormality
9	M	6 h		34				Respiratory distress	
11	F	1 h	3·1	38		+	+	Cerebral haemorrhage	Bilateral talipes; born severely asphyxiated; extensive tentorial tear and cerebral haemorrhage; no gross abnormality of other internal organs
11	F	3 d	2·7	36			+	Respiratory distress syndrome	Apnoea at birth; died on respirator; lungs completely unexpanded, congested; other organs normal
15	M	Few hours						Uncertain	
15	F	Few hours						Uncertain	
17	M	1¼ h	2·2	34			+	Tentorial tear: atelectasis	Lungs atelectatic, two small tentorial tears without bleeding; other organs normal
17	F	Few hours	2·0	34			+	Prematurity; atelectasis	Lungs imperfectly expanded; other organs normal
19	F	15 min	1·4	32	+	+	+	Cerebral haemorrhage; atelectasis	Small left-sided intraventricular haemorrhage, pulmonary atelectasis; normal placenta
19	F	10 h	2·0	37	+	+	+	Respiratory distress	
19	F	24 h	2·5	36	+	+	+	Cerebral haemorrhage; hypoxia	Small tentorial tear, slight bleeding
23	M	4 h	3·2	40				Cerebral haemorrhage	
27	M	24 h	3·3	40	+		+	Respiratory distress syndrome	Severe hydramnios; difficult forceps delivery; incomplete aeration of lungs; brain normal; no note of muscle abnormality
28	M	11 d	3·2	43	+	+	+	Congenital eventration of diaphragm	Limp and cyanosed at birth, postural talipes, unable to suck; progressive respiratory deterioration; dome of right diaphragm raised with reduced muscle; lungs poorly aerated, other organs normal; including motor nerve end-plates
28	F	6 h	4·0	40				Respiratory failure	
30	M	2 d	1·6	27				Prematurity	
38	F	45 min	1·6	34				Uncertain	
39	F	1½ h		32				Respiratory distress	
40	F	5 d						Respiratory failure	
42	M	3 min	3·4	40			+	Crib death	
53	F	3 d	1·8	36				Prematurity	

*From Harper, 1975a.

Once beyond the neonatal period, the prognosis for life is good. The mean age at examination in the author's study was 9 years, with only two deaths occurring after the neonatal period; even allowing for possible lack of ascertainment of other fatal cases, the series of 70 patients represents a total of 650 years of patient survival. The tendency to improvement of hypotonia and motor function during early childhood has already been mentioned, and for most affected children performance is limited more by mental capacity than by physical handicap. Unfortunately the longer outlook is less satisfactory, for during late childhood and adolescence the "adult" features of myotonic dystrophy appear. The relationship of myotonia to age has already been shown in Table 9–4; lens opacities can usually be detected by the second decade, and progressive weakness and wasting may also be noted from this stage. No case of truly transient congenital myotonic dystrophy has ever been recorded and, despite the striking improvement of some patients during childhood, all cases followed long enough have gradually developed the classical features of the adult disease. At present there is no evidence as to whether such patients have a downhill course that is more, or less, rapid than the disease with onset in adult life, but it seems improbable that any child who successfully survives the neonatal hazards of myotonic dystrophy can look forward to a normal adult life.

DIFFERENTIAL DIAGNOSIS*

Congenital myotonic dystrophy may present as any one of a variety of paediatric problems, including generalised hypotonia, motor delay, mental retardation, respiratory distress, feeding difficulties and unexplained facial weakness. Clearly, the only way to ensure that the diagnosis is made is to be aware of the syndrome and its characteristic features, and in particular to consider the child in relation to its family, not in isolation. The differential diagnosis of the various presenting syndromes of neuromuscular disease in childhood has been well reviewed elsewhere, notably by Dubowitz (1978), so that only a small number of disorders particularly likely to be confused with it will be mentioned here, in particular the Möbius syndrome and the heterogeneous group of congenital myopathies.

Möbius Syndrome

For many years a specific disorder has been considered to exist resulting from agenesis of specific cranial nerve nuclei, and with facial

---

*See Figure 9–7.

diplegia, ptosis and paralysis of external ocular muscles as the main clinical features. The clinical features were collected by Henderson (1939) and Evans (1955); Pitner et al (1965) have reviewed autopsy studies. Although such an entity does seem to exist, and possibly to have a genetic basis (Hannisian et al, 1970), there is no doubt that a heterogeneous group of conditions has been classed under this name. Both Vanier (1960) and Dodge et al (1966) note that Möbius syndrome had been an initial diagnosis in their cases of myotonic dystrophy, and one patient studied by the author had been included in a published series of cases of this syndrome (Wallis, 1960). The term "Möbius syndrome" should be confined to those cases in which there is definite evidence of a nuclear lesion rather than primary muscle disease. In myotonic dystrophy the ocular muscle palsies and ptosis are less marked or absent, and careful study of the other clinical features and the family should resolve the situation.

Congenital Myopathies

This confusing and still incompletely delineated group of disorders contains many of those cases of infants formerly labelled "benign congenital hypotonia" or "amyotonia congenita", terms now best avoided. Hypotonia and motor delay are common features of the group, but clinical signs are often insufficient to distinguish the conditions from each other, and from the equally heterogeneous group of anterior horn cell disorders that may present in a similar way. When a number of generalised metabolic disorders, notably Pompe's disease (glycogenosis type II), are added, it can be seen that careful studies are required if some cases of congenital myotonic dystrophy are not to be confused with these conditions. In particular the less severe cases of congenital myotonic dystrophy, in which the facial diplegia is less obvious and hypotonia and developmental delay are the principal features, may be difficult to distinguish.

Fortunately, muscle biopsy provides a specific diagnosis in most of the congenital myopathies, provided it is taken, processed and interpreted by experts, using histochemistry and electron microscopy in addition to conventional stains. Dubowitz and Brooke (1973) give a clear description of the changes, as well as those in congenital myotonic dystrophy (Chapter 12); the clinical features have been well reviewed by Gardner-Medwin (1977).

Four types of congenital myopathy have been sufficiently well defined to warrant mention here.

Nemaline (Rod Body) Myopathy.* Severe infantile hypotonia is common, with muscle hypoplasia, respiratory problems and progressive

---

*Shy et al, 1963; Engel et al, 1964; Hudgson et al, 1967.

scoliosis; facial weakness may resemble myotonic dystrophy. There are also skeletal changes similar to those of the Marfan syndrome. Inheritance is autosomal dominant, with transmission frequently through a mildly, even subclinically affected parent. Muscle biopsy shows the characteristic rods within muscle fibres, from which the disease derives its name.

Central Core Disease. Hypotonia is again the most conspicuous feature, and there is considerable variation in severity of symptoms; selective weakness of trunk and other proximal muscles is usual, but not facial weakness. There may be improvement during childhood and some cases are extremely mild. Most reported families have followed autosomal dominant inheritance, but with marked variation in severity. The "central cores" seen on muscle biopsy are characterised by lack of mitochondria and their associated oxidative enzymes.

Centronuclear Myopathy. Originally termed "myotubular myopathy" by Spiro et al (1966), the main clinical features include facial weakness, ophthalmoplegia and ptosis in addition to hypotonia and motor delay, a combination which may be confused with congenital myotonic dystrophy, although in the latter condition ptosis and ocular weakness are rarely prominent. Hawkes and Absolon (1975) have described an unusual patient in whom this myopathy was accompanied by cataract and by myotonic discharges on electromyography, although there was no clinical myotonia.

Congenital Fibre Type Disproportion. This is essentially a biopsy diagnosis (Brooke, 1973), with hypertrophy of type 2 fibres contrasting with atrophy of type 1 fibres, and no other specific changes. The clinical features are non-specific, with hypotonia a general finding; various skeletal problems have been noted including arthrogryposis, congenital dislocation of the hip and progressive scoliosis. Prognosis for life appears to be good. Inheritance is uncertain and the condition may well prove to be heterogeneous.

Table 9-7. DIFFERENTIAL DIAGNOSIS OF CONGENITAL MYOTONIC DYSTROPHY

Congenital myopathies
    Nemaline myopathy
    Central core disease
    Centronuclear (myotubular) myopathy
    Congenital fibre type disproportion
Congenital myasthenia gravis
Spinal muscular atrophies (severe and intermediate types)
Möbius syndrome
Primary cerebral disorders
    Anoxic brain damage
    Metabolic cerebral degenerations (e.g., type II glycogenosis)

Table 9–8. CONGENITAL MYOTONIC DYSTROPHY AND MYOTONIA
CONGENITA: DISTINGUISHING FEATURES IN INFANCY AND
EARLY CHILDHOOD

	Congenital Myotonic Dystrophy	Myotonia Congenita
Myotonia — clinical	Absent	Frequent
EMG	Slight — usually detectable	Conspicuous
Hypotonia	Frequent, severe	Absent
Weakness	Severe	Slight or absent
Muscle bulk	Hypoplasia	Normal or hypertrophy
Mental retardation	Frequent	Absent
Inheritance	Autosomal dominant	Autosomal dominant or recessive
	Mother almost always affected	Sporadic cases frequent

Congenital Myotonic Dystrophy and Myotonia Congenita

Myotonia congenita has deliberately been omitted from the differential diagnosis of congenital myotonic dystrophy in Table 9–7, since the two conditions are quite dissimilar in infancy. Confusion of nomenclature, together with widespread ignorance of the fact that myotonic dystrophy can occur in infancy, frequently results in misunderstanding, and to help avoid this the main distinguishing features are summarised in Table 9–8. A clear distinction is of great importance in genetic counselling, in view of the different prognosis of the two disorders.

AETIOLOGY AND GENETIC BASIS OF CONGENITAL MYOTONIC DYSTROPHY

The recognition of the clinical syndrome of congenital myotonic dystrophy, the features of which have been described above, has raised a number of questions concerning its pathogenesis, inheritance and other possible aetiological factors, including the following:

1. Why are the clinical features in neonatal cases so different from those seen in adult life?.

2. What is the relationship between the congenital form and the adult disease? Are different genes involved?

3. What is the explanation for the almost exclusively maternal transmission of the congenital form? Can this be reconciled with the autosomal dominant inheritance occurring in the adult disease?

In the author's opinion the key to the first two questions lies in the third, and the problem of maternal transmission will therefore be considered first.

It has already been mentioned that cases of congenital myotonic

Table 9-9. CONGENITAL MYOTONIC DYSTROPHY:
SEVERITY OF PARENTAL DISEASE*

	No.
Asymptomatic (1)	20
Minor symptoms, medical attention not sought (2)	14
Symptoms sufficient to require medical attention (3)	8
Moderately disabled (4)	5
Severely disabled (5)	1
Uncertain	4
Parent not identified	2
Total	54

*From Harper, 1975b.

dystrophy were noted to have affected mothers from the time of the earliest reports, but only with the accumulation of large series did it become apparent that the maternal transmission was so overwhelming as to demand a special explanation. The full data on parental transmission are shown later in Table 10–2, but taking cases with onset under 5 years of age the combined series of published cases gives 118 instances of maternal transmission and only six paternally transmitted cases out of a total of 132. When strictly congenital cases are considered, only two paternally transmitted cases remain, neither of which had severe problems at birth or evidence of intrauterine abnormalities.

A maternal transmission of this type does not fit with autosomal dominant inheritance, and prompted a full genetic study of the families of patients with congenital onset (Harper, 1975b). The first question to be answered was whether the affected mothers were themselves particularly severely affected or had any special features. This proved not to be the case; when severity of muscle disease was graded from 1 to 5, over half the affected mothers were either asymptomatic or had symptoms not requiring medical attention (Table 9–9). None had congenital onset themselves, and the clinical picture was essentially that of the normal adult disease.

Turning to the sibs of the cases with congenital onset, the data are summarised in Table 9–10. This shows that although most affected sibs also have congenital onset, or at least severe childhood disease, over half (ignoring the propositi) are entirely unaffected, with no hint of neonatal or other problems. This strongly suggests that to have congenital myotonic dystrophy a child must have inherited the myotonic dystrophy gene, but that the maternal transmission has in some way affected the mode of onset. Further support for this view comes from the finding, given in detail in the next chapter, that series of adult cases show an excess of *paternally* transmitted cases and that transmission by the sexes is equal when considered over the entire age range.

Table 9–10.   GENETIC DATA ON SIBSHIPS OF PATIENTS WITH CONGENITAL MYOTONIC DYSTROPHY*

	Total	Male	Female
Congenital cases			
Total	70	40	30
Propositi	56	27	29
Non-propositi	14	12	2
Other affected sibs	9	5	4
Unaffected sibs	46	22	24
Neonatal deaths			
(1 sex uncertain)	24	10	13
Total liveborn	149	77	71

*From Harper, 1975b.

The genetic data thus support the view that congenital myotonic dystrophy results from a combination of the gene causing the normal form of the disease together with some maternally transmitted factor. Returning to the clinical features it can now be seen that this hypothesis explains a number of otherwise puzzling facts; in particular it would account for the onset in utero with effects most marked immediately after birth, but with a tendency to improve during childhood, only to deteriorate gradually during adolescence and adult life. The essential defect in congenital myotonic dystrophy is a widespread intrauterine hypoplasia of muscle, and its distinctive features can all be explained by the extent and distribution of this hypoplasia. The absence of myotonia and other typical "adult" features is also easier to explain on the basis of a maternally transmitted factor than on the basis of the action of the myotonic dystrophy gene being brought forward into intrauterine life.

The hypothesis has been challenged by Bundey and Carter (1972) who prefer to explain the congenital form by the existence of genetic heterogeneity. The arguments for and against such heterogeneity in myotonic dystrophy are given in Chapter 10, but as regards the congenital form it fails to explain the existence of all grades of severity in the same family, and the complete lack of congenital cases arising as new mutations without an affected parent. The maternal transmission has been attributed to relative male infertility in families with congenitally affected children, but the fact that this form does not occur at all among the offspring of affected males in these families makes this argument unacceptable. Finally, the suggestion that congenital myotonic dystrophy might be recognised only when the mother is known to be affected is not borne out by many of the author's cases, in which the infant was diagnosed first and the mother only subsequently found to be affected.

In the author's view the evidence for the action of a maternal environmental factor as well as the abnormal gene is overwhelming; the unsolved problem is, what is the nature of the factor? This remains entirely unknown, the evidence being at present negative and circumstantial, but several possibilities come to mind.

The first is an immunological disturbance comparable to that of rhesus haemolytic disease, which also requires a specific genotype together with an intrauterine factor for its production. Against this is the lack of any evidence of immune phenomena, together with a lack of the birth order effect (Harper, 1975b) that is seen in rhesus haemolytic disease. The condition of congenital myasthenia gravis provides a parallel situation now known to result from passive transfer of antibodies against acetycholine receptor protein, but there is no evidence in this disorder that the genotype of the fetus plays a role, and the myasthenic state is a temporary phenomenon, with no subsequent predisposition to myasthenia in later life.

A second possibility is the action of some metabolite in the mother that might pass transplacentally to affect the fetus. This is made more plausible by the existence of myotonia caused by drugs interfering with cholesterol synthesis (see Chapter 14), although present evidence is against myotonic dystrophy being due to a metabolic disturbance of this type. A good example of an intrauterine metabolic defect is seen in maternal phenylketonuria (Mabry et al, 1962) in which cerebral damage to the non-phenylketonuric fetus results from the transplacental effects of phenylalanine and other metabolites from the affected mother. Again, the situation is different from myotonic dystrophy in that all offspring of a phenylketonuric mother are affected, whereas in myotonic dystrophy the genetically normal offspring are in no way damaged.

A variety of maternal effects in man and other species results from infective agents whose effect may be genotype specific. Slow viruses such as scrapie (Dickinson et al, 1974) or more conventional agents such as hepatitis B virus (Blumberg, 1977) are examples. A search for conventional viral agents by electron microscopy and culture of a placenta giving rise to a congenital case in the author's series proved negative; examination of viral titres for ten common viruses on sera of the mothers of congenital cases studied by the author showed no difference from those of control sera.

It can be concluded that congenital myotonic dystrophy is a syndrome with a number of unique features which are diagnostically highly distinctive once one is familiar with the disorder. Not only are there striking clinical differences between this form of the disease and the classical picture of myotonic dystrophy with onset in adolescence or adult life, but there is strong evidence for aetiological differences also, even though the two forms occur within the same family and appear to involve the same abnormal gene. The fact that the almost exclusively maternal transmission of congenital myotonic dystrophy occurs within a disorder that in general clearly follows autosomal dominant inheritance should serve as a reminder that intrauterine and other non-mendelian influences may play an important role in disorders following mendelian inheritance (Harper, 1977). It will be interesting to see if comparable effects are observed in conditions other than myotonic dystrophy, and of even greater interest to elucidate the basis of the maternal effect in myotonic dystrophy itself.

REFERENCES

Aicardi J., Conti D. and Goutières F. (1974): Les formes néo-natales de la dystrophie myotonique de Steinert. J. Neurol. Sci. 22:149–164.

Bell D. B. and Smith D. W. (1972): Myotonic dystrophy in the neonate. J. Pediatr. 81:83–86

Bell J. (1948): The Treasury of Human Inheritance. 4. Nervous Diseases and Muscular Dystrophies. Part V. Dystrophia Myotonica and Allied Diseases. Cambridge University Press.

Blumberg B. S. (1977): Australia Antigen and the Biology of Hepatitis. Nobel Foundation, Stockholm.

Bossen E. H., Shelburne J. D. and Verkauf B. S. (1974): Respiratory muscle involvement in infantile myotonic dystrophy. Arch. Pathol. 97:250–252.

Brooke M. H. (1973): A neuromuscular disease characterised by fibre type disproportion. In Clinical Studies in Myology (Ed.: B. A. Kakulas). Excerpta Medica, Amsterdam.

Bundey S. and Carter C. O. (1972): Genetic heterogeneity for dystrophia myotonica. J. Med. Genet. 9:311–315.

Calderon R. (1966): Myotonic dystrophy: a neglected cause of mental retardation. J. Pediatr. 68:423–431.

Caughey J. E. and Barclay J. (1954): Dystrophia myotonica and the occurrence of congenital physical defects in affected families. Australas. Ann. Med. 3:165–170.

Dickinson A. G., Stamp J. T. and Renwick C. C. J. (1974): Maternal and lateral transmission of scrapie in sheep. J. Comp. Pathol. 84:19–25.

Dodge P. R., Gamstorp I., Byers R. K. and Russell P. (1966): Myotonic dystrophy in infancy and childhood. Pediatrics 35:3–19.

Dubowitz V. (1978): Muscle Disorders in Childhood. W. B. Saunders Co., London, Philadelphia.

Dubowitz V. and Brooke M. H. (1973): Muscle Biopsy: A Modern Approach. W. B. Saunders Co., London, Philadelphia.

Dunn L. J. and Dierker L. J. (1973): Recurrent hydramnios in association with myotonia dystrophica. Obstet. Gynecol. 42:104–106.

Dyken P. R. and Harper P. S. (1973): Congenital dystrophia myotonica. Neurology (Minneap.) 23:465–473.

Engel W. K., Wanko T. and Fenichel G. M. (1964): Nemaline myopathy, a second case. Arch. Neurol. 11:22–39.

Evans P. R. (1955): Nuclear agenesis, Möbius syndrome: the congenital facial diplegia syndrome. Arch. Dis. Child. 30:237–243.

Farkas E., Tomé F. M. S., Fardeau M., Arsenio-Nunes M. L., Dreyfus P. and Diebler M. F. (1974): Histochemical and ultrastructural study of muscle biopsies in 3 cases of dystrophia myotonica in the newborn child. J. Neurol. Sci. 21:273–288.

Fried K., Payewski M., Mundel G., Casp E. and Spira R. (1975): Thin ribs in neonatal myotonic dystrophy. Clin. Genet. 7:417–420.

Gardner-Medwin D. (1977): Children with genetic muscular disorders. Br. J. Hosp. Med. 17:314–316, 321–324, 326.

Giovanucci M. L., Calabri G. and Paoli A. (1970): Su di caso di distrofia miotonica in una bambina con ritardo mentale. Haematologica 54:849.

Gordon N. and Hilson D. (1967): Myotonic dystrophy—its occurrence in childhood. Br. J. Clin. Pract. *21*:537–540.

Hanissian A. S., Fuste F., Hayes W. T. and Duncan J. M. (1970): Möbius syndrome in twins. Am. J. Dis. Child. *120*:472–475.

Harper P. S. (1972): Genetic studies in myotonic dystrophy. Thesis for degree of D. M., University of Oxford, U. K.

Harper P. S. (1975a): Congenital myotonic dystrophy in Britain. 1. Clinical aspects. Arch. Dis. Child. *50*:505–513.

Harper P. S. (1975b): Congenital myotonic dystrophy in Britain. 2. Genetic basis. Arch. Dis. Child. *50*:514–521.

Harper P. S. (1977): Mendelian inheritance or transmissable agent?—the lesson of Kuru and the Australia antigen. J. Med. Genet. *14*:389–398.

Harper P. S. and Dyken P. R. (1972): Early onset dystrophia myotonica—evidence supporting a maternal environmental factor. Lancet *2*:53–55.

Hawkes C. H. and Absolon M. J. (1975): Myotubular myopathy associated with cataract and electrical myotonia. J. Neurol. Neurosurg. Psychiatry *38*:761–764.

Henderson J. L. (1939): The congenital facial diplegia syndrome: clinical features, pathology and aetiology. Brain *62*:381–403.

Hudgson P., Pearce G. W. and Walton J. N. (1967): Preclinical muscular dystrophy: histopathological changes observed in muscle biopsy. Brain *90*:565–576.

Jean B., Bouchard M., Laberge C., Lemieux L., Coulombier J., and Gauzere R. (1968): Dystrophie myotonique dans une institution Canadienne Francaise. Rev. Neuropsychiatr. Infant. *16*:701–707.

Karpati G., Carpenter S., Watters G. V., Eisen A. E. and Andermann F. (1973): Infantile myotonic dystrophy. Histochemical and electron microscopic features in skeletal muscle. Neurology *23*:1066–1077.

Klein D. (1958): La dystrophie myotonique (Steinert) et la myotonie congenitale (Thomsen) en Suisse. J. Genet. Hum. (Suppl.) *7*.

Lenard H. G., Goebel H. H. and Weigel W. (1977): Smooth muscle involvement in congenital myotonic dystrophy. Neuropaediatrie *8*:42–52.

L'Hirondel J., Guihard J., Velotlerou A., and Orange C. (1970) La maladie de Steinert néonatale: à propos d'une observation. Sem. Hop. Paris *46*:1867–1874.

Maas O. (1937): Observations on dystrophia myotonica. Brain *60*:498–524.

Mabry C. C., Denniston J. C., Nelson T. L. and Son C. D. (1962): Maternal phenylketonuria. A cause of mental retardation in children without metabolic defect. N. Engl. J. Med. *269*:1404–1408.

Messer J., Brochard A., Willard D. and Jesel M. (1973): Myotonic dystrophy in the neonate. Acta Paediatr. Belg. *27*: Fasc 4.

Mundler F. (1970): Forme néonatale et infantile précoce de la dystrophie myotonique (maladie de Steinert). Pediatrie *25*:865–872.

Parker N. (1963): Dystrophia myotonica presenting as congenital facial diplegia. Med. J. Aust. *2*:939–944.

Pitner S. E., Edwards J. E., and McCormick W. F. (1965): Observations on the pathology of the Möbius syndrome. J. Neurol. Neurosurg. Psychiatry *28*:362–374.

Pruzanski W. (1965): Congenital malformations in myotonic dystrophy. Acta Neurol. Scand. *41*:34–38.

Rosman N. P. and Kakulas B. A. (1966): Mental deficiency associated with muscular dystrophy—a neuropathological study. Brain *89*:769–788.

Sarnat H. B., O'Connor T. and Byrne P. A. (1976): Clinical effects of myotonic dystrophy on pregnancy and the neonate. Arch. Neurol. *33*:459–465.

Sarnat H. B. and Silbert S. W. (1976): Maturational arrest of fetal muscle in neonatal myotonic dystrophy. Arch. Neurol. *33*:466–474.

Serradell A. (1972): La enfermedad de Steinert neonatal. A proposito de una observation. Med. Clin. *58*:3.

Shy G. M., Engel W. K., Somers J. E. and Wanko T., (1963): Nemaline myopathy: new congenital myopathy. Brain *86*:793–810.

Simpson K. (1975): Neonatal respiratory failure due to myotonic dystrophy. Arch. Dis. Child. *50*:569–571.

Spiro, A. J., Shy G. M. and Gonotas N. K. (1966): Myotubular myopathy. Arch. Neurol. *14*:1–14.

Swift T. R., Ignacio O. J. and Dyken P. R. (1975): Neonatal dystrophia myotonica: electrophysiologic studies. Am. J. Dis. Child. *129*:734–737.

Thomasen E. (1948): Myotonia. Universitetsforlaget Aarhus.

Vanier T. M. (1960): Dystrophia myotonica in childhood. Br. Med. J. *2*:1284–1288.

Verger P., Guillard J. M. and Eschapasse P. (1967): La maladie de Steinert (myopathie myotonique) a debut précoce (dans la petite enfance). Ann. Pédiatr. *14*:745–749.

Wallis P. G. (1960): Creatinuria in Moebius syndrome. Arch. Dis. Child. *35*:393–395.

Watters G. V. and Williams T. W. (1967): Early onset myotonic dystrophy. Arch. Neurol. *17*:137–152.

Zellweger H. and Ionasescu V. (1973): Early onset of myotonic dystrophy. Am. J. Dis. Child. *125*:601–604.

CHAPTER TEN

The Genetic Basis of Myotonic Dystrophy

Thomsen's original description of the striking hereditary pattern of myotonia congenita in his own family resulted in a similar hereditary nature being considered likely for the other myotonic disorders as they became distinguished. The cases of myotonic dystrophy reported by Batten and Gibb (1909) included an affected brother and sister, but even from this study it was clear that the familial pattern was less regular than in myotonia congenita, and when Rohrer (1916) analysed a series of 92 published cases he could find affected relatives in less than half. He proposed that a proportion of cases were not hereditary, but this was soon refuted by the remarkable studies of Fleischer (1918) in Germany, who not only examined all available relatives, but painstakingly searched the church records of their ancestors. Fleischer found numerous relatives with minor features of the disease, notably cataract, so that only five of his 38 patients remained isolated cases. He further showed that several of his families were related through distant common ancestors not known to have been affected. His conclusion that the disorder showed regular dominant inheritance, but might vary greatly in the degree of expression, was generally accepted and has been amply confirmed by subsequent studies.

The meticulous nature of Fleischer's work led some investigators to the extreme view that true isolated cases could not exist. Thus, Adie and Greenfield (1923) considered that a general rule existed whereby, if a disorder was familial, every case must show affected relatives if sufficiently careful study was made. This view, although clearly erroneous in general, is certainly less far from the truth for myotonic dystrophy than for most inherited disorders. Maas (1937) searched with great enthusiasm for minor signs of the disease in relatives and claimed that stigmata of the condition could be identified in almost all children of affected individuals, not just the 50 percent expected on the basis of dominant inheritance. The minor"stigmata" which he considered as evidence of the disease have not been generally accepted as reliable diagnostic features.

The view that myotonic dystrophy did in fact conform to the criteria for autosomal dominant inheritance was placed beyond doubt by the extensive studies of Bell (1948) and Thomasen (1948), and subsequently by those of Lynas (1957) and Klein (1958). The first of these was compiled largely from the literature, together with families previously studied by Maas in London. The other three were essentially clinical and epidemiological surveys based on defined areas, Denmark, Northern Ireland and Switzerland respectively. Most of the evidence to be discussed here is based on these valuable studies.

MODE OF INHERITANCE

A number of criteria must be fulfilled before autosomal dominant inheritance can be accepted; in particular the disorder should occur in 50 percent of the offspring of an affected person, but not be transmitted by an unaffected individual, and incidence in the sexes and transmission of the condition by them should be equal. These criteria will be considered in turn, but first it may be asked whether there is evidence to support any other mode of inheritance operating in myotonic dystrophy, either in the disorder as a whole or in a subgroup of families.

X-linked inheritance can be immediately ruled out by the frequent observation of male-to-male transmission, as well as by the equal incidence in the sexes. A family consisting of affected females only has been briefly reported (Pierson et al, 1975), but occasional chance occurrences of this type are to be expected and bear little on the mode of inheritance. Autosomal recessive inheritance is equally improbable in myotonic dystrophy, for not only is there regular transmission from one generation to the next, but multiple affected sibs with definitely unaffected parents are not seen. Apparent instances of such a situation are not infrequent (see Fig. 10–1), but critical examination of the parents shows signs of the disease in one of them, and the fact that the affected sibs transmit the disorder to their own offspring further serves to exclude autosomal recessive inheritance. The fact that no individual pedigrees supporting this form of inheritance have ever been reported despite the abundant literature on the condition makes it most unlikely that a subgroup following autosomal recessive inheritance exists, as in myotonia congenita, and this is supported by a notable lack of consanguinity (*see below*).

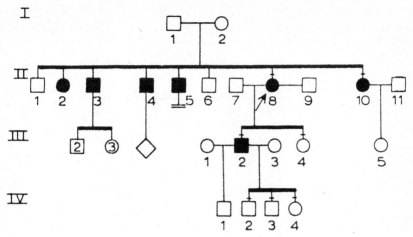

Figure 10–1. INHERITANCE PATTERN OF MYOTONIC DYSTROPHY.

The occurrence of multiple affected sibs born to apparently unaffected parents is suggestive superficially of autosomal recessive inheritance, but the fact that the disorder has been transmitted to individual III-2 strongly favours autosomal dominant inheritance; one of the deceased grandparents is likely to have been mildly affected. (Family 37 of Harper, 1972.)

Turning to positive evidence for regular autosomal dominant inheritance, an important point in its favour is the absence of "skipped generations" in pedigrees of the disease. In the few instances in which this appears to occur examination of the supposedly unaffected individual has shown clear evidence of the disease, as in the family described below and illustrated in Figure 10–2.

The propositus, born in 1918, developed weakness of the hands at age 42 years, and when examined in 1970 showed generalised muscle weakness, myotonia and early cataracts. His three children were stated to be healthy, and permission to interview them was refused. The following year the eldest daughter gave birth to a son with profound hypotonia, feeding difficulty and facial weakness. The diagnosis of congenital myotonic dystrophy was made only after the history of the affected paternal grandfather was obtained. The mother denied symptoms, but examination showed unequivocal myotonia and early limb and facial weakness.

The most important test of autosomal dominant inheritance is whether the first-degree relatives of affected individuals show the expected 50 percent ratio of affected members. Data from the major genetic studies are shown in Table 10–1, and it can be seen that, although the 50 percent ratio is often exceeded when propositi are included in the calculations, almost all fall short of 50 percent affected after deduction of the propositi. Among these studies, only that of Klein (1958) approached complete ascertainment of the disease in the population; deduction of the propositi in this case probably overcompensates for bias of ascertainment. Klein's data were subjected to more detailed segregation analysis

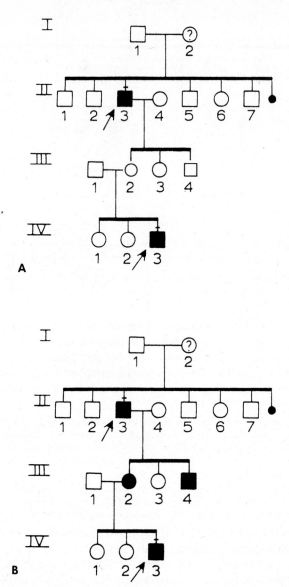

Figure 10–2. Apparent "skipped generation" in myotonic dystrophy.

A, Pedigree before investigation of generation III.

B, Pedigree after full investigation. There is no skipping of generations and the pattern of transmission is compatible with autosomal dominant inheritance. (Family 14 of Harper, 1972.)

**Table 10–1. MYOTONIC DYSTROPHY – PROPORTION
AFFECTED IN SIBSHIPS**

Source	Type of Relative	Total Members	Affected	Propositi	% Affected Propositi Included	Propositi Excluded
Thomasen (1948)	Sibships of propositi	76	42	17	55.3	42.5
	Children of propositi	56	26	1	46.4	45.5
	Other sibships	71	36	0	50.7	50.7
Lynas (1957)	Combined sibships	109	42	18	38.6	26.4
Klein (1958)	Combined sibships	717	362	182	50.5	33.6
Harper (1972)	Sibships of propositi	142	87	47	61.3	42.1

by Todorov et al (1970), who found them to be compatible with autosomal dominant inheritance, but with a reduced penetrance of the gene and an excess of sporadic cases.

The conclusion that can be drawn from the combined data is that they fit well with autosomal dominant inheritance and are quite incompatible with any other form of inheritance, but that fewer than the expected 50 percent of first-degree relatives show the disease — i.e., the gene is not fully penetrant. This is examined further in the following section.

PENETRANCE OF THE MYOTONIC DYSTROPHY GENE

With a disorder so variable in both severity and age at onset as myotonic dystrophy, it is reasonable to ask whether some individuals might show complete lack of penetrance — i.e., fail to develop any features of the disease — throughout their life. The answer to this question will clearly depend in part on how thoroughly signs of the disorder are sought, and on the age of the individual; these factors have not always been taken into account in genetic analysis of the problem. The practical significance of the degree of penetrance is considerable, and is discussed fully in relation to preclinical detection of the disorder in Chapter 11. If all those carrying the myotonic dystrophy gene can be shown to have recognisable abnormalities by a particular age, more definite genetic advice can be given regarding the risk of transmitting the disorder than is the case if a significant proportion of gene carriers remains undetectable.

One simple but powerful argument in favour of near-complete penetrance of the myotonic dystrophy gene in older age groups is the lack of "skipped generations" referred to above. In other individuals, however, particularly older members with mild ocular and muscle abnormalities, there is a strong presumption that nothing abnormal would have been detected had they been examined earlier in adult life. Thus, the woman described in Figure 10–4 showing lens opacities and slight myotonia as the only abnormalities at age 61 years had a normal slit-lamp examination at age 50.

In the younger age groups there are patients in whom initial assessment has been normal but in whom abnormalities subsequently develop. Polgar et al (1972) record a 9 year old girl in whom clinical and electromyographic myotonia developed a year after all investigations had previously been negative. A 25 year old man with an affected father studied by the author was found to be normal clinically and by slit-lamp and electromyographic examination, but two years subsequently had developed multiple lens opacities, not in themselves diagnostic, but sufficiently abnormal to classify him as equivocally affected.

Some information can be obtained from the curves for age at onset of the disease already shown in Figure 2–17. The various studies agree in demonstrating that 50 percent of patients have developed the disorder by around 20 years of age, and that a significant number do not develop it until after 50 years of age. This approach is limited by two sources of bias. First, since the curves are based on definite cases of the disease, they inevitably reach 100 percent of manifestation and would not include any individuals who carry the gene but never develop the disorder. Second, they are based on age of development of the symptoms, and do not take into account the possibility of presymptomatic detection at an earlier age. The finding in the author's study (Harper, 1973) that 18 percent of asymptomatic first-degree relatives showed unequivocal abnormalities on clinical and slit-lamp investigation (Table 11–1) illustrates the inaccuracy of relying on age at symptomatic onset as a basis for penetrance analysis.

The same defects apply to the studies of the proportion of affected members in sibships already discussed, in which it is rarely made clear on what criteria members were scored as unaffected, and what range of age groups was included. These can be overcome in part by grouping individuals by age, and data from the author's studies treated in this way are shown in Figure 10–3, which includes only offspring of patients who had been fully examined; sibships ascertained through an affected sib or child are excluded.

Several conclusions can be drawn from these data: under 10 years of age the penetrance is clearly far from complete, but a rapid rise to the expected 50 percent ratio is seen in the 10 to 14 year old group, suggesting that penetrance is essentially complete by this age even though many of the individuals are asymptomatic. There are two possible sources of bias, however, that may result in overestimation of completeness in penetrance. First, the inclusion only of examined individuals may exaggerate the proportion of members affected by preferential ascertainment of such individuals — the finding of more than 50 percent affected in young adult age groups, where a number of unaffected members had moved to other localities as the result of work or marriage, suggests that this is indeed

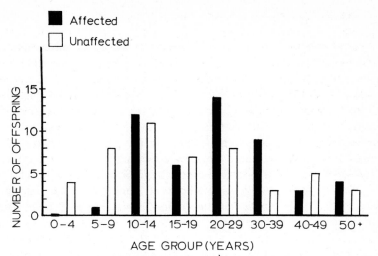

Figure 10-3. Myotonic dystrophy: gene penetrance in relation to age (from Harper, 1973).

happening. A reverse effect from increased mortality of affected individuals might be expected in older age groups, but is not seen in Figure 10-3.

Bundey (1974), reanalysing previous data (Bundey et al, 1970) in a similar way, found that in families in which the propositus developed myotonic dystrophy before 20 years of age penetrance appeared to be complete by age 14, but that this was not the case in families in which the propositus showed late onset; this suggested that in such later-onset families healthy members cannot be reassured with so high a degree of confidence that they are not later going to develop the disorder. Likewise, the data on congenital myotonic dystrophy (Harper, 1975b) suggest that in such sibships other children carrying the abnormal gene are also likely to develop this form of the disease and that, conversely, healthy children will remain free from it. Whether this will invariably prove to be the case will require prospective study.

The main practical conclusion to be drawn from studies of penetrance in myotonic dystrophy is that the great majority of individuals carrying the abnormal gene can be detected in early adult life by careful clinical examination combined with the other preclinical tests discussed in Chapter 11. Since this is the stage at which genetic counselling is generally sought, it is possible to give much more definite advice to such individuals regarding the risk of developing or transmitting the disorder than for some other dominantly inherited disorders, notably Huntington's chorea, in which the penetrance of the gene, however studied, remains low throughout the years of reproductive life.

TWIN STUDIES

In a disorder such as myotonic dystrophy showing simple mendelian inheritance, a monozygotic twin pair should always be concordant for the disorder, and dizygotic twins should show discordance in 50 percent of cases, as in sibs. The most valuable information provided by twins in this situation is the variation in clinical picture seen between a pair of monozygous twins, since differences in age at onset, in severity, and in systems principally affected must indicate the action of environmental factors. Unfortunately, there are few reports of twins with myotonic dystrophy; Klein (1958) mentions monozygous twin brothers who both showed mild muscle changes and who were identified by the characteristic lens opacities. His series also contained three dizygous pairs, two of whom were discordant for the disease, and a concordant dizygous pair was recorded by Thomasen. The author's study of the adult disease (Harper, 1972, 1973) contained no twins, but a discordant dizygotic pair was found in the study of congenital myotonic dystrophy in Britain (Harper, 1975a). Since it is likely that a maternal environmental factor is involved in this form of disease, this provides evidence that possession of the abnormal gene is a necessary factor in addition to any maternal environmental influence. Further twin data of this nature would be particularly valuable.

CONSANGUINITY

There is general agreement that consanguinity is not a feature of marriages resulting in offspring with myotonic dystrophy. No consanguinity was found in the study of Thomasen (1948), nor is it recorded in the other major genetic studies. Todorov et al (1970) calculated the coefficient of consanguinity for the Swiss families and compared it with the extensive data available for the various Swiss regions. They found no increase over the general population level either in the present or in previous generations. The author's data (Harper 1972, 1975b) show no consanguinity either in the American families principally with the adult form of myotonic dystrophy, or in the British survey of families with congenital myotonic dystrophy.

The lack of consanguinity in myotonic dystrophy contrasts sharply with the situation for myotonia congenita, where Becker (1971) found a tenfold increase in consanguinity in West Germany, and where consanguinity was one of the factors that led to recognition of a separate recessively inherited form. There is no evidence of a comparable situation in myotonic dystrophy, and the absence of consanguinity in the congenital form of the disease argues strongly against the involvement of recessive inheritance in the causation of this.

SEX-RELATED EFFECTS

A disorder showing autosomal dominant inheritance would not be expected to show significant differences between the sexes either in the frequency of the disease or in the frequency of transmitting it. Such findings would not necessarily exclude this mode of inheritance, but would require the action of special factors, such as limitation of expression of the gene to one sex, relative diminution of fertility in one sex, or effects of the intrauterine environment. In myotonic dystrophy sex differences in general had been found to be relatively slight until the recent demonstration that the congenital form of the disorder is almost invariably transmitted by the female. This finding is such a striking deviation from what is expected on genetic grounds that it becomes important to reassess the data on other age groups to see whether similar unrecognised differences may exist here also.

The incidence of myotonic dystrophy in adults has been found by all workers to be equal in the two sexes. The study of Klein (1958) showed 48.5 percent of males in a total of 717 members of affected sibships, although some bias may have resulted from the propositi being included in the estimate. Thomasen (1948), after removing propositi, also found a near-equal sex ratio of 48.5 percent of males (68 out of 138 total). The author's study of congenital myotonic dystrophy (Harper, 1975b) showed a slight excess of affected males in the sibships (45 out of 79), which was more marked when propositi were removed (19 out of 23).

Severity of muscle symptoms was found by Thomasen to be greater in males. He noted 71 percent of males but only 49 percent of females to have a disability rated at greater than two-thirds. Klein by contrast found no difference in disability between the sexes, and attributed this to the greater tendency of Swiss women to undertake manual work. Neither author encountered differences in age at onset, and Klein's data showed age at death to be similar, although Bell (1948) found males to die on average six years earlier than females, a comparable situation to that of the general population.

Studies on transmission of the disease by the sexes show differences that at first sight appear contradictory. Table 10–2 summarizes the results of the main studies, all of which agree in finding a marked increase in the number of sibships in which transmission was through an affected male parent, with the exception of the author's own study, in which transmission by the sexes was equal, and those of childhood disease which show predominantly maternal transmission. Even allowing for the sibships in which the transmitting parent was unknown it is difficult to ignore this increased male transmission, and although it could be explained on the basis of a relative reduction in fertility of affected women, this is the reverse of what has been found, as discussed later in the chapter.

Table 10–2.   PARENTAL TRANSMISSION OF MYOTONIC DYSTROPHY

	Sex of Affected Parent			TOTAL	% MALE (UNKNOWNS OMITTED)
	MALE	FEMALE	UNKNOWN		
Mainly Adults Studied					
Bell (1948): collected cases	300	146	131	577	67.3
Thomasen (1948)	30	24	not recorded	54	55.6
Klein (1958)	92	59	31	182	60.9
Combined series	422	229	162	813	64.8
All Age Groups Studied					
Harper (1972)	53	54	42	149	49.6
Childhood Onset					
Harper and Dyken (1972) and Dyken and Harper (1973) – onset under 5 years	4	28	2	34	12.5
Harper (1975b) – onset at birth personal cases	1	51	2	54	1.92
Previous cases in literature	1	39	4	44	2.50

The earlier genetic studies were all concerned principally with affected adults, and were performed at a time when the congenital form of the disease had not been clearly recognised; it is apparent from the clinical descriptions that affected infants would rarely if ever have been included in the data. Following the recognition by Vanier (1960) of the disease in infancy and early childhood, it came to be realised that myotonic dystrophy could present in infancy with features quite unlike those associated with the classical adult disease, and that most of these cases appeared to be maternally transmitted.

The author's study (Harper, 1972) was done at a time when the disorder in childhood was recognised, although not its maternal transmission. Thus, in contrast to the previous genetic studies, a representative sample of the disease across all age groups was obtained, and the equality of transmission by the sexes suggests that overall there is no excess of male transmission in myotonic dystrophy. When the childhood cases are more closely analysed, however, a striking difference is seen: there is not merely an excess of maternal transmission, but it is almost invariable. Separation of cases with onset under 5 years of age in the author's American study (Harper and Dyken, 1972) showed maternal transmission in 16 out of 17 cases (13 out of 14 sibships). The later survey of congenital myotonic dystrophy in Britain revealed that there was definite maternal transmission in 51 out of 54 sibships in which onset of the disease was at birth, only one case being paternally transmitted. Collected case reports in the literature confirm the pattern (Table 10–2).

The possible reasons for the maternal transmission of congenital myotonic dystrophy are discussed in Chapter 9; but it is clear that we have here the reason for the apparent preferential male transmission noted by earlier studies of adults. If, as seems probable, the disease shows equal transmission by the sexes when all age groups are included, omission of the maternally transmitted congenital cases would inevitably produce an apparent male excess of transmission in studies based mainly on the adult disease, and this is what is seen. The factor requiring explanation is thus not a primary inequality of transmission, but why a proportion of the maternally transmitted cases should show the severe congenital form of the disease. The clinical and genetic evidence favouring operation of an unidentified intrauterine factor has already been argued, and it can be seen from the overall genetic data that none of the evidence is incompatible with the existence of autosomal dominant inheritance as the basis for the disease as a whole.

CYTOGENETIC STUDIES

A disorder showing simple mendelian inheritance, such as myotonic dystrophy, would not be expected to exhibit a visible chromosomal abnormality, and the numerous reports of chromosome analysis in this condition probably reflect misunderstanding of this fundamental point. Not surprisingly some abnormalities have appeared among these patients, but whether they are of significance is difficult to say in view of the likelihood that normal results would not have been reported. Several males with both myotonic dystrophy and Klinefelter's syndrome have been recorded (Grumbach et al, 1957; Teter et al, 1960; Fiol et al, 1975). It is of interest that in the last of these patients the hypogonadism had been noted to be much more marked than is usually the case in myotonic dystrophy. Despite the similarity of the testicular histology of the two conditions it seems unlikely that there is any true relationship, and it is probable that the concidence of the two conditions, rather more often than might have been expected, is the result of both disorders being causes of male hypogonadism, in which chromosomal studies are a commonly performed investigation.

Other families have been described in which myotonic dystrophy has been associated with a balanced translocation. In one of these families with a D — D translocation (Bowen et al, 1968), neurologically normal individuals also showed the chromosome abnormality, making any causal relationship unlikely. Such families are nevertheless important in that they might allow location of the myotonic dystrophy gene by linkage analysis. The family of Bowen et al was restudied by the author (family 8 of Harper et al, 1972) with this in view, but the finding that the chromosome abnormality originated from the unaffected grandparent made this impossible.

An interesting suggestion was made by Fitzgerald and Caughey (1962) that a true chromosomal defect might be present in the severely affected individuals with congenital myotonic dystrophy. The occurrence of other congenital abnormalities in such patients and the probable involvement of an intrauterine maternal factor make this a more likely possibility than in the disease as a whole; Fitzgerald and Caughey found a small additional acrocentric chromosome in three such patients and suggested that it might be of causal significance. This has not been confirmed, and studies on the author's series of patients with congenital myotonic dystrophy (performed by Dr. George Conner) were essentially normal. These are summarised in Table 10–3.

Only one example of meiotic chromosome studies is known to the author. This was performed on a testicular biopsy from a boy with congenital myotonic dystrophy (family 1 in Harper and Dyken, 1972) and was entirely normal.

Most cytogenetic studies in myotonic dystrophy were performed before the introduction of new banding techniques that allow recognition of greater detail of chromosome structure, but no abnormalities have been reported using such techniques, nor are they likely. The original conclu-

Table 10–3. CHROMOSOME ANALYSIS IN CHILDREN WITH CONGENITAL MYOTONIC DYSTROPHY AND THEIR AFFECTED MOTHERS*

Children CASE	SEX	AGE AT STUDY (YEARS)	Chromosome Distribution									
			40	41	42	43	44	45	46	47	48	49
1	M	2½						5	55			
2	F	1½						4	93	2		
3	M	4					1	6	92	1		
4	F	6				2	9	8	79	2		
5	M	6		2		3	7	18	70			
Mothers												
1		24						5	53			
2		26			1	2	1	2	94			
3		30		1	1	2		11	81	3		1
4		32					1	10	84	5		
5		36		1			9	15	75			
6		44				2	5	19	71			
			(2 cells 46+ fragment; 1 cell 45+ fragment)									
7		30			2		1	14	81	1		
			(1 cell 46+ fragment)									

*Unpublished data of Dr. George Conner on patients studied by Professor A. E. H. Emery, Edinburgh, and the author.

sion stated at the beginning of this section remains valid: as a mendelian disorder a specific biochemical basis rather than a chromosomal defect is to be expected in myotonic dystrophy.

GENETIC HETEROGENEITY

Myotonic dystrophy traditionally has been regarded as a single entity, but as with many other inherited disorders this view has come under critical scrutiny. The existence of genetic heterogeneity, in which what appears to be a single clinical entity proves to be composed of two or more fundamentally different disorders, has proved to be so common in medical genetics that it is important to ask whether the immense variability of myotonic dystrophy could result in part from such heterogeneity. The problem of the relationship between myotonic dystrophy and the other myotonic disorders has already been discussed.

It is essential first to differentiate clearly between the concept of multiple mutations at a single locus, and the existence of more than one locus. Studies on biochemically understood loci — such as the β chain of haemoglobin — have shown that mutations may occur at numerous points along the nucleic acid chain that determines the amino acid sequence. There is no reason to suppose that this is not true for other loci, although our lack of understanding may prevent its precise documentation. Such mutations at different points in the same locus might be expressed clinically as showing different grades of severity or age at onset. It is likely that such processes are responsible for the observed similarities of the course of the disease within a family that are seen in most genetic conditions.

Heterogeneity due to more than one locus is a fundamentally different situation, since it implies that more than one basic defect is involved. Nevertheless, such heterogeneity is common, as for instance in the mucopolysaccharidoses, in the X-linked muscular dystrophies in which the Duchenne and Becker types have been shown to be controlled by different loci, and in many other groups of genetic diseases.

For myotonic dystrophy the evidence is somewhat in favour of the former, but strongly against the latter form of heterogeneity. Bundey and Carter (1972) analysed the correlation of age at onset of the disease within and between families, and found high correlation coefficients for age at onset between sibs and between parents and offspring (0.81 and 0.80 respectively). They have suggested that their findings support the existence of two, maybe three different forms of myotonic dystrophy, possibly allelic, producing different though overlapping age at onset and severity. A similar situation in Huntington's chorea has been postulated by Went et al (1975) on the basis of study of two very large Dutch kindreds showing significantly different mean age of onset and death.

Bundey and Carter's (1972) suggestion is weakened by several factors: first, their data conflict with the earlier study of Bell (1948), who found a high correlation coefficient between sibs (0.67) but a low parent-child correlation (0.32). Second, age at onset in myotonic dystrophy is notably difficult to score precisely. An individual diagnosed at age 40 years may have had symptoms that could have been recognised ten years previously, and if preclinical features had been sought as part of a family study the diagnosis might have been made at age 20 years. A further drawback is that these authors' "early-onset" group contains all those with onset under the age of 20 years, and does not differentiate the congenital cases, in which there is strong evidence for other factors being involved (see Chapter 9). When these are removed the correlation coefficient of 0.64 no longer differs significantly from 0.5, the value to be expected if the factors influencing variation were primarily from other loci.

Evidence regarding the existence of multiple loci is bound to remain circumstantial until we have more precise knowledge of the biochemical basis, but no biochemical heterogeneity at any level has so far been shown, nor does the genetic evidence support it. The mode of inheritance of myotonic dystrophy is invariably autosomal dominant, in contrast to myotonia congenita, in which the existence of both autosomal dominant and recessive forms of the disorder provides clear evidence of heterogeneity (Becker, 1966; Harper and Johnston, 1972). Genetic linkage studies likewise give no evidence suggesting multiple loci; in some other disorders, e.g., hereditary elliptocytosis, families have fallen into two distinct groups, one showing close linkage to a genetic marker (the Rh blood group system), the other showing absence of linkage. The extensive linkage data for myotonic dystrophy (Mohr, 1954; Renwick et al, 1971; Harper et al, 1972) reveal no such heterogeneity, and are described fully in the following chapter.

The author's opinion is that myotonic dystrophy is indeed a single genetic and biochemical entity, albeit a remarkably variable one. The one group clearly separable on clinical grounds — those patients with congenital onset — occurs within families containing the more usual form, and as discussed earlier may be explicable in terms of the maternal environment. Otherwise the intriguing problem is not so much the difference between affected families, but how to explain the extraordinary clinical variation within a family, notably between generations. It is likely that both genetic and environmental factors are involved in this, but so far their nature remains unknown.

ANTICIPATION

The term anticipation has been used to denote the progressively earlier appearance of a disease in successive generations, generally with increasing severity. Figure 2–4 shows such a family, and such a pattern has frequently been recorded from the time of the earliest family studies on myotonic dystrophy. There is no disagreement regarding the observations, but there remains an unresolved conflict as to whether they represent a true biological phenomenon or merely result from biases that favour the recording of families of this type. In general, neurologists have accepted anticipation as a genuine event whereas geneticists have not. The dichotomy is seen most clearly in the monograph of Caughey and Myrianthopoulos (1963) in which the two authors held opposite opinions on the subject.

Penrose (1948) cogently set out the biases that might be involved, which are summarised in Table 10–4. They arise partly from the fact that reproduction is reduced in the severe cases of early onset, so that these are less likely than late-onset cases to be seen in the parental (or grandparental) generations. In addition, the fact that family studies are generally done at a single point of time rather than over many years likewise means that only late-onset cases in the older generation will be alive for

**Table 10–4.   ANTICIPATION IN MYOTONIC DYSTROPHY;
FACTORS PRODUCING BIAS**

Older Generation	
SEVERE	MILD
Less likely to be ascertained directly (probably dead)	More likely to be ascertained directly (alive and with symptoms at time of observation)
Less likely to be ascertained indirectly (less likely to have reproduced)	More likely to be ascertained indirectly (more likely to have children)
Younger Generation	
SEVERE	MILD
More likely to be ascertained directly (referred because of symptoms)	Less likely to be ascertained directly (symptoms mild or absent)
More likely to be ascertained indirectly (will show disease while parent is alive)	Less likely to be ascertained indirectly (may not be able to be scored as affected)

examination, and only early-onset cases in the childhood generation will yet have developed signs of the disease allowing them to be observed as affected. Clearly, the net result of these biases will be to favour the observation of families in which the disease appears to be mild and late-onset in earlier generations, but severe and early-onset in later generations. Penrose also pointed out that such an effect could only be produced by a disorder showing high intrinsic variability, and that the apparent anticipation was the product of the biases acting on this variability. A low parent-child correlation for age of onset would add to the effect, although the existence of this is in doubt, as discussed above.

Since Penrose's publication few arguments have been raised against it, particularly since no convincing explanation of how a gene could "worsen" in successive generations was ever forthcoming, but the discovery of the almost exclusive maternal transmission of the severe infantile and congenital cases and the likely existence of a maternal environmental factor (Harper and Dyken, 1972) raise the question whether this might not provide a genuine biological basis for anticipation. In the author's series (Harper, 1975a) none of the congenital cases had reproduced or was likely to do so, and none was the result of a new mutation; thus, all such cases were inevitably represented in the childhood generation. The affected mothers, by contrast, often were mildly affected, as were affected grandparents.

It thus seems likely that the phenomenon of anticipation in myotonic dystrophy can be satisfactorily explained on the basis of a situation in which both bias and a true biological factor are acting, and in the author's opinion the likely factors are as follows:

1. Myotonic dystrophy is a highly variable genetic disorder, probably as the result of influence of other loci, possibly due to heterogeneity.

2. Biases exist, as set out by Penrose, which act on this variability.

3. The most severe cases of congenital onset result from a maternal environmental factor, and generally are seen only at the "bottom" of the pedigree.

OTHER GENETIC INFLUENCES IN MYOTONIC DYSTROPHY

We have seen that there is no convincing evidence for more than one genetic locus being responsible for myotonic dystrophy, and that evidence for multiple alleles is not strong. Is it possible to explain some of the remarkable phenotypic variability of the disease in terms of the rest of the genome? An additive effect of numerous other loci would tend to produce a continuous variation in expression of the disorder, together with individuals in whom effects of the abnormal gene had been entirely suppressed (lack of penetrance). The fact that myotonic dystrophy invariably shows clear autosomal dominant inheritance, and that skipped generations are never found in thoroughly investigated families, suggests that other loci can at most modify the disorder, not suppress it entirely as may occur with some other genetic disorders such as retinoblastoma. Nor has any instance been recorded of a child developing the disorder before the parent (although diagnosis not infrequently is made first in the child). Significant influences of other loci would be expected to result in a correlation coefficient of 0.5 between sibs, and between parents and offspring, since each group has on average half its genes in common with the other. The observed correlation coefficients, discussed above, differ greatly, but are certainly compatible with this hypothesis.

Penrose (1948), analysing the data of Bell (1948), suggested that a variant "normal" allele might exist at the myotonic dystrophy locus which modified its effect. Since an affected parent possessing this allele clearly could not transmit both it and the myotonic dystrophy allele to a child, this would account for the low correlation between parent and offspring observed by Bell. This ingenious hypothesis is made unlikely by the failure of others to find a low parent-offspring correlation, and by the likely existence of a maternal factor that could also produce the observed effect.

MUTATION RATE

A knowledge of the proportion of cases of myotonic dystrophy resulting from new mutations is important to the clinician as well as to the geneticist. If an individual represents a new mutation his brothers and sisters have no risk of developing or transmitting the disorder, whereas if he has received the gene from a parent his sibs have a 50 percent prior risk of also inheriting it.

The mutation rate for an autosomal dominant disorder may be estimated either directly or indirectly. The direct method, theoretically simple, consists simply of recording the frequency of those cases of the disease in which neither parent is affected, as opposed to those in which a parent is affected. This can give an accurate value for a condition such as achondroplasia, which is unlikely to be overlooked, and in which there is little difficulty in deciding whether or not a parent is affected. For myotonic dystrophy, however, not only is the total incidence likely to be underestimated, but it may be difficult to decide whether a parent has been affected, especially if one or both parents are dead. To accept a case as a new mutation just because the parents are not known to have been affected will give a gross overestimate of the proportion of new mutations, and of the mutation rate.

The indirect method of calculating the mutation rate assumes that the disorder is neither increasing nor decreasing in frequency, and that the tendency for abnormal genes to be lost owing to relative reduction in fertility is balanced by an equal number of new mutations. Thus, if the genetic fitness (F) of the individual with myotonic dystrophy is 75 percent of normal (see Table 10–8), 25 percent of the abnormal genes will be lost per generation, and 25 percent of cases should be the result of new mutations. The absolute mutation rate can be readily calculated as $(1-F) \times$ the population incidence (i), which is of the order of 5×10^{-5}. Since the mutation rate (μ) is generally expressed per gamete, not per individual, the final rate will be half this figure.

$$\mu = \frac{1}{2}(1 - F) \times i$$
$$= \frac{1}{2} \times 0.25 \times 5 \times 10^{-5}$$
$$= 0.625 \times 10^{-5}$$

Unfortunately this figure depends on the accuracy of the fitness estimate of 0.75, which may well be too low; μ is thus likely to be an overestimate, as has already been discussed. Some recorded estimates using this approach are given in Table 10–5A. Do these agree with direct estimations of the mutation rate? Here the evidence is contradictory. Bundey et al (1970) estimated that one-quarter of cases resulted from new mutations, and

Table 10–5A. MUTATION RATE IN MYOTONIC DYSTROPHY*

Lynas (1957)	0.5×10^{-5}
Klein (1958)	1.6×10^{-5}
Todorov et al (1970)	1.1×10^{-5}
Grimm (1975)	1.3×10^{-5}

*Calculated by indirect method (see text).

Lynas (1957) in Northern Ireland estimated an even higher proportion. The author by contrast found no instance of a proved new mutation in 48 families containing 150 affected individuals (Table 10–5B). In all cases in which it was possible to examine the supposedly normal parents, one parent was found to be unequivocally affected, usually with lens changes and mild but definite myotonia. Five instances in which the parents could not be examined represent possible new mutations, but comprise only 11 percent of the total, and could well have proved to be transmitted cases had full investigation been possible. Similarly, a study of congenital myotonic dystrophy (Harper, 1975b) showed no definite new mutations in 54 kindreds, there being only two instances in which the parents could not be examined. It is likely that if the other studies had accepted as new mutations only those cases in which the parents had been examined personally, they would have found a much lower proportion of mutations.

From the practical viewpoint of genetic counselling the proportion of cases due to new mutation is more important than the absolute mutation rate. If an isolated case is the result of a new mutation, only the descendants of that individual and not his sibs will be at risk, whereas sibs will be at 50 percent prior risk if the case is a transmitted one. There can be no

Table 10–5B. FREQUENCY OF POSSIBLE NEW MUTATIONS IN 48 KINDREDS WITH MYOTONIC DYSTROPHY

One parent of propositus affected	previously diagnosed	23
	not previously diagnosed	5
Parent not known to be affected but not available for study	more than one child affected (mutation excluded)	15
	one affected child (mutation possible but not proved)	5
Parents examined — both normal	(mutation proved)	0
		48

doubt that the proportion of new mutations is very low, so the author's policy is always to assume that an apparently isolated case is a transmitted one until definite objective evidence can be obtained of neither parent being affected. How mild the condition may be is illustrated by the following example (family 2 in Harper, 1972; Fig. 10–4).

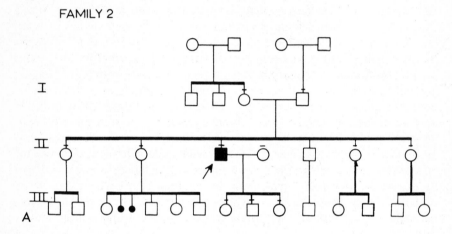

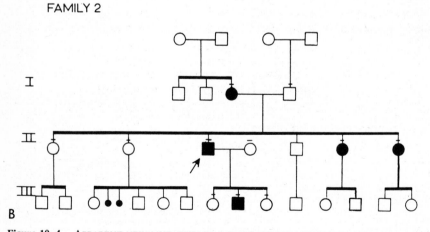

Figure 10–4.   APPARENT NEW MUTATION IN A FAMILY WITH MYOTONIC DYSTROPHY.

A, Pedigree on initial investigation. The propositus appears to be the result of a new mutation.

B. Pedigree after full investigation of asymptomatic members.

A 40 year old man from Maryland, U.S.A. was diagnosed as having myotonic dystrophy, with cataracts, myotonia and moderate muscle weakness. Family studies showed a son also to be affected, but the parents of the propositus were both stated to be in good health at over 60 years of age, and a new mutation was thought to be likely. When examined the father, aged 70, was normal; the mother, aged 61, was symptomless but showed slight myotonia of grip and thenar percussion. Slit-lamp examination revealed numerous coloured and white lens opacities, and ophthalmic examination had documented similar opacities at a routine consultation 11 years previously. Six years before this, slit-lamp examination had been normal. Examination of the sibs of the propositus, all considered to be healthy and not at risk, showed two out of five to be definitely affected, with both lens opacities and clinical myotonia.

It is clear from the evidence discussed in this section that the mutation rate expected from indirect calculations based on reduction in genetic fitness is not seen in direct observation of families. One reason for this may be that the patients on whom fertility studies are based are not typical of the entire population of individuals with the myotonic dystrophy gene, many of whom are almost or entirely symptomless and are only ascertained through family studies. It seems likely that such mildly affected individuals with near-normal reproductive capacity form a largely unnoticed source of transmission of the myotonic dystrophy gene.

INCIDENCE AND GEOGRAPHICAL DISTRIBUTION

Myotonic dystrophy is not a rare disorder, and is without doubt the commonest muscular dystrophy of adult life. Precise figures are few, however, and are all likely to be underestimates owing to the numerous cases that do not come to medical attention or are misdiagnosed. Distinction must be made between estimates of prevalence, showing the number of affected individuals at a given time in relation to a total population, and estimates of incidence that record the number of individuals genetically affected in relation to total births, regardless of whether the disease was present at the time of study. For a disease that shortens lifespan, prevalence estimates will naturally be lower than incidence estimates. Of the estimates shown in Table 10–6, that of Klein (1958) is likely to be most accurate, being made in a country (Switzerland) with good medical services and a well-documented, relatively static population. Even here ascertainment was not complete, as Klein admits that new families were coming to his attention after he had completed his study. This frequency of 4.9 per 100,000 population is similar to that of 5.5 per 100,000 population recorded by Grimm (1975) for West Germany. Further geographical details are given by Grimm (1975), based on the extensive data (1,036 patients) of the Göttingen Institut für Humangenetik. The data of Kurland (1958) are likely to be an underestimate, being based on a general survey of neurological disorders in a population.

Table 10-6. PREVALENCE OF MYOTONIC DYSTROPHY

Source	Place	Frequency per 100,000
Klein (1958)	Switzerland	4.9
Lynas (1957)	Northern Ireland	2.4
Kurland (1958)	Rochester, Minnesota, USA	3.3
Grimm (1975)	West Germany	5.5
Todorov et al (1970)	Switzerland	13.5*

*Gene frequency, not disease frequency.

The figures given above represent the frequency of the disease rather than that of the abnormal gene. The gene frequency will be higher, since only a proportion of gene carriers will be showing signs of the disease at any particular time. Todorov et al (1970) have estimated the incidence of the myotonic dystrophy gene, using the data of Klein, supplemented by further data from French-speaking Switzerland; taking into account the overall penetrance and pattern of age at onset, they arrived at a value of 13.5 per 100,000 births.

Geographical variation in the incidence of myotonic dystrophy is not marked, and the disorder has been reported from many countries and all races including Japan, China, India and Africa as well as in black American families (Harper, 1972). Population studies have shown a relatively even distribution within individual countries such as Denmark (Thomasen, 1948) and Switzerland (Klein, 1958), and the disorder has not been noted with particular frequency in inbred or isolated populations. The presence of an enthusiastic investigator is probably the major influence on whether the disease appears to be common in a particular area, although, as with other dominantly inherited disorders such as Huntington's chorea, the presence of one or two large and fertile families can exert a disproportionate influence within a locality.

Table 10-7. APPROXIMATE INCIDENCE AND PREVALENCE OF DIFFERENT MUSCULAR DYSTROPHIES (per 100,000)

Type	Prevalence	Incidence	Source
Myotonic dystrophy	2.4–5.5	13.5	See above
Duchenne*	2.8	16.8	Gardner-Medwin (1970)
Becker	1.8	2.8	Kloepfer and Emery (1974)
Facio-scapulo-humeral	0.56	0.92	Morton and Chung (1959)
Limb-girdle	1.0	3.3	Morton and Chung (1959)
Myotonia congenita	0.54	0.54	Becker (1971)

*Data for male population and births.
Mean incidence for 10 studies 21.1 ± 1.2 (Emery, 1977).

The frequency of myotonic dystrophy is compared with data for other dystrophies in Table 10–7, and it can be seen that myotonic dystrophy is commoner than the other dystrophies of adult life, even though the data should be regarded as approximate. Only Duchenne dystrophy has a higher birth incidence, its prevalence being reduced by early mortality.

FERTILITY

A reduced fertility has been found by most workers, and the principal data are summarised in Table 10–8. Although a marked difference in fertility between the sexes might be expected in view of the high incidence of testicular atrophy in males (see Chapter 6), this is not the case, a slight relative infertility of males being found by Harper (1972), no difference by Bell (1948) and a relatively higher fertility by Klein (1958). Taken together these data suggest a reduction to about 75 percent of normal fertility, but it must be emphasised that the true fertility of all individuals in the population carrying the abnormal gene is likely to be considerably closer to normal, since any study inevitably tends preferentially to recognise the more severely affected and less fertile members. An indication of this bias at work is seen in the fact that fertility is increased when the more severely affected propositi are excluded. The increased abortion rate and other problems of pregnancy in myotonic dystrophy have already been considered in Chapter 6.

Table 10–8.   FERTILITY IN MYOTONIC DYSTROPHY

| | | Affected Patients and Unaffected Sibs: Children per Parent | | | |
		BELL (1948) SERIES "A" ENGLAND	KLEIN (1958) SWITZERLAND	THOMASEN (1948) DENMARK	HARPER (1972) USA
Males	affected	2.49	2.3		1.73
	unaffected	2.64			
Females	affected	2.52	1.5		2.09
	unaffected	2.81			
Both Sexes	affected		1.9	1.5	1.92
	unaffected		2.5	2.2	2.88
Relative Fertility (= F)	affected / unaffected	0.90	0.76	0.68	0.67

REFERENCES

Adie, W. J. and Greenfield J. G. (1923): Dystrophia myotonica (mytonia atrophica). Brain 46:73–127.

Batten F. E. and Gibb H. P. (1909): Myotonia atrophica. Brain 33:187–205.

Becker P. E. (1966): Zur Genetik der Myotonien. In Progressive Muskeldystrophie, Myotonie, Myasthenie. Springer, Berlin, pp. 247–255.

Becker P. E. (1971): Paramyotonia congenita (Eulenburg). Adv. Hum. Genet. 3:1–134.

Becker P. E. (1971): Genetic approaches to the nosology of muscle disease. Myotonias and similar disorders. Birth Defects Original Articles Series: 7, 52–62.

Bell J. (1948): Dystrophia myotonica and allied diseases. In Treasury of Human Inheritance. Cambridge University Press, London.

Bowen P., Lee C. S. N. and Harvey J. C. (1968): Balanced reciprocal translocation between two D group chromosomes in a family with myotonic dystrophy. Am. J. Med. Sci. 255:368–375.

Bundey S. (1974): Detection of heterozygotes for myotonic dystrophy. Clin. Gen. 5:107–109.

Bundey S., Carter C. O. and Soothill J. F. (1970): Early recognition of heterozygotes for the gene of dystrophia myotonica. J. Neurol. Neurosurg. Psychiatry 33:279–293.

Bundey S. and Carter W. (1972): Genetic heterogeneity for dystrophia myotonia. J. Med. Genet. 9:311–315.

Caughey J. E. and Myrianthopoulos N. C. (1963): Dystrophia Myotonica and Related Disorders. Charles C Thomas, Springfield, Ill.

Dyken P. R. and Harper P. S. (1973): Congenital dystrophia myotonica. Neurology (Minneap.) 23:465–473.

Emery A. E. H. (1977): Genetic considerations in the X-linked muscular dystrophies. In Pathogenesis of Human Muscular Dystrophies (Ed.: L. P. Rowland). Excerpta Medica, Amsterdam.

Fiol M. E., Daly R. F. and Osborne R. M. (1975): Dystrophia myotonica in a 47 XXY male. Neurology 25:472–476.

Fitzgerald P. H. and Caughey J. E. (1962): Chromosome and sex chromatin studies in cases of dystrophia myotonica. N. Z. Med. J. 61:410–412.

Fleischer B. (1918): Über myotonischer Dystrophia mit Katarakt. Albrecht von Graefes Arch. Klin. Ophthalmol. 96:91–133.

Gardner-Medwin D. (1970): Mutation rate in Duchenne type of muscular dystrophy. J. Med. Genet. 7:334.

Grimm T. (1975): Thesis. University of Göttingen.

Grimm T. (1975): Inst. Human-Genet., Univ. Göttingen. The age of onset and the age at death in patients with dystrophia myotonica. J. Genet. Hum. 23:301–308.

Grumbach M. M., Blanc W. A. and Engle E. T. (1957): Sex chromatin pattern in seminiferous tubule dysgenesis and other testicular disorders: relationship to true hermaphroditism and to Klinefelter's syndrome, with a review of gonadal ontogenesis. J. Clin. Endocrinol. Metab. 17:703–736.

Harper P. S. (1972): Genetic studies in myotonic dystrophy. Thesis for degree of D. M., Oxford, U. K.

Harper P. S. (1973): Pre-symptomatic detection and genetic counselling in myotonic dystrophy. Clin. Gen. 4:134–140.

Harper P. S. (1975a): Congenital myotonic dystrophy in Britain. 1. Clinical aspects. Arch. Dis. Child. 50:505–513.

Harper P. S. (1975b): Congenital myotonic dystrophy in Britain. 2. Genetic basis. Arch. Dis. Child. 50:514–521.

Harper P. S. and Dyken P. R. (1972): Early onset dystrophia myotonica. Evidence supporting a maternal environmental factor. Lancet 2:53–55.

Harper P. S. and Johnston D. M. (1972): Recessively inherited myotonia congenita. J. Med. Genet. 9:213–215.

Harper P. S., Penny R., Foley T., Jr., Migeon C. J. and Blizzard R. M. (1972): Gonadal function in males with myotonic dystrophy. J. Clin. Endocrinol. Metab. 35:852–856.

Harper P. S., Rivas M. L., Bias W. B., Hutchinson J. R., Dyken P. R. and McKusick V. A.

(1972): Genetic linkage confirmed between the locus for myotonic dystrophy and the ABH-secretion and Lutheran blood group loci. Am. J. Hum. Genet 24:310–316.

Klein D. (1958): La dystrophie myotonique (Steinert) et la myotonie congenitale (Thomsen) en Suisse. J. Genet. Hum. (Suppl.)7:1–328.

Kloepfer H. W. and Emery A. E. H. (1974): Genetic aspects of neuromuscular disease. In Disorders of Voluntary Muscle (Ed.: J. N. Walton). Churchill Livingstone, Edinburgh.

Kurland L. T. (1958): Descriptive epidemiology of selected neurologic and myopathic disorders with particular reference to a survey in Rochester, Minnesota. J. Chronic Dis. 8:378–418.

Lynas M. A. (1957): Dystrophia myotonica, with special reference to Northern Ireland. Ann. Hum. Genet. 21:318–351.

Maas O. (1937): Observations on dystrophia myotonica. Brain 60:498–524.

Mohr J. (1954): A Study of Linkage in Man. Munskgaard, Copenhagen.

Morton N. E. and Chung C. S. (1959): Formal genetics of muscular dystrophy. Am. J. Hum. Genet. 11:360–379.

Penrose L. S. (1948): The problem of anticipation in pedigrees of dystrophia myotonica. Ann. Eugen. (Lond.) 14:125–232.

Pierson M., Saborio M., Schmitt J., André J. M. and Fortier G. (1975): Une famille de dystrophie myotonique de Steinert, forme congénitale n'affectant que les filles. J. Genet. Hum. 23 (Suppl): 180.

Polgar J. G., Bradley W. G., Upton A. R. M., Anderson J., Howat J. M. L., Petito F., Roberts D. F. and Scopa J. (1972): The early detection of dystrophia myotonica. Brain 95:761–776.

Renwick J. H., Bundey S. E., Ferguson-Smith M. A. and Izatt M. M. (1971): Confirmation of the linkage of the loci for myotonic dystrophy and ABH secretion. J. Med. Genet. 8:407–416.

Rohrer K. (1916): Über Myotonia atrophica (Dystrophia myotonica). Dtsch. Z. Nervenheilkd. 55:242.

Teter J., Saper J. and Janczewski Z. (1960): Disturbances of somato-sexual development in cases of dystrophia myotonica and congenital myotonia. Endokrynol. Pol. 11:1.

Thomasen E. (1948): Myotonia. Universitetsforlaget Aarhus.

Todorov A., Jéquier M., Klein D. and Morton N. E. (1970): Analyse de la ségrégation dans la dystrophie myotonique. J. Genet. Hum. 18:387–406.

Vanier T. M. (1960): Dystrophia myotonica in childhood. Br. Med. J. 2:1284–1288.

Went L. N., Vegter van der Vlis M., Volkers W. and Collewijn H. (1975): Huntington's chorea. In Early Diagnosis and Prevention of Genetic Diseases (Eds.: L. N. Went, Chr. Vermeij-Keers and A. G. J. M. van der Linden). Leiden University Press, Leiden, pp. 13–25.

CHAPTER ELEVEN

Preclinical Detection and Preventive Genetic Measures

Once the diagnosis of myotonic dystrophy is suspected in a family it is not difficult to establish the diagnosis in symptomatic family members. It is considerably harder, however, to be sure that the disorder is *not* present in a member of the family at risk, particularly in childhood and early adult life. Genetic advice is similarly straightforward for an affected individual, whose offspring run a 50 percent risk of inheriting the disorder, but much more difficult for the apparently healthy member in whom the possibility of later development of the disease must be considered.

A variety of approaches have been applied to the detection of the presymptomatic carrier of the myotonic dystrophy gene; the large number reflects the fact that none has proved entirely satisfactory, a situation likely to continue until the basic biochemical defect in the disorder is understood. Nevertheless, the existing tests, when used with discrimination and in combination, give valuable help in many cases. Our present knowledge is based principally on such studies aimed specifically at the preclinical detection of the disease, in particular those of Bundey et al (1970), Polgar et al (1972) and Harper (1972, 1973).

CLINICAL EXAMINATION

Many patients with myotonic dystrophy are remarkably uncomplaining, even when obvious clinical abnormalities are present. Absence of symptoms should never be relied on and careful examination is mandato-

232

Table 11-1. RESULTS OF CLINICAL AND SLIT-LAMP EXAMINATION
OF 131 ASYMPTOMATIC FIRST-DEGREE RELATIVES OF
PATIENTS WITH MYOTONIC DYSTROPHY*

Total examined	131	
Definitely abnormal	23	(17.6%)
Equivocally abnormal	14	(10.7%)
Definitely normal	94	(71.7%)

*After Harper, 1972.

ry. In some such individuals the characteristic facies, the muscle weakness and wasting and the myotonia will all be found; in others myotonia may be the only abnormality. Myotonia of grip and percussion myotonia of the thenar muscles have been found by the author to be the most satisfactory tests. The results of clinical examination of a personal series of asymptomatic first-degree relatives of patients with myotonic dystrophy are given in Table 11-1.

Two clinical features that were rejected in this study as too non-specific when present as the only abnormality were baldness and cataract. Baldness is much too common a characteristic to warrant its use in diagnosis, and its acceptance as such in the study of Lynas (1957) may well have resulted in an overestimate of affected individuals, living and dead. Cataract is a valuable diagnostic sign when supported by the specific slit-lamp appearance, but is too common in old age to be used as a criterion alone, when the latter is non-specific or when the lens is either totally opaque or has been removed.

SLIT-LAMP EXAMINATION

Examination of the lenses with the slit-lamp biomicroscope is an essential part in the exclusion of myotonic dystrophy in the individual at risk, particularly when the lenses appear normal ophthalmoscopically. The characteristic multicoloured appearance of the early opacities has already been described in Chapter 8, but it must be re-emphasised that these are invisible with the ophthalmoscope and frequently are present in patients with no ocular symptoms. When the individual at risk for myotonic dystrophy is seen in the hospital it is preferable for the examination to be done by an experienced ophthalmologist using a fixed instrument, but the author has found a portable instrument (KOWA Ltd.) of great value in allowing examination in the home of asymptomatic relatives for whom hospital attendance might have been impossible. In either case full dilatation of the lenses is essential, but the clinician who is not an ophthalmologist would do well to bear in mind the following potential problems:

Table 11–2.   LENS CHANGES IN OTHERWISE UNAFFECTED FIRST-DEGREE RELATIVES OF PATIENTS WITH MYOTONIC DYSTROPHY*

Changes of myotonic dystrophy	4
Non-specific changes	11
Senile cataract	3
Advanced cataract, type uncertain	1
Pigment spots on lens surface	1
Total abnormalities	19
Total examined by slit-lamp	96
Total individuals studied	112

*From Harper 1972.

1. Always use short-acting mydriatics (such as cyclopentolate), or reverse the action of the longer-acting homatropine.

2. Do not dilate both eyes in a patient who has to drive a car immediately afterwards.

3. Use caution in elderly people and enquire as to the existence of glaucoma.

The results of slit-lamp and ophthalmoscopic examination in a personal series of 150 patients with myotonic dystrophy were given in Table 8–2 and Figure 8–3. The results in asymptomatic first-degree relatives are shown in Table 11–2, and are correlated with the presence of myotonia in Table 11–3. It can be seen that, of those individuals who did not show myotonia, four revealed specific multi-coloured lens opacities, and a further 12 showed whitish opacities that were normal but not diagnostic of myotonic dystrophy. Similar results were obtained in the study of Bundey et al (1970) in which EMG was also employed. In this study seven out of 93 clinically normal relatives showed diagnostic lens opacities, electrical myotonia being absent in three of these; in the study of Polgar et al (1972) only one out of 22 clinically normal relatives exhibited lens opacities.

The significance of the "non-specific" lens opacities seen with the slit-lamp in these and other studies remains to be established. At present

Table 11–3.   LENS OPACITIES AND MYOTONIA IN ASYMPTOMATIC FIRST-DEGREE RELATIVES OF PATIENTS WITH MYOTONIC DYSTROPHY

		Slit-lamp Examination				
		SPECIFIC ABNORMALITY	NON-SPECIFIC ABNORMALITY	NORMAL	NOT PERFORMED	TOTAL
Clinical myotonia	present	8	4	3	4	19
	absent	4	12	80	16	112
	TOTAL	12	16	83	20	131

the author is hesitant in making the diagnosis of myotonic dystrophy in a person in whom this is the only abnormality, but is equally reluctant to ignore these appearances in view of the frequency with which they are seen in established cases of the disease. Until evidence is provided by long-term follow-up of such patients one has to admit that one does not know for certain whether such individuals are carriers of the myotonic dystrophy gene. The following example illustrates this problem.

C. P., a 24 year old man whose father was affected with myotonic dystrophy, sought genetic advice before marriage. Two of his sisters were affected and had had congenitally affected children. Neurological and slit-lamp examination and EMG were all normal. Two years later he requested reassessment, having meanwhile had a healthy daughter. Clinical examination was again negative, as was EMG; however, slit-lamp examination now showed scattered whitish opacities in both lenses, but no coloured opacities. Repeat examination a year later was unchanged.

A quantitative approach to this problem has been made by Pescia and Emery (1976) which may prove valuable in the correct identification of gene carriers without typical lens opacities. They performed a total count of lens opacities in a series of healthy controls and compared the results with the counts in patients with myotonic dystrophy and their first-degree relatives. The controls showed a mean total opacity count for the two eyes of 14.65 ± 18.43, and the opacity count in almost all the neurologically affected individuals was greatly increased. Among those neurologically normal there were two with opacity counts of 98 and 99, strongly suggesting that they were gene carriers. It will be important for such studies to be extended on larger numbers and to be repeated serially, and it would certainly seem wise for quantitative studies to be performed on any family member in whom the presence of atypical lens opacities is the only recognisable feature of the disease.

ELECTROMYOGRAPHY

Although electromyography (EMG) is not essential for diagnosis in most patients with obvious clinical myotonia, it is valuable in the small number in whom clinical myotonia is equivocal or absent. The author's study, based on home visits, did not use EMG, but Bundey et al (1970) found electrical myotonia in four out of 44 neurologically normal first-degree relatives; all four also had diagnostic slit-lamp abnormalities. Polgar et al (1972) found electrical myotonia in three family members with equivocal and one with no clinical myotonia out of 23 examined. A further electrophysiological test that has been claimed to be of value is the estimation of motor units in a muscle such as extensor digitorum brevis of the foot. McComas et al (1971) found the number of motor units to be reduced early in the disease, and Polgar et al (1972) using this test found 10 out of 24 asymptomatic relatives to be abnormal. Unfortunately, this approach has been criticised both because of the tendency for extensor digitorum brevis to sustain secondary changes from trauma and other factors, and because the method of McComas may exaggerate the normal number of motor units in the muscle. These considerations, together with the finding that changes in peripheral nerve are not constant features of the disease, make it unwise for preclinical myotonic dystrophy to be diagnosed solely on the basis of studies of extensor digitorum brevis.

ELECTRORETINOGRAPHY

The finding of abnormalities of the electroretinogram in a high proportion of early cases of myotonic dystrophy has been mentioned in Chapter 8, but has not yet been explored as a possible method of preclinical detection. A first step in its assessment should be the investigation of a series of asymptomatic relatives shown definitely to be affected by other criteria; if a high proportion of these prove to be abnormal, a series of first-degree relatives at risk should be studied prospectively.

SERUM CREATINE KINASE ACTIVITY

This test, so valuable in the detection of the carrier state in Duchenne muscular dystrophy, is of little value in myotonic dystrophy. A moderate elevation is frequent in established cases (Goto, 1974), but levels commonly are normal in early cases, even though definite clinical abnormalities are present, and have not been shown to be elevated in clinically normal carriers of the gene (Emery and Walton, 1967). Similarly, most cases of congenital myotonic dystrophy show normal levels; in the author's series, in which patients were studied by a variety of different hospitals and methods, most individuals had activity within the normal range for the particular laboratory.

Unfortunately, there is a widespread misapprehension among clinicians that the SCK activity is equally valuable diagnostically in all muscle dystrophies. The author has seen both adults and children at risk for myotonic dystrophy diagnosed as being affected solely on the basis of a single, slightly elevated SCK without any other supporting evidence, as well as others with definite clinical abnormalities given false reassurance on the basis of normal values. It cannot be emphasised too strongly that an abnormal SCK without other abnormalities is not adequate evidence for the diagnosis of myotonic dystrophy, nor does a normal level exclude the disorder. The problem is compounded by the lack of an established normal range in many laboratories, and by the variation of enzyme activity with exercise and other factors.

SERUM FOLLICLE STIMULATING HORMONE (FSH)

Harper et al (1972) showed a marked elevation of serum FSH, measured by radioimmunoassay, in all of a series of 39 males with myotonic dystrophy. This is discussed in relation to other endocrine abnormalities in Chapter 6. Some of these patients were asymptomatic, but this measurement has yet to be fully explored as a predictive test. Increasing availability of radioimmunoassay may make this a useful test in males if the separation between normal and abnormal proves to be as clear-cut in asymptomatic as in established cases. Estimation of gonadotrophins is less likely to be of help in females owing to the marked variations in relation to the menstrual cycle; no data so far have been reported from children of either sex, but the normally low gonadotrophins during childhood are likely to rule out the use of this approach before puberty.

ABNORMAL INSULIN RESPONSE TO GLUCOSE

The finding of an increased insulin secretion in response to a glucose load and other stimuli is discussed fully in Chapter 6. Walsh et al (1970) and Barbosa et al (1974) have attempted to apply this as a preclinical test in relatives at risk, but at present it appears to be insufficiently sensitive and possibly not specific enough to be of use except in an auxiliary capacity. Whether an individual at risk who shows a raised insulin response as the only abnormality should be regarded as carrying the myotonic dystrophy gene is doubtful.

SERUM IMMUNOGLOBULINS

The reported abnormalities in serum immunoglobulins and their possible relationship to the underlying cause of myotonic dystrophy are discussed in Chapter 14. Bundey et al (1970) were the first to attempt to use them in preclinical detection; they found significantly reduced IgG serum level in affected patients as well as a reduction in IgM, but there was no correlation with severity of disease, and levels in asymptomatic but neurologically abnormal relatives had levels of IgG and IgM similar to those of the normal controls. Roberts and Bradley (1977), using samples from the patients of Polgar et al (1972), also found a reduced IgG (but not IgM) level and have attempted to give odds influencing the probability of being affected based on the level of IgG. This seems unwise; not only was the difference between affected and normal controls slight (log values of 2.935±0.148 mg/100 dl compared with 3.005±0.084 mg/100 dl), but no attempt was made to see if the values for the asymptomatic but neurologically abnormal members could be distinguished. In the author's opinion levels of immunoglobulins do not give sufficient discrimination to be of value in preclinical detection.

ABNORMALITIES OF THE ERYTHROCYTE MEMBRANE

Throughout this book emphasis has been laid on the fact that myotonic dystrophy is a generalised disease, and that any primary metabolic defect is likely to be expressed in tissues other than muscle. The red blood cell, although itself a specialised cell type lacking some enzyme systems, has the advantage of ready availability in large numbers, and reports of abnormalities in the red cell membrane are thus of considerable potential importance both from the viewpoint of preclinical detection and from that of the understanding of the basic biochemical defect. These studies will be discussed fully in Chapter 14 but their implications for preclinical detection require mention here.

Roses, Appel and colleagues in a series of reports (Roses and Appel, 1973, 1974; Roses et al, 1975) have described abnormal phosphorylation of membrane proteins prepared from red cell ghosts in patients with myotonic dystrophy. This phosphorylation is dependent on membrane-bound protein kinases, and a significantly diminished protein kinase activity was found in myotonic dystrophy red cells compared with normal. Initially the difference could be shown only in stored material, but later work demonstrated the reduction in fresh red cells also. Electrophoresis of membrane protein components showed phosphorylation of band III to be most reduced, and further work on muscle membranes (Roses and Appel, 1974) revealed similar changes in this tissue. Biophysical changes have also been shown in the red cell membrane, using the technique of electron spin resonance as a measure of membrane fluidity (Roses et al, 1974; Butterfield et al, 1976, 1977). A significant difference in membrane fluidity of myotonic dystrophy and normal red cell membranes was found, and it was suggested that this technique might prove suitable for preclinical detection.

So far no systematic evaluation of these approaches in comparison with other preclinical tests for myotonic dystrophy has been published, and indeed no other group has yet fully confirmed the findings. The situation has been complicated further by the claim that abnormalities of red cell membrane phosphorylation occur in Duchenne dystrophy (Roses et al, 1975) and that these provide a more sensitive method of carrier detection than does the SCK activity (see Chapter 14). The fact that the findings in Duchenne dystrophy are in total disagreement with both genetic evidence and previous work on carrier detection raises very real doubts as to the significance of the changes, and in turn means that the abnormalities reported in myotonic dystrophy must be treated with caution until independent confirmation is obtained. If they do indeed prove to be as specific as originally suggested, this will prove to be a major advance in preclinical detection and will be the first test to be based on a biochemical abnormality related directly to the primary defect. At present it seems more likely that they are a relatively non-specific indicator of generalised membrane involvement in myotonic dystrophy.

PREDICTION OF SEVERITY

When an individual is definitely affected with myotonic dystrophy, there is little difficulty in quoting the 50 percent genetic risk of transmitting the disorder to any offspring; however, this information in itself is inadequate, for it leaves unanswered the important question of how severe the condition is likely to be in those 50 percent of offspring that are affected. This is particularly relevant in those instances in which the disease is mild in the potential parent; in such a situation a couple might wish to have children if they knew the disease was likely to be mild also in offspring, whereas if a more severe form of the disease were likely they might well be deterred from reproducing.

Unfortunately, the extreme degree of variability of myotonic dystrophy makes this question difficult to answer with certainty, and the maternal transmission of congenital cases is a further factor that must be considered. The degree of variation seen within individual families means that, despite the correlation of age at onset within families found by some authors, a mildly affected individual cannot be reassured that the disorder will not be more severe in the subsequent generation. Indeed, since the group of patients for whom this advice is required are likely to be milder than average in the severity of their disease, one might expect the offspring to be more severely affected purely on statistical grounds, leaving aside any possibility of "anticipation" and the congenital form of the disease. This same situation is seen in other variable dominantly inherited disorders, such as tuberous sclerosis.

The risks to mildly affected women require special consideration, and although published data are scanty it is possible to estimate the risks of such a person having a child with severe childhood disease. For those women who already have one child with congenital myotonic dystrophy there is little doubt that other affected offspring will be likely to have the same form of the disease. Table 11–4 shows the risks based on the

Table 11–4. GENETIC RISKS IN FAMILIES WITH CONGENITAL
MYOTONIC DYSTROPHY

Affected	Propositi (congenital)	56
	Other congenital cases	14
	Severe childhood disease (not congenital)	9
	Total affected (less propositi)	23
	Neonatal deaths	24
	Unaffected	46
	Total (less propositi)	93

author's study of congenital myotonic dystrophy (Harper, 1975b). When the propositi (through whom the families were ascertained) are removed, it can be seen that (1) half the offspring appear to be unaffected; (2) one-quarter die neonatally; and (3) the remaining quarter survive, but are severely affected in childhood (although not all of these have symptoms dating from birth). It seems probable, as discussed in Chapter 9, that most of the neonatal deaths in this situation are of infants with congenital myotonic dystrophy, even though they were not diagnosed as such in the author's retrospective study. With improved neonatal resuscitation it is likely that a proportion of such infants would now move out of the neonatal death category into the "surviving, severely affected" group. The possibility also cannot be excluded that some of the children classed as normal might later develop symptoms. Faced with this situation it seems most unwise for women who have had a congenitally affected child to reproduce further in the absence of reliable methods of prenatal detection.

The risk of a severely affected child being born to an affected parent who has not yet reproduced is much less easy to determine, for there are no published data on how common congenital myotonic dystrophy is in relation to the disease as a whole. The rapidly increasing number of reports once the clinical syndrome is recognised by paediatricians indicates it is far from rare, but all series, including those of the author (Harper and Dyken, 1972; Harper, 1975a) are selected because of the occurrence of congenital cases in the families, and thus cannot be used to estimate the incidence of this form of the disease. As yet, no prospective unselected study has been undertaken of the outcome of pregnancies of affected women, and until such data are available only an approximate estimate is possible.

Two approaches can be used to provide a solution to the problem. First, unselected series of patients can be classified by symptoms, and the proportion presenting with "severe childhood disease" calculated. Table 11–5 (based on Figure 2–18) shows the author's data, based on a study of

Table 11–5. PRESENTING FEATURES OF MYOTONIC DYSTROPHY*

		Number	*%*
All Cases	Neonatal complications	5	2.9
	Mental retardation	20	11.8
	Other presentations	145	85.3
	TOTAL	170	100.0
Severe Childhood Disease	Total	25	14.7
	Maternally transmitted	20	11.8
	Paternally transmitted	5	2.9

*Based on data from Harper (1972).

all age groups, before the special significance of the childhood form was recognised. Almost 15 percent of cases could be classed as having "severe childhood disease", most of which were maternally transmitted. Since overall transmission of the disease by the sexes was equal in this series, the risk of an affected child of an affected woman having "severe childhood disease" is thus 23.6 percent, whereas the corresponding risk for the affected child of an affected man is only 5.8 percent.

These data exclude abortions, stillbirths and neonatal deaths, and it has already been shown (Table 6–4) that these are extremely common in the pregnancies of women with myotonic dystrophy, stillbirths and neonatal deaths having an excess of 12 percent over a control group.

If these data are taken along with those on the outcome of survivors, the approximate risks for a pregnancy in a woman with myotonic dystrophy (ignoring abortions) are seen in Table 11–6. The combined risk of such a pregnancy ending in a death or a severely affected child is 21 percent; as already stated, it is likely that a proportion of infants who would have died will now survive.

An independent approach to calculating the risks can be made by utilising the discrepancies in parental sex ratio discussed in Chapter 10. It

Table 11–6. RISKS FOR OFFSPRING OF WOMEN WITH MYOTONIC DYSTROPHY*

	%
Normal	50.0
Neonatal deaths and stillbirths	12.0
Severely affected—surviving	9.0
Later affected	29.0
Combined severely affected + deaths	21.0

*Based on data from Harper (1972).

has been mentioned that the excess of paternally transmitted cases found by earlier investigators was almost certainly the result of the maternally transmitted congenital cases that were then unrecognised. The data already given in Table 10–2 have shown that in these series there were only 229 maternally transmitted cases compared with 422 paternally transmitted, a deficiency of 193 (45.7) percent over what would be expected. Although this seems a high proportion to attribute to unrecognised or fatal maternally transmitted cases, it corresponds to 23 percent of all maternally transmitted births, a figure agreeing closely with that of 21 percent derived from the other approach.

Thus, although there is still need for an unbiased prospective study of the risks, there seems little doubt that women with myotonic dystrophy in general run a high risk of a severely affected child, and that 20 to 25 percent of births will result in either a death or a severely affected child.

GENETIC LINKAGE

Two genes (or more correctly, their loci) are said to be linked when they are located on the same chromosome within measurable distance of each other. Until very recently little was known of the human gene map except for a few genetic markers such as blood groups; myotonic dystrophy was the first serious autosomal genetic disease for which genetic linkage was established, and the first, and so far only, one for which it has been shown possible to use this information to make a prenatal prediction of the disease. (The linkage between the HLA system and congenital adrenal hyperplasia (Dupont et al, 1977) may prove to be a second).

A variety of techniques now exists for the detection of genetic linkage, but in the case of myotonic dystrophy it was the use of classical family studies that established the genetic linkage with two other loci — those controlling the Lutheran blood group antigens and the secretion of ABH blood group substances. The study of Mohr (1954) in Denmark showed that these two marker loci were themselves closely linked, and Mohr's data suggested that the myotonic dystrophy locus might also be on the same chromosome. Renwick et al (1971) reanalysed Mohr's data and added additional British data that greatly increased the likelihood of linkage. Harper et al (1972), studying families from the USA, reached similar conclusions, and the combined results make the existence of the linkage virtually certain.

The subject of genetic linkage is often confusing to the non-geneticist but can be simply illustrated by the families shown in Figures 11–1 and 11–2 (data from Harper, 1972). Figure 11–1 shows linkage between the myotonic dystrophy and Lutheran blood group loci; it can be seen that in

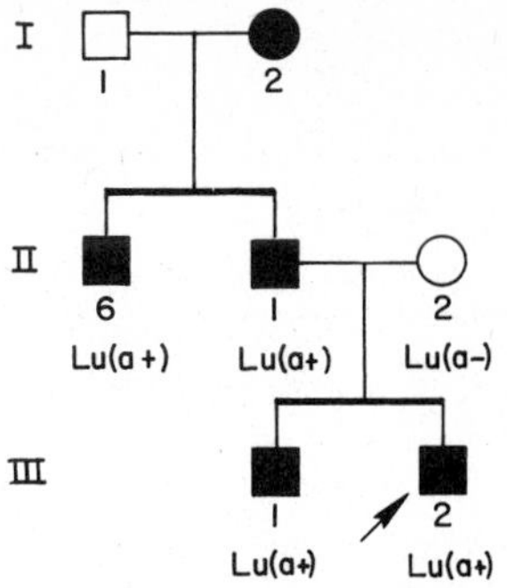

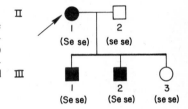

Figure 11-1. Genetic linkage between myotonic dystrophy and Lutheran blood group loci. In all instances the myotonic dystrophy gene and that for the Lutheran a+ antigen have been passed on together.

Figure 11-2. Genetic linkage between the myotonic dystrophy and secretor loci. In all instances the myotonic dystrophy and secretor (*Se*) genes have been handed on together. The non-secretor (*se*) gene has been transmitted to the unaffected child.

each case the gene for myotonic dystrophy has been inherited along with the Lutheran "a" antigen, whereas those individuals without this antigen have not received the dystrophy gene. Cumulative evidence from a number of such families establishes the existence of the linkage; the distance apart on the chromosome of the two loci is directly related to the frequency of recombination, i.e., the separation of the genes during transmission from parent to child. In the absence of linkage such recombination would occur with a frequency of 50 percent.

The family in Figure 11-2 illustrates linkage of the myotonic dystrophy and secretor loci; in each case the gene for myotonic dystrophy has been transmitted together with the "secretor" allele. Conversely, in Figure 11-3 the myotonic dystrophy gene is transmitted along with the non-secretor allele in all cases. In this situation linkage may be less obvious, since the secretor phenotype is dominant to the non-secretor phenotype, so that some affected individuals may be secretors, others non-secretors. Both families are equally indicative of linkage, and illustrate the fact that linkage between two loci does not imply association. Myotonic dystrophy patients are neither more nor less likely to be secretor or non-secretor than the rest of the population; it is the pattern of transmission of the two characters in an individual family that indicates linkage.

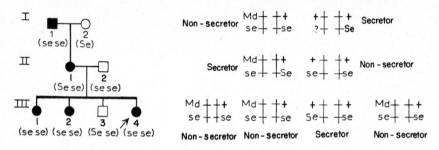

Md–Myotonic Dystrophy

+ – Normal allele at myotonic dystrophy locus

Se – Secretor allele

se – Non–secretor allele

Figure 11–3. Genetic linkage between the myotonic dystrophy and secretor loci. In all instances the myotonic dystrophy and non-secretor (*se*) genes have been handed on together.

Since a single family rarely gives sufficient information on its own to establish firmly the existence of genetic linkage, the evidence has to be compiled from numerous small and often fragmentary pieces of family data, each contributing information on the probability of the linkage and the most likely distance between the loci. When such probability estimates are expressed logarithmically as log of the odds or "LODs" they can be simply added or subtracted, so that data from separate families or separate studies can readily be combined. The use of computer techniques (Renwick, 1969a) and in particular the three-point analysis programme (Bolling and Renwick, 1971) also increases the information that can be extracted from complex pedigrees.

Our present knowledge of the linkage relations of myotonic dystrophy is summarised in Figure 11–4; the distances given are based on the combined data of the studies already mentioned. The order of the loci on the chromosome is still open to question, but that shown (myotonic dystrophy — secretor — Lutheran) is the most probable.

Although we know that the genes for myotonic dystrophy, secretor status and the Lutheran blood group are on the same chromosome, we do

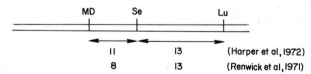

Figure 11–4. Genetic map distances (centimorgans) of the myotonic dystrophy, secretor and Lutheran loci.

not yet know which chromosome this is. There are several ways in which this might be established. First, inheritance of the myotonic dystrophy gene might be correlated in a family with inheritance of a recognisable structural variation of a particular chromosome; this is how the first gene was assigned to an autosome in man (the Duffy blood group to chromosome 1, Donohue et al, 1968). The balanced D group translocation reported by Bowen et al (1968) in a family with myotonic dystrophy provided such an opportunity, but although linkage data were obtained (Harper et al, 1972) the chromosome abnormality was found to have originated from the unaffected side of the family and could give no information on the location of the myotonic dystrophy gene.

A second approach will become feasible if the underlying biochemical defect in the disease is discovered and is expressed in cultured cells. The technique of cell hybridisation to produce hybrid cells between different species allows a correlation to be sought between a particular enzyme and a particular human chromosome. This results from the progressive loss of human chromosomes that occurs in such hybrid cells, which allows loss of retention of a specific human enzyme to be correlated with loss or retention of a specific human chromosome. Thus, it has been suggested that myotonic dystrophy might be the result of failure of conversion of desmosterol to cholesterol. The particular enzyme responsible for this, sterol Δ [24]reductase, is present in the cultured fibroblast and has been assigned by hybridisation techniques to chromosome 20. Unfortunately, it does not seem likely that this step is really the primary defect in human myotonic dystrophy, since Thomas and Harper (1978) have shown no abnormality in desmosterol — cholesterol conversion in the myotonic dystrophy fibroblast (see Chapter 14).

The third, and most likely, way in which the myotonic dystrophy gene will be placed on a specific chromosome is the discovery of linkage between the secretor or Lutheran loci and some other marker whose chromosome location is already known, or which can be directly tested by the methods described above. The increasing number of marker genes is resulting in numerous instances of previously isolated loci being joined up to form a recognisable portion of the human gene map, and there can be little doubt that the precise location of the myotonic dystrophy gene will become known in the near future.

Practical Applications of Genetic Linkage: Prenatal Prediction

The geneticist is interested in gene mapping in its own right, but most clinicians will wish to know whether it has anything to offer in the management of a particular family. The answer at present is a qualified "yes". Although the linkage with the Lutheran blood group system is too loose to be of practical help, the existence of close linkage with the secretor locus may allow one to infer whether the myotonic dystrophy gene has or has not been inherited in a particular patient at risk. This is of particular value since at present no direct biochemical test for the disorder exists that will identify affected individuals before clinical features develop.

The family shown in Figure 11–3 will serve as an example. Since the myotonic dystrophy gene in the mother is clearly inherited on the same chromosome as the non-secretor gene, non-secretor children must also have the dystrophy gene and secretor children should be unaffected. Given a recombination rate of about 10 percent, such a prediction should be 90 percent accurate, and could have been made at birth for all the children in generation III.

The above family was studied during the survey that established genetic linkage, but the family shown in Figure 11–5 represents a practical counselling problem. Here the proposita wished to know the risk of myotonic dystrophy in her children. Since her healthy mother was nonsecretor, the proposita must have inherited her secretor allele from her father, along with the gene for myotonic dystrophy. Since she was marrying a non-secretor individual, any secretor children would thus have a chance of around 90 percent of also having inherited myotonic dystrophy, and non-secretor offspring would have a similar chance of being free of the disease.

Prenatal prediction is also possible in such a situation (Renwick 1969b). Harper et al (1971) showed that the secretor status of the fetus can be determined in early pregnancy by the presence or absence of ABH blood group substances in the amniotic fluid. This can be done reliably by the 15th week of pregnancy, the stage at which most amniocenteses are performed, giving adequate time for termination of a pregnancy predicted to be affected.

Figure 11–6 shows a family in which this approach was used to make

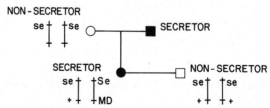

Figure 11–5. Use of the myotonic dystrophy — secretor linkage in genetic counselling. The proposita has received both a secretor gene and a myotonic dystrophy gene from her affected father; since her husband is non-secretor, any secretor offspring would be expected to be affected, in the absence of crossing-over. (Family studied by courtesy of Professor C. O. Carter.)

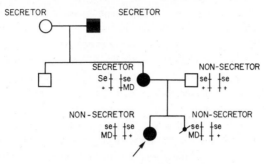

Figure 11-6. Prenatal prediction in myotonic dystrophy using the secretor linkage. After Insley et al, 1976 (see text).

a prenatal prediction (Insley et al, 1976). The secretor typing of the family from saliva showed that, as in the previous family, the myotonic dystrophy and non-secretor alleles were likely to be on the same chromosome, although the fact that both grandparents were secretor made the situation less simple than in the family previously discussed. Typing of amniotic fluid at 14 weeks' gestation was undertaken by the author and independently by Drs. Race and Sanger, and the fetus was shown to be non-secretor; a prediction of around 85 percent likelihood of being affected was given and the pregnancy terminated.

Schrott et al (1973) have also described a pregnancy that was allowed to continue after prenatal prediction suggested that it was likely to be unaffected, and their report and a subsequent paper (Schrott and Omenn, 1975) discuss some of the difficulties and limitations of the linkage approach.

Further details of prediction risk for different values of recombination have been given by Spence et al (1976) and Fenger and Hilden (1977). Some of the factors needing consideration are summarised below.

1. The test gives a prediction, not a diagnosis, with an error of around 7 to 10 percent owing to recombination; since the recombination rate is higher in females than in males for most loci, the accuracy of prediction is likely to be somewhat greater than 90 percent when a male is the affected parent, and somewhat less in the case of females.

2. The test can only be used when the affected parent is heterozygous at the secretor locus (Se se). If this parent is shown on saliva testing to be non-secretor, nothing further can be done; if secretor, this requires the previous generation to be tested to determine whether the myotonic dystrophy allele is on the same chromosome as the secretor or the non-secretor alleles. Referring again to Figure 11-3, it can be seen that

typing of I-I was essential to know this. At most one-fifth of matings are of the maximally informative type.

3. Any prenatal prediction should be confirmed on the abortus — since myotonic dystrophy has no biochemical or structural marker detectable in early fetal life, this cannot be done at present. No histological abnormality was found in the muscle of the fetus reported above.

For those clinicians who remain confused about this subject, some consolation can be given. All that is needed to determine whether linkage can be applied to a particular family is a pedigree and saliva samples from the relevant members and spouses. A geneticist colleague can work out whether the family is suitable, and amniocentesis need only be considered in those instances in which it is known that an informative answer can be obtained.

REFERENCES

Barbosa J., Nuttall F. Q., Kennedy W. and Goetz F. (1974): Plasma insulin in patients with myotonic dystrophy and their relatives. Medicine 53:307–323.

Bowen P., Lee C. S. N., Harvey J. C. and McGregor J. R. (1968): Chromosome counts in myotonic dystrophy. Am. J. Med. Sci. 255:385–367.

Bundey S., Carter C. O. and Soothill J. F. (1970): Early recognition of heterozygotes for the gene for dystrophia myotonica. J. Neurol. Neurosurg. Psychiatry 33:279–293.

Butterfield D. A., Chesnut D. B., Appel S. H. and Roses A. D. (1976): Spin label study of erythrocyte membrane fluidity in myotonic and Duchenne dystrophy and congenital myotonia. Nature 263:159–161.

Donahue R. P., Bias W. B., Renwick J. H. and McKusick V. A. (1968): Probable assignment of the Duffy blood group locus to chromosome 1 in man. Proc. Nat. Acad. Sci. USA 61:949–955.

Dupont B., Oberfeld S. E., Smithwick E. M., Lee T. D. and Levine L. S. (1977): Close genetic linkage between HLA and congenital adrenal hyperplasia (21 hydroxylase deficiency). Lancet 2:1309–1311.

Emery A. E. H. and Walton J. N. (1967): The Genetics of muscular dystrophies.

Fenger K. and Hilden J. (1977): Recurrence risk of myotonic dystrophy. Lancet 1:1011.

Goto I. (1974): Creatine phosphokinase isozymes in neuromuscular disorders. Arch. Neurol. 31:116–119.

Harper P. S. (1972): Genetic studies in myotonic dystrophy. Thesis for degree of D.M., University of Oxford, U.K.

Harper P. S. (1973): Presymptomatic detection and genetic counselling in myotonic dystrophy. Clin. Genet. 4:134–140.

Harper P. S. (1975a): Congenital myotonic dystrophy in Britain. 1. Clinical aspects. Arch. Dis. Child. 50 505–513.

Harper P. S. (1975b): Congenital myotonic dystrophy in Britain. 2. Genetic basis. Arch. Dis. Child. 50:514–521.

Harper P. S., Bias W. B., Hutchinson J. R. and McKusick V. A. (1971): ABH secretor status of the foetus: a genetic marker identifiable by amniocentesis. J. Med. Genet. 8:438–440.

Harper P. S. and Dyken P. R. (1972): Early onset dystrophia myotonica. Evidence supporting a maternal environmental factor. Lancet 2:53–55.

Harper P. S., Rivas M. L., Bias W. B. M., Hutchinson J. R., Dyken P. R. and McKusick V. A. (1972): Genetic linkage confirmed between the locus for myotonic dystrophy and the ABH secretion and Lutheran blood group loci. Am. J. Hum. Genet. 24:310–316.

Insley J., Bird G. W. G., Harper P. S. and Pearce G. W. (1976): Prenatal prediction of myotonic dystrophy. Lancet *1*:806.

Lynas M. A. (1957): Dystrophia myotonica, with special reference to Northern Ireland. Ann. Hum. Genet. *21*:318–351.

McComas A. J., Campbell M. J. and Sica R. E. P. (1971): Electrophysiological study of dystrophia myotonica. J. Neurol. Neurosurg. Psychiatry *34*:132–139.

Mohr J. (1954): A Study of Linkage in Man. Munskaard, Copenhagen.

Pescia G. and Emery A. E. H. (1976): The importance of biomicroscopic examination of the lens in the detection of heterozygotes for certain hereditary diseases, in particular myotonic dystrophy. J. Genet. Hum. *24*:227–234.

Polgar J. G., Bradley W. G., Upton A. R. M., Anderson J., Howat J. M. L., Petito F., Roberts D. F. and Scopa J. (1972): The early detection of dystrophia myotonica. Brain *95*:761–766.

Renwick J. H. (1969a): Progress in mapping human autosomes. Br. Med. Bull. *25*:65–73.

Renwick J. H. (1969b): Widening the scope of antenatal diagnosis. Lancet *2*:386.

Renwick J. H. and Bolling D. R. (1971): An analysis procedure illustrated on a triple linkage of use for prenatal diagnosis of myotonic dystrophy. J. Med. Genet. *8*:399–406.

Renwick J. H., Bundey S. E., Ferguson-Smith M. A. and Izatt M. M. (1971): Confirmation of the linkage of the loci for myotonic dystrophy and ABH secretion. J. Med. Genet. *8*:407–416.

Roberts D. F. and Bradley W. G. (1977): Immunoglobulin levels in dystrophia myotonica. J. Med. Genet. *14*:16–19.

Roses A. D. and Appel S. H. (1973): Protein kinase activity in erythrocyte ghosts of patients with myotonic muscular dystrophy. Proc. Natl. Acad. Sci. USA *70*:1855–1859.

Roses A. D. and Appel S. H. (1974): Muscle membrane protein kinase in myotonic muscular dystrophy. Nature *250*:245–247.

Roses A. D., Butterfield D. A., Appel S. H. and Chesnut D. B. (1975): Phenytoin and membrane fluidity in myotonic dystrophy. Arch. Neurol. *32*:535–538.

Schrott H. G., Karp L. and Omenn G. S. (1973): Prenatal diagnosis of myotonic dystrophy. Clin. Genet. *4*:38–45.

Schrott H. G. and Omenn G. S. (1975): Myotonic dystrophy: opportunities for prenatal prediction. Neurology *25*:789–791.

Spence M. A., Lange K. and Crandall B. F. (1976): Computations for prenatal prediction of myotonic dystrophy. Lancet *2*:1198–1199.

Thomas N. S. T. and Harper P. S. (1978): Myotonic dystrophy: studies on the lipid composition and metabolism of erythrocytes and skin fibroblasts. Clin. Chim. Acta *83*:13–33.

Walsh J. C., Turtle J. R., Miller S. and McLeod J. G. (1970): Abnormalities of insulin secretion in dystrophia myotonica. Brain *93*:731–742.

CHAPTER TWELVE

Muscle Pathology in Myotonic Dystrophy

The existence of characteristic changes in the muscles of patients with myotonic dystrophy has been known since the earliest autopsy reports (Steinert, 1909; Adie and Greenfield, 1923) and has been well documented in both autopsy and biopsy studies of a variety of different muscles (Wohlfart, 1951; Greenfield et al, 1957; Berthold, 1958), but the study of muscle tissue in this disorder until recently has contributed relatively little to our fundamental understanding of the disease. In part this is because muscle biopsy is rarely needed diagnostically; unlike many other neuromuscular diseases in which the clinical picture may be indeterminate and biopsy is essential for a specific diagnosis to be reached, most adult cases of myotonic dystrophy can be diagnosed with clinical certainty and biopsy serves only to confirm what is already known. A further factor has been the prevalence of inadequate methods of taking and preparing biopsies, and a dearth of expert interpretation of the changes. Although modern techniques of preparation (Dubowitz and Brooke, 1973) and the application of histochemistry (Engel and Brooke, 1966; Dubowitz, 1974) and electron microscopy (Neville, 1973) have revolutionised the situation for this and other muscle diseases, it unfortunately remains a fact that relatively few centres have the expertise to process and interpret biopsy samples adequately; if muscle biopsy is to be done at all it should be done by, or in collaboration with, such a centre. The introduction of needle biopsy (Edwards, 1971) is likely to facilitate study of muscle in situations in which there is reluctance to undertake open biopsy, and should also allow serial studies to be performed. Samples obtained in this way have been shown to provide adequate tissue for a wide variety of histological and biochemical investigations.

250

DIAGNOSTIC FEATURES

It has already been mentioned that muscle biopsy is rarely needed to establish the diagnosis of myotonic dystrophy, but there are several clinical situations in which there may be real doubt and where the finding of the typical changes of the disorder in a muscle biopsy is of considerable help. Conversely, the finding of a different histological picture may help to eliminate myotonic dystrophy from the differential diagnosis of a puzzling clinical picture. These situations include the following:

1. Patients with progressive muscle wasting or weakness in whom there is evidence of a primary myopathic process, but who show only minimal or equivocal myotonia. Here the distinction is principally from other primary muscle disorders of adult life such as facio-scapulo-humeral dystrophy, polymyositis and other acquired myopathies.

2. Patients with definite myotonia, but only minimal muscle weakness and wasting, in whom the distinction from myotonia congenita may be difficult, particularly if there are no other family members with more typical disease.

3. Children with congenital myotonic dystrophy in whom hypotonia rather than myotonia is the predominant feature, and in whom a variety of congenital myopathies and anterior horn cell disorders have to be considered in the differential diagnosis.

Table 12–1 summarises the principal biopsy changes in myotonic dystrophy (excluding the congenital form), and in Table 12–2 these are compared with those seen in other major dystrophies and in myotonia congenita. For a more detailed comparative review of the histological features of these other disorders the reader is referred to the monograph of Dubowitz and Brooke (1973).

None of the features listed in Table 12–1 is in itself diagnostic of myotonic dystrophy, but their presence in combination allows the diagno-

Table 12–1. MUSCLE HISTOLOGY IN MYOTONIC DYSTROPHY

Characteristic Features
  Increased central nuclei
  Nuclear chains
  Ringed fibres
  Sarcoplasmic masses
  Type 1 fibre atrophy
  Muscle spindles: increased fibre splitting
  Terminal innervation: increased arborisation

Less Prominent Features
  Small angular fibres
  "Moth-eaten" fibres
  Type 2 fibre hypertrophy
  Increased fibrosis

Table 12-2.   MYOTONIC DYSTROPHY: COMPARATIVE FEATURES OF MUSCLE HISTOLOGY

	Myotonic Dystrophy	Myotonia Congenita	Duchenne Dystrophy	Autosomal Recessive Limb-girdle Dystrophy
Central nuclei	Abundant	Uncommon	Moderate	Common
Ringed fibres	Common	Absent	Uncommon	Common
Fibre size	Type 1 fibre atrophy	Hypertrophy	Hypertrophy frequent (all fibre types)	Increased variation + hypertrophy
Fibre distribution	Normal	Type 2 fibre deficiency	Type 2 fibre deficiency	Type 2 fibre deficiency
Fibre splitting	Uncommon (except spindles)	Absent	Uncommon	Marked
Necrosis and phagocytosis	Slight	Absent	Marked	Moderate
Regenerative activity	Absent	Absent	Marked	Moderate
Fibrosis	Slight	Absent	Marked	Marked

sis to be made with a high degree of probability. Likewise, it can be seen from Table 12–2 that some of the most striking features of other myopathies are lacking in myotonic dystrophy, notably the active necrosis, phagocytosis, regenerative activity and fatty infiltration so characteristic of Duchenne dystrophy; other abnormalities such as fibre splitting and fibrosis are also much less prominent except in severely involved muscle. Thus, even in clinically doubtful cases, a careful comparison of these features should allow a clear confirmation or exclusion of the diagnosis of myotonic dystrophy in relation to other dystrophies and as distinct from acquired myopathies and polymyositis.

In myotonia congenita, the changes in muscle histology are minimal or absent apart from fibre hypertrophy (see Chapter 3), and the finding of a significant degree of the changes in Table 12–1 is strong evidence that the disorder is myotonic dystrophy, not myotonia congenita, even in the absence of muscle wasting or other diagnostic clinical features.

Changes in Fibre Size and Architecture

Even in mildly affected patients an increased variation of fibre size is seen in conventional haematoxylin-eosin preparations. A high proportion of fibres may have a "moth-eaten" appearance, and small angular fibres, uncommon in most primary muscle disorders, are frequent. By contrast there are few changes of active degeneration and necrosis except in severely involved muscles, nor is fibrosis a prominent early feature. Several additional changes, although not totally specific for myotonic dystrophy, are sufficiently common to be conspicuous and diagnostically important features.

Central Nuclei*

An increased number of centrally placed nuclei is one of the most characteristic changes of myotonic dystrophy, and occurs at an early stage, often before other significant changes in the muscle can be recognised. Initially, the numbers are small, but they increase progressively with severity of involvement, and on longitudinal section can be seen to lie in chains, each of which may contain up to 20 nuclei (Fig. 12–1A). Although this appearance is suggestive of continuing division of the centrally placed nuclei, there is in fact no evidence as to whether this or continued inward migration is principally responsible for the increase. The nuclei themselves vary in size and appearance, some being pyknotic, others enlarged and pale. These changes are seen even more clearly with

---

*See Figure 12–1.

the electron microscope, which shows irregularity of the nuclear membrane and inclusion bodies within the nuclei.

Although an increased number of central nuclei occurs in many muscle disorders, the central nuclear chains of myotonic dystrophy are rarely seen to any significant extent in other dystrophies, and are perhaps the most important single diagnostic feature.

Only in some of the congenital myopathies, notably myotubular (centronuclear) myopathy (Spiro et al, 1966), do similar changes occur; this disorder requires careful distinction from the congenital form of myotonic dystrophy (see Chapter 9) but is unlikely to be a problem in relation to myotonic dystrophy in adult life. The central nuclei in myotubular myopathy (and possibly in congenital myotonic dystrophy also) presumably reflect an immaturity of development rather than a secondary inward migration of nuclei.

Ringed Fibres*

This term is applied to fibres seen running circumferentially in a cross-section of muscle. They have also been referred to as striated annulets or "ringbinden". In fact, they run a spiral course rather than forming a true ring, and have been the subject of considerable debate as to whether they represent a natural phenomenon or whether they result from artefacts of preparation. Heidenhain (1918) first described ringed fibres in patients with myotonic dystrophy, although they had been recognised both before and subsequently in other dystrophies, as well as in a variety of other muscle disorders, and occasionally in normal muscle.

Bethlem and Wijngaarden (1963) examined the incidence of ringed fibres in 200 biopsies from patients with a number of muscle diseases, and found them to occur in five out of seven cases of myotonic dystrophy and in almost one-third of other dystrophies. Dubowitz and Brooke (1973) likewise showed ringed fibres in 70 percent of biopsies from myotonic dystrophy patients, and found that in other dystrophies their frequency was related directly to the chronicity of the disorder.

Why ringed fibres should occur is poorly understood. Although they can undoubtedly be produced as artefacts of preparation, their occurrence in muscle disease, particularly myotonic dystrophy, cannot satisfactorily be attributed to this. Bethlem and Wijngaarden (1963) were able to produce them experimentally following tendon section in animals, and suggested that they might be formed when contact between origin and insertion had been interrupted. Support for this view comes from the electron-microscopic studies of Schotland et al (1966), who considered

---

*See Figure 12–7.

that the fibres were formed in the abnormal position rather than adopting it after rupture. The electron micrographs shown in Figure 12–7 support this view, and also reveal that the ringed fibre and the fibre enclosed by it are in fact portions of a single fibre, enclosed by the same basement membrane. The initimate relationship of the two portions certainly excludes artefact in this situation. Nevertheless, a more direct relationship to the myotonic process with its repeated prolonged contractions in muscle affected by the dystrophic process cannot be ruled out, and it remains a fact that ringed fibres are seen more frequently in myotonic dystrophy than in any other disorder.

Sarcoplasmic Masses

These are homogeneous areas of sarcoplasm, often adjacent to a ringed fibre, that are another characteristic feature of myotonic dystrophy. Histochemical studies (Engel, 1962) have shown them to consist of disorganised but normally staining intermyofibrillary material with a complete absence of myofibrils and their associated enzymes. Electron microscopy reveals aggregations of tubules with numerous free ribosomes and scattered bundles of myofilaments (Fardeau et al, 1964; Mussini et al, 1970).

Changes in Fibre Type*

The development of a variety of histochemical techniques has allowed the division of muscle fibres into two major types according to staining properties; type 1 fibres are rich in oxidative enzymes, but weak in myosin ATPase activity, whereas the converse is the case for type 2 fibres. Subdivision of type 2 fibres is possible by preincubation of the sections in an acid medium before staining for myosin ATPase activity. Under these conditions type 1 fibres show high activity. Although this classification does not fully correspond to others based on speed of contraction and colour, it has added a range of valuable distinguishing features and made it mandatory for muscle biopsies to be taken and processed in a way that allows these techniques to be used.

In myotonic dystrophy the earliest change is an inequality of size of types 1 and 2 fibres, with a tendency to reduction in size of type 1. Later there is marked atrophy of type 1, whereas type 2 fibres show a tendency to hypertrophy (Engel and Brooke, 1966). Brooke and Engel (1969) have performed a detailed quantitative analysis of the changes in fibre type

*See Figures 12–2 and 12–4.

based on a series of 36 biopsies from patients with myotonic dystrophy. For biceps muscle biopsies from males, the mean type 1 fibre diameter was 44 ± 17 μm compared with a normal value of 65 ± 11 μm. By contrast the type 2 fibre diameter was 77 ± 17 μm in the myotonic dystrophy group, slightly greater than the normal value of 73 ± 12 μm. This combination of changes is highly specific for myotonic dystrophy, and is rarely seen in other dystrophies or other myotonic disorders. The deficiency of type 2B fibres, almost the only change seen in myotonia congenita (Dubowitz and Brooke, 1973), is less common in myotonic dystrophy, and the non-progressive myotonic disorders fail to show the selective type 1 fibre atrophy.

Ultrastructural Changes

A number of electron-microscopic studies have been performed on muscle biopsies in myotonic dystrophy, and consistent abnormalities have been found. The early studies (Wechsler and Hager, 1961; Aleu and Afifi, 1964; Klinkerfuss, 1967) showed degenerative changes in the myofibrils, with the Z line and I band particularly affected. Further work has confirmed this (Schroder and Adams, 1968; Johnson, 1969) and has also shown important negative findings, including absence of significant changes in blood vessels, largely normal innervation and lack of abnormality in the basement membrane. Abnormally-shaped and degenerating mitochondria have also been a prominent finding in most studies.

Abnormalities of the sarcotubular system have been particularly sought in view of the relationship between myotonia and membrane function, and there is some doubt as to how significant such changes are in myotonic dystrophy. Samaha et al (1967) found patchy changes in the sarcoplasmic reticulum with considerable areas entirely normal. Schotland (1970), however, noted a marked proliferation of the sarcotubular system, with a lattice-like network of tubules, a finding confirmed by Mussini et al (1970), who considered the changes to arise from infolding of the limiting membrane. Schroder and Becker (1972) found similar proliferative changes in myotonia congenita as well as in myotonic dystrophy.

None of the electron-microscopic changes in myotonic dystrophy is specific, all being found to some extent in other muscle dystrophies and in some denervating disorders as well. It is also far from clear which of the changes are the primary ones. In general, the severity of changes has paralleled the degree of muscle involvement. The studies of Mussini et al (1970) suggest that the sarcotubular abnormalities are seen earlier than the degeneration of myofibrils, but at present no single abnormality or combination of changes can be said to be either diagnostic or a primary finding in the disorder.

The electron microscope has recently been applied in conjunction with other experimental techniques that promise to give considerably more specific information. So far, Duchenne dystrophy has been the main target of these studies, but it is likely that they will provide equally valuable data in myotonic dystrophy.

Freeze fracture techniques have recently been developed which allow the splitting of cell membranes and the study of both surfaces by electron microscopy. This approach was first applied to normal muscle by Raynes et al (1968), and human dystrophic muscle has been examined by Ketelsen (1975) and Schotland et al (1977); abnormalities would be of considerable relevance to any possible functional membrane defect in muscular dystrophies. The characteristic appearance of normal muscle is a regular distribution of spherical particles, and observations so far suggest an increased density of these in Duchenne dystrophy and a decrease in denervating disorders. A preliminary report in six patients with myotonic dystrophy (Schotland et al, 1977) has shown an increased particle density on both faces of the muscle plasma membrane.

Mokri and Engel (1976) have also applied electron microscopy to study of the plasma membrane of muscle in Duchenne dystrophy. They paid particular attention to those fibres that appeared free from dystrophic changes and showed a consistent focal disruption of the plasma membrane. They also demonstrated these fibres to be abnormally permeable to peroxidase, suggesting that the membrane defect was a functional one as well as structural. Myotonic dystrophy has not yet been studied in this way.

These experimental electron-microscopic approaches give a clear indication that there may be a fundamental defect of membrane structure in the muscular dystrophies, and provide a link with the electrophysiological and biochemical evidence for a membrane abnormality, to be discussed in subsequent chapters.

The Muscle Spindle

The first note of an abnormality in the muscle spindle in myotonic dystrophy was made by Steinert himself (1909), who found fibrosis of spindles in his autopsied case.

Although early studies of autopsy material did not show definite abnormalities (Wohlfart, 1951), Daniel and Strich (1964) made a special study of the muscle spindles and found unusual and characteristic changes since confirmed and further documented by Swash (1972) and Swash and Fox (1975). Daniel and Strich studied spindles from the lumbrical muscles of five autopsied patients and showed that the intrafusal muscle fibres were unusually small and greatly increased in number when viewed on cross-section; longitudinally they appeared tangled with an increase of fibrous tissue. Some of the fibres had central nuclei, some of which were pyknotic, suggesting involvement by the dystrophic process. Swash (1972) examined a large number of spindles (192 from seven patients) and found similar changes, but by using silver stains was also able to show abnormalities of motor innervation to the intrafusal fibres. Terminal branches of motor nerves showed increased numbers of abnormally-shaped end-plates with nerve endings placed over a considerable part of the intrafusal fibre. Swash initially interpreted these findings as evidence for a neural basis of the disease, but further work using serial sections (Swash and Fox, 1975) showed that the increased number of intrafusal fibres was in fact the result of splitting and refusion, the fibres being relatively normal at their ends and at the equatorial region, where sensory innervation appeared entirely normal. Marked degenerative changes were seen in the intrafusal fibres on electron microscopy, even in fibres appearing normal otherwise. Further evidence that the changes resulted from splitting has come from histochemistry which shows uniform fibre types, suggesting origin from a single fibre (Heene, 1973). Figures 12–9 to 12–12, kindly supplied by Dr. Michael Swash, illustrate some of the principal changes.

The most likely sequence of events thus seems to be that relatively normal intrafusal muscle fibres undergo a process of splitting in response to the mechanical stresses resulting from myotonic after-discharges. The changes in terminal innervation may be a secondary response of reinnervation of the split fibres.

Changes in Innervation

The evidence for and against a significant neural abnormality in myotonic dystrophy has already been discussed in Chapter 7, and attempts have been made to correlate the observed functional changes with specific histological abnormalities. The only constant neural abnormality to be documented is the occurrence of elongated and unusually extensive terminal arborisations found by Coers (1955), Coers and Woolf (1959) and MacDermot (1961), but it seems distinctly possible that these are secondary changes in response to recurrent mechanical stress (Harriman, 1976) analogous to changes in the muscle spindle, and that they do not represent a primary defect of innervation. The fact that electron microscopy has clearly shown normal innervation of degenerating fibres (Engel et al, 1975), and the lack of type grouping and other features of denervation, make it difficult to avoid the conclusion that changes in nerve are subsidiary, if not secondary, to those in the muscle itself. Further evidence for this view has come from a different approach: Drachman and Fambrough (1975) studied the number and distribution of acetylcholine receptors using α-bungarotoxin, and found no change in myotonic dystrophy, in contrast to the marked increase in such receptors occurring in muscle from patients with myasthenia gravis.

Muscle Changes in Congenital Myotonic Dystrophy

The early reports on muscle biopsies from children with the severe congenital form of myotonic dystrophy suggested that abnormalities were slight compared with those found in affected adults (Vanier, 1960; Dodge et al, 1965). A series of more recent investigations based both on biopsy studies (Karpati et al, 1973; Dubowitz and Brooke, 1973; Farkas et al, 1974) and on autopsies of fatal neonatal cases (Bossen et al, 1974; Sarnat and Silbert, 1976) has shown that a number of unusual and distinctive changes can be demonstrated with the use of histochemistry and electron microscopy, and that these differ in many respects from the changes seen in adult myotonic dystrophy.

All studies agree in finding a striking hypoplasia of muscle, evident macroscopically in the respiratory muscles as well as those of the limbs (Bossen et al, 1974), and accounting for the clinical features of respiratory distress, thin ribs (Fried et al, 1975) and probably for the common occurrence of arthrogryposis. Microscopically, fibres are reduced both in number and in size; Sarnat and Silbert (1976) found a range of 5 to 13 μm diameter and noted the cross-sectional shape to be round rather than having the normal polygonal appearance. Although the reduction in muscle fibres gives a relative prominence of fibrous tissue, all authors agree on the complete lack of necrosis and active degenerative changes, with a lack of the moth-eaten and pyknotic fibres commonly seen in the adult disease, and with ringed fibres and sarcoplasmic masses absent in neonatal cases. Sarnat and Silbert also noted the muscle spindles to be normal, thus supporting the view of Swash and Fox (1975) that the splitting of these in adults with myotonic dystrophy is a response to mechanical stress. The one feature similar to the adult disease is the high proportion of central nuclei.

Histochemical studies have shown a lack of fibre type distinction in some cases, with type 1 fibre hypotrophy in others, together with a peripheral ring devoid of oxidative enzymes (Farkas et al, 1974). Electron microscopy has shown this to correspond to absence of mitochondria in this region, and other ultrastructural changes include persistence of myofibrils in the periphery, disorganisation of the Z band of the myofibrils, and dilated tubular systems. Nerve endings appear normal. Figures 12–3 to 12–7 illustrate some of these changes in one of the author's patients with congenital myotonic dystrophy. A feature recently recognised as particularly characteristic is an increase in the number of "satellite cells", believed to be the source of newly developing or regenerating myoblasts. These can be seen in the author's case and are even more marked in a fatal neonatal case studied by Dr. V. Sahgal (Fig. 12–8). In most other congenital myopathies satellite cells are reduced in number.

Taken as a whole the changes are those of a failure of development of muscle rather than an active degeneration, and Sarnat and Silbert (1976) suggest that a primary defect in the muscle cell membrane may produce a failure of response to neural influences during development. The muscle changes must also be considered in the light of the maternal transmission of congenital myotonic dystrophy and the likely involvement of an intrauterine factor (Harper and Dyken, 1972). It is possible that muscle cell culture might throw light on these intriguing problems.

DEVELOPMENTAL AND TISSUE CULTURE STUDIES

Considerable progress has been made in understanding the early development of muscle, and both structural aspects (Webb, 1972) and biochemistry (Perry 1971) have been studied. Most of the work has utilised animal material, but information is now available for normal human fetal muscle (Webb, 1972; Toop and Emery, 1974). "Dystrophic" animal models such as mouse and chicken have also been examined, but in human dystrophies appreciable numbers of fetuses at risk have been examined only for Duchenne dystrophy. The changes reported for such fetuses have been minimal; increased numbers of hyaline fibres and variability of fibre size have been noted (Toop and Emery, 1974; Emery, 1977), but consistent changes have not been seen even with the electron microscope. Emery and McGregor (1977) saw no abnormalities at all in cultured fetal muscle. This suggests that in myotonic dystrophy only congenital cases would be likely to show changes in early fetal life. One such case at risk (Insley et al, 1976) exhibited no definite changes, but no detailed study has been performed on fetal material in myotonic dystrophy.

Tissue culture techniques have allowed aspects of growth and development of muscle to be studied in adult muscle, and even though such processes may not be identical to those of normal muscle development they provide a powerful experimental tool. Not only may changes in histochemistry and ultrastructure be examined, but also the processes of cell fusion and myotube development, as well as the relationship of muscle development to innervation. So far most work has concentrated on delineating the normal patterns of development, and changes in the dystrophies have been few or absent. Kakulas et al (1968) found abnormally-shaped myoblasts and delayed myotube formation in Duchenne dystrophy, the latter also being detected by Bateson et al (1972);

Text continued on page 270

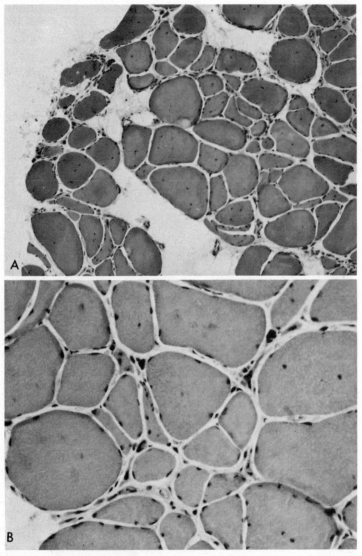

Figure 12-1. Muscle histology in adult myotonic dystrophy. Haematoxylin and eosin preparations, courtesy of Dr. E. Bossen, Dept. of Pathology, Duke University Medical Center, Durham, N.C. (From Roses, A. D., Harper, P. S. and Bossen, E. H.: Handbook of Clinical Neurology, Vol. 40, 1979, in press.)

A, Transverse section showing variation in fibre size and numerous internal nuclei.

B, Higher power transverse section showing atrophic fibres with clumped nuclei.

Illustration continued on following page.

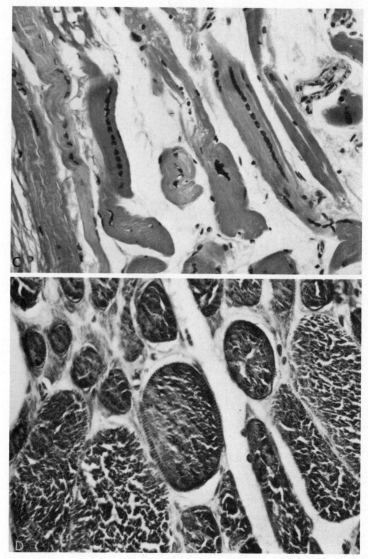

Figure 12–1. *Continued*
C, Longitudinal section showing long chains of internal nuclei (× 250).
D, Transverse section showing ringed fibres.

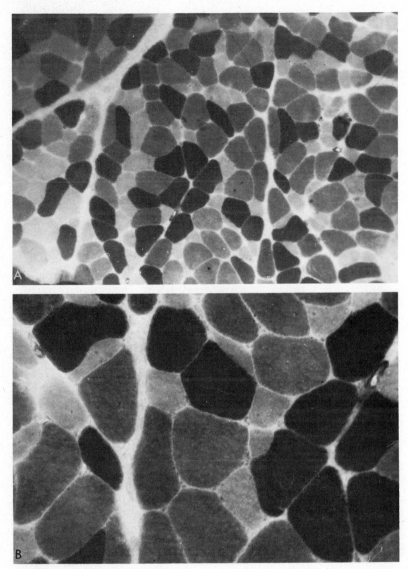

Figure 12-2. Histochemical study of muscle biopsy (deltoid) from 46 year old male with myotonic dystrophy (patient J.G.). Cryostat transverse sections stained with ATPase at pH 9.4, showing moderate type 1 fibre atrophy (*darkly stained fibres*) with inequality of fibre size (courtesy of Dr. P. Hudgson, Regional Neurology Center. Newcastle on Tyne, England).

A, × 125.

B, × 350.

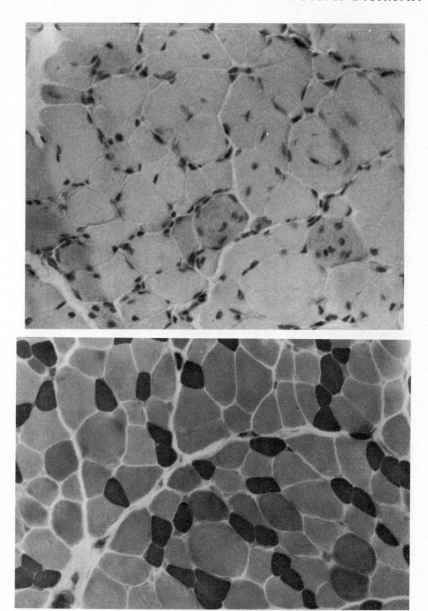

Figures 12–3 to 12–7. Histological changes in childhood myotonic dystrophy (patient G.H.; see Chapter 9 for full clinical details). The patient presented at birth with congenital myotonic dystrophy, but was aged 7 years when this biopsy was taken, at the time of tendon transplant surgery (tibialis posterior muscle). Micrographs by courtesy of Mrs. Caroline Sewry (formerly Maunder), The Jerry Lewis Muscle Research Centre, Hammersmith Hospital, London.

12–3, Cryostat section stained with haematoxylin and eosin, showing internal nuclei, basophilic fibres, and increased variability in fibre size. There is no excess of connective tissue and no inflammatory response in this or other sections (× 420).

12–4, Cryostat section stained with myosin ATPase after acid preincubation, showing

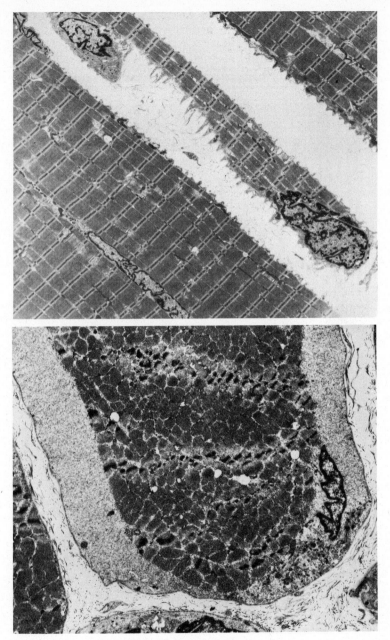

Figures 12–3 to 12–7. *Continued*

marked atrophy of type 1 fibres (*darkly staining*) with some hypertrophy of type 2 fibres (× 265).

    12–5, Electron micrograph of longitudinal section showing an atrophic fibre and an adjacent fibre with a central nucleus and focal loss of myofibrils (× 4,500).

    12–6, Electron micrograph of transverse section showing an outer zone devoid of myofibrillar material or other organelles. This appearance is particularly characteristic of congenital myotonic dystrophy (× 4,600).

Illustration continued on following page.

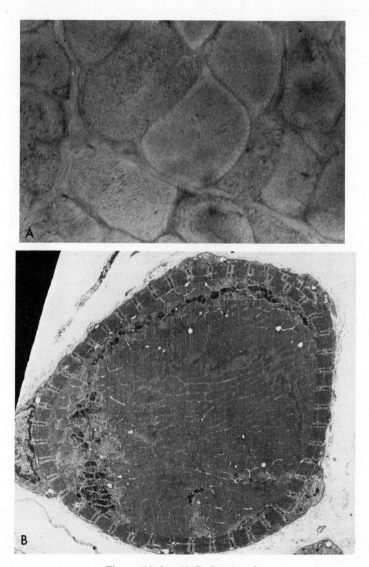

Figures 12–3 to 12–7. *Continued*

12–7, Ringed fibres in myotonic dystrophy.

A, Cryostat section stained with periodic acid Schiffs showing several ringed fibres (× 900).

B, Electron micrograph of a ringed fibre, showing outer zone at right angles to inner zone. Both components are enclosed within the same plasma membrane, indicating their common origin from a single fibre (× 2,900).

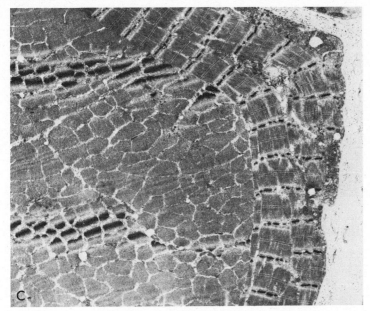

Figures 12–3 to 12–7. *Continued*

C, Higher-powered electron micrograph of similar fibre. The close relationship of the two components argues strongly against this being artefactual (× 7,400).

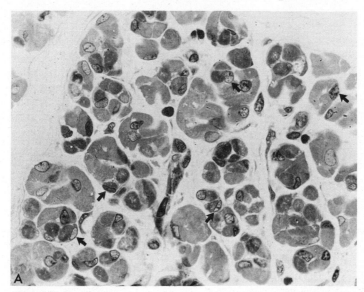

Figure 12–8. SATELLITE CELLS IN CONGENITAL MYOTONIC DYSTROPHY.

An increased number of satellite cells is a characteristic feature of congenital myotonic dystrophy, and contrasts with other congenital myopathies. These preparations, provided by courtesy of Dr. V. Sahgal, are taken from a fatal neonatal case of the disease.

A, × 1,100, showing abundant satellite cells (*arrowed*).

Illustration continued on following page.

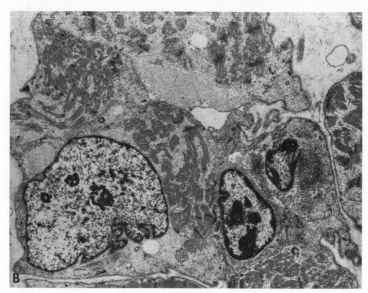

Figure 12–8. *Continued*

B, Electron micrograph (× 15,000), showing a satellite cell and five myoblasts in various stages of development under the same basement membrane. Each myoblast has its own plasma membrane.

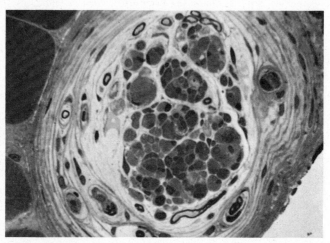

Figures 12–9 to 12–12. Changes in muscle spindles in myotonic dystrophy. Photo micrographs from Swash and Fox, 1975, by courtesy of Dr. Michael Swash and the Journal of Neurology, Neurosurgery and Psychiatry.

12–9, Toluidine blue semi-thin section. Mid polar region to show extensive fibre splitting in a muscle spindle (× 350).

12–10, Electron micrograph of plasma membranes delineating fragments of varying maturity. The fragment to the right is undergoing regeneration; to the left a hemidesmosome links the apposed plasma membranes.

12–11, Electron micrograph of section through nuclear bag region of one intrafusal fibre. Splitting is not present; primary sensory nerve terminals are indicated by the arrows (× 9,000).

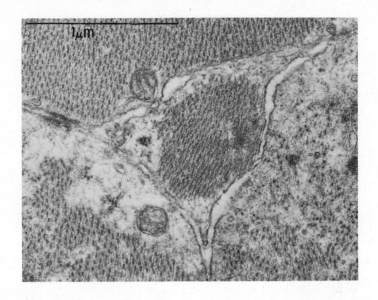

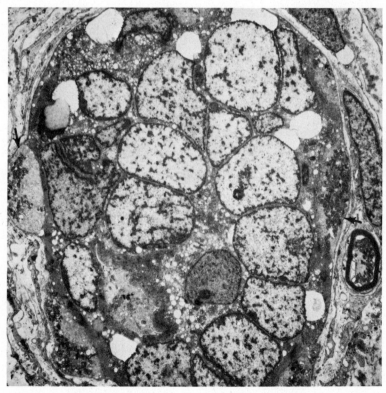

Figures 12–9 to 12–12.   *See legend on opposite page.*

Illustration continued on following page.

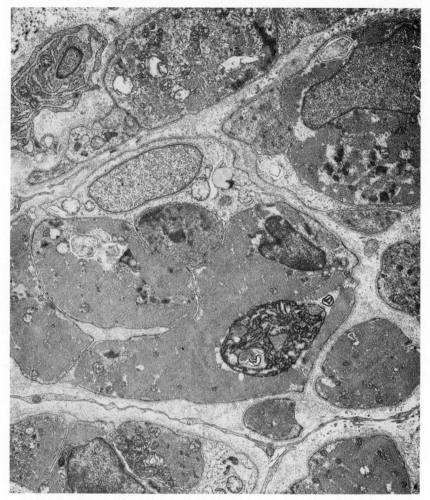

Figures 12–9 to 12–12 *Continued*

12–12. Electron micrograph to show variable morphology in splitting fibre fragments (× 15,000).

Bishop et al (1971) found no qualitative or quantitative changes in morphology or growth rate. Their study included muscle from one patient with myotonic dystrophy, and that of Bateson et al two such patients; no abnormality was noted. Subsequent muscle cultures in myotonic dystrophy have likewise failed to show anything abnormal, including muscle from a congenital case of the author, the biopsy of which is illustrated (Witkowski, personal communication).

The lack of obvious abnormalities in dystrophic human muscle in culture has been used as an argument that muscular dystrophies are primarily neurogenic in origin, but it is more likely that it simply reflects the early stage of techniques for studying muscle in culture. Already these are improving, and specific changes have been shown in culture in some metabolic and congenital myopathies (Askansas and Engel, 1977). It should not be long before they become fruitful in other dystrophies, including myotonic dystrophy.

REFERENCES

Adie W. J. and Greenfield J. G. (1923): Dystrophia myotonica (myotonia atrophica). Brain 46:73-127.

Aleu F. P. and Afifi A. K. (1964): Ultrastructure of muscle in myotonic dystrophy. Preliminary observations. Am. J. Pathol. 45:221-231.

Askansas V. and Engel W. K. (1977): Diseased human muscle in tissue culture. In Pathogenesis of Human Muscular Dystrophies. (Ed.: L. P. Rowland). Excerpta Medica, Amsterdam, pp. 856-871.

Bateson R. G., Warren J. and Hindle D. (1972): Growth pattern in vitro of normal and diseased adult human skeletal muscle. J. Neurol. Sci. 15:183-191.

Berthold H. (1958): Zur pathologischen Anatomie der Dystrophia Myotonica. Dtsch. Z. Nervenheilkd. 178:394-412.

Bethlem J. and Van Wijngaarden G. K. (1963): The incidence of ringed fibres and sarcoplasmic masses in normal and diseased muscle. J. Neurol. Neurosurg. Psychiatry 26:326-332.

Bishop A., Gallup B., Skeate Y. and Dubowitz V. (1971): Morphological studies on normal and diseased human muscle in culture. J. Neurol. Sci. 13:333-350.

Bossen E. H., Shelburne J. D. and Verkauf B. S. (1974): Respiratory muscle involvement in infantile myotonic dystrophy. Arch. Pathol. 97:250-252.

Brooke M. H. and Engel W. K. (1969): The histographic analysis of human muscle biopsies with regard to fibre types. I. Adult and male and female. Neurology (Minneap.) 19:221-233.

Brooke M. H. and Engel W. K. (1969): The histographic analysis of human muscle biopsies with regard to fibre types — children's biopsies. Neurology (Minneap.) 19:591-605.

Coers C. (1955): Etude histologique et histochimique de la jonction neuro-musculaire dans les syndromes myotoniques. Acta Neurol. Pychiat. Belg. 55:18-22.

Coers C. and Woolf A. L. (1959): The innervation of muscle. Oxford.

Daniel P. M. and Strich S. J. (1964): Abnormalities in the muscle spindles in dystrophia myotonica. Neurology 14:310-316.

Dodge P. R., Gamstorp I., Byers R. K. and Russell P. (1965): Myotonic dystrophy in infancy and childhood. Pediatrics 35:3-19.

Drachman D. B. and Fambrough D. M. (1976): Are muscle fibres denervated in myotonic dystrophy? Arch. Neurol. 33:485-488.

Dubowitz V. (1974): Muscle biopsy — technical and diagnostic aspects. Ann. Clin. Res. 6:69-79.

Dubowitz V. and Brooke M. H. (1973): Muscle Biopsy: A Modern Approach. W. B. Saunders Co., London, Philadelphia.

Edwards R. H. T. (1971): Percutaneous needle-biopsy of skeletal muscle in diagnosis and research. Lancet 2:593-595.

Emery A. E. H. (1977): Muscle histology and creatine kinase levels in the foetus in Duchenne muscular dystrophy. Nature 266:472-473.

Emery A. E. H. and McGregor L. (1977): The foetus in Duchenne muscular dystrophy: Muscle growth in tissue culture. Clin. Genet. 12:183-187.

Engel A. E., Jerusalem F., Tsojihata M. and Gomez M. R. (1975): The neuromuscular junction in myopathies. A quantitative ultrastructural study. In Recent Advances in

Myology (Eds.: W. G. Bradley, D. Gardner-Medwin and J. N. Walton). Excerpta Medica, Amsterdam.

Engel W. K. (1962): Chemocytology of striated annulets and sarcoplasmic masses in myotonic dystrophy. J. Histochem. Cytochem. 10:229–230.

Engel W. K. and Brooke M. H. (1966): Histochemistry of the myotonic disorders. From Symposion über Progressive Muskeldystrophie (Ed.: E. Kuhn).

Fardeau M., Lapresle J. and Milhaud M. (1964): Contribution à l'étude ultrastructurale des plaques motrices du muscle squelettique: ultrastructure des masses sarcoplasmiques laterales. C. R. Soc. Biol. (Paris) 159:15–17.

Farkas É., Tomé F. M. S., Fardeau M., Arsenionunes M. L., Dreyfuss P. and Doebler M. F. (1974): Histochemical and ultrastructural study of muscle biopsy in three cases of dystrophia myotonica in the newborn child. J. Neurol. Sci. 21:273–288.

Fried K., Payewski M., Mundel G., Caspie E. and Spira R. M. (1975): Thin ribs in neonatal myotonic dystrophy. Clin. Genet. 7:417–420.

Greenfield J. G., Shy G. M., Alvord E. C. and Berg L. (1957): An Atlas of Muscle Pathology in Neuromuscular Disease. Livingstone, Edinburgh.

Harper P. S. and Dyken P. R. (1972): Early onset dystrophia myotonica. Evidence supporting a maternal environmental factor. Lancet 2:53–55.

Harriman D. G. F. (1976): In Greenfield's Neuropathology (Eds.: W. Blackwood and J. A. N. Corsellis).

Heene R. (1973): Histological and histochemical findings in muscle spindles in dystrophia myotonica. J. Neurol. Sci. 18:369–372.

Heidenhain H. (1918): Über progressive Verebung der Muskulatur bei Myotonia Atrophica. Beitr. Pathol. Anat. 64:198–225.

Insley J., Bird G. W. G., Harper P. S. and Pearce G. W. (1976): Prenatal prediction of myotonic dystrophy. Lancet 1:806.

Johnson A. G. (1969): Alteration of the Z lines and I-band myofilaments in human skeletal muscle. Arch. Neuropathol. (Berlin) 12:218–226.

Kakulas B. A., Papadimitriou J. M., Knight J. O. and Mastaglia F. L. (1968): Normal and abnormal human muscle in tissue culture. Proc. Aust. Assoc. Neurol. 5:79–85.

Karpati G., Carpenter S., Watters G. V., Eisen A. A. and Andermann F. (1973): Infantile myotonic dystrophy. Histochemical and electron-microscopic features in skeletal muscle. Neurology 23:1066–1077.

Ketelsen U. P. (1975): The plasma membrane in human skeletal muscle cells in the pathological state. Freeze-etch studies. In Recent Advances in Myology (Eds.: W. G. Bradley, D. Gardner-Medwin and J. N. Walton). Excerpta Medica, Amsterdam, pp. 446–454.

Ketelsen U. P. and Schmidt D. (1972): Augensymptome und elektronenmikroskopische Befunde des M. orbicularis oculi bei dystrophischer Myotonie (Curschmann-Steinert). Albrecht von Graefes Arch Klin. Ophthalmol. 185:245–268.

Klinkerfuss G. H. (1967): An electron-microscopic study of myotonic dystrophy. Arch. Neurol. 16:181–193.

MacDermot V. (1961): The histology of the neuromuscular junction in dystrophia myotonica. Brain 84:75–84.

Mokri B. and Engel A. G. (1976): Duchenne dystrophy: electron-microscopic findings pointing to a basic or early abnormality in the plasma membrane of the muscle fibre. Neurology 25:1111–1120.

Mussini I., Di Mauro S. and Angelini C. (1970): Early ultrastructural and biochemical changes in muscle in dystrophia myotonica. J. Neurol. Sci. 10:585–604.

Neville H. E. (1973): Ultrastructural changes in muscle disease. In Muscle Biopsy: A Modern Approach. (Eds.: V. Dubowitz and M. H. Brooke). W. B. Saunders Co., London, Philadelphia.

Perry S. V. (1971): Development and specialization in muscle and the biochemistry of the dystrophies. J. Neurol. Sci. 12:289–306.

Samaha F. J., Schroder J. M., Rebeiz J. and Adams R. D. (1967): Studies on myotonia. Biochemical and electron-microscopic studies on myotonia congenita and myotonia dystrophica. Arch. Neurol. 17:22–33.

Sarnat H. B. and Silbert S. W. (1976): Maturational arrest of fetal muscle in neonatal myotonic dystrophy. Arch. Neurol. *33*:466–474.

Schotland D. L. (1970): An electron-microscopic investigation of myotonic dystrophy. J. Neuropathol. Exp. Neurol. *29*:241–253.

Schotland D. L., Bonilla E. and Van Meter M. (1977): Duchenne dystrophy: alteration in muscle plasma membrane structure. Science *196*:1005–1007.

Schotland D. L., Spiro D. and Carmel P. (1966): Ultrastructural studies of ring fibers in human muscle disease. J. Neuropathol. Exp. Neurol. *25*:431.

Schroder J. M. and Adams R. (1968): The ultrastructural morphology of the muscle fibre in myotonic dystrophy. Acta Neuropathol. (Berlin) *10*:218–241.

Schroder J. M. and Becker P. E. (1972): Anomalien des T-Systems und des sarkoplasmatischen Reticulums bei der Myotonie, Paramyotonie und Adynamie. Virchows Arch. Pathol. Anat. *357*:319–344.

Spiro A. J., Shy G. M. and Gonotas N. K. (1966): Myotubular myopathy. Persistence of fetal muscle in an adolescent boy. Arch. Neurol. *14*:1–14.

Steinert H. (1909): Myopathologische Beitrage. 1. Über des klinische und anatomische Bild des Muskelschwunds der Myotoniker. Dtsch. Z. Nervenheilkd. *37*:38–104.

Swash M. (1972): The morphology and innervation of the muscle spindle in dystrophia myotonica. Brain *95*:357–368.

Swash M. and Fox K. P. (1975): Abnormal intrafusal muscle fibres in myotonic dystrophy: a study using serial sections. J. Neurol. Neurosurg. Psychiatry *38*:91–99.

Swash M. and Fox K. P. (1975): The fine structure of the spindle abnormality in myotonic dystrophy. Neuropathol. Appl. Neurobiol. *1*:171–187.

Toop J. and Emery A. E. H. (1974): Muscle histology in fetuses at risk for Duchenne muscular dystrophy. Clin. Genet. *5*:230–233.

Vanier T. M. (1960): Dystrophia myotonica in childhood. Br. Med. J. *2*:1284–1288.

Webb J. N. (1972): The development of human skeletal muscle with particular reference to muscle cell death. J. Pathol. *106*:221–228.

Wechsler W. and Hager H. (1961): Elektronenmikroskopische Untersuchungen bei myotonischer Muskeldystrophie. Arch Psychiatr. Nervenkr. *201*:668–690.

Wohlfart G. (1951): Dystrophia myotonica and myotonia congenita: histopathologic studies with special reference to changes in the muscles. J. Neuropathol. Exp. Neurol. *10*:109–124.

CHAPTER THIRTEEN

The Electrophysiological Basis of Myotonia

Electrophysiological studies in myotonic dystrophy and allied disorders can give important information on a wide variety of topics. First, practical diagnostic information can be obtained enabling the distinction to be made between myotonic dystrophy and other myotonic disorders, as well as distinguishing other neuromuscular conditions with a superficial clinical resemblance. Second, studies on neuromuscular conditions can provide evidence as to whether the defect lies entirely within the muscle fibre itself or whether abnormalities of innervation also play a part. Finally, studies of individual fibres allow detailed analysis of the phenomenon of myotonia itself and its response to a variety of experimental conditions.

DIAGNOSTIC ASPECTS

It must be admitted from the outset that, although electromyography and allied investigations are always of interest in myotonic dystrophy, they are not necessary for diagnosis in the great majority of cases. It is rare for clinical myotonia to be lacking in symptomatic cases of the disease, and its apparent absence is much more likely to be due to failure to look for it than to its not being there. There are, however, a number of circumstances in which electromyography can be extremely helpful in resolving an otherwise inconclusive diagnostic situation, and these are summarised below.

1. The investigation of asymptomatic at-risk relatives. This has been discussed fully in Chapter 11, but it must be re-emphasised that no individual should be considered unaffected until thoroughly studied.

274

2. The diagnosis in infancy. Clinical myotonia is not usually present in congenital myotonic dystrophy until well after infancy (Chapter 9), but myotonia can generally be detected electromyographically even in the neonatal period. It may require a careful search, and more information may come from discovery of myotonia in the mother.

3. The distinction of myotonic dystrophy from non-dystrophic myotonias. This distinction may not be easy, especially in early cases of myotonic dystrophy without wasting or obvious systemic features, and with no clear family history of dystrophic problems. The finding of reduced size of action potentials and other "myopathic" features on electromyography in addition to myotonia favours a diagnosis of myotonic dystrophy rather than myotonia congenita. It is not infallible evidence, however, and must be taken in the context of the clinical picture as a whole.

4. The distinction of true myotonia from non-myotonic disorders producing muscle stiffness. This is of particular importance in the differential diagnosis of the non-dystrophic myotonias. Disorders to be distinguished include the syndromes of continuous muscle fibre activity, hypothyroidism, and conditions such as the McArdle syndrome in which the muscle contractures are electrically silent. The only certain way of avoiding confusion between these conditions and true myotonic disorders is by electrophysiological studies.

ELECTROMYOGRAPHY

Two principal types of abnormality are seen on electromyography in typical cases of myotonic dystrophy, myotonia, and "dystrophic"

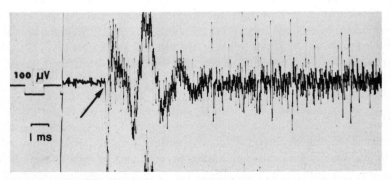

Figure 13–1. Electromyogram from patient with myotonic dystrophy to show increased irritability in response to a mechanical stimulus. Persistent electrical activity is seen following movement of the recording electrode at the point arrowed. (Study performed by Dr. J. Graham, Cardiff.)

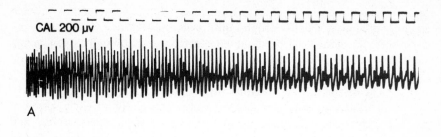

A

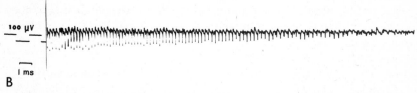

B

Figure 13–2. *A* and *B*, Myotonic potentials in two patients with myotonic dystrophy, illustrating the repetitive discharges with gradual decay of amplitude. (Courtesy of Dr. J. Graham.)

changes indicating damage to and loss of muscle fibres. Their relative prominence depends on the stage of the disease and on the site chosen for study; in general it is more informative if a relatively unaffected muscle is studied in a patient with advanced disease, whereas in a minimally affected individual changes will be seen more readily in a muscle showing clinical involvement. The first feature usually seen is a marked increase over normal of insertion activity when the needle is introduced or moved subsequently (Fig. 13–1). This reaction in response to mechanical irritation is characteristic, and initially may mask the presence of myotonia.

Once the insertion activity has settled, which may take as long as 1 minute, electrical silence is usually obtainable with the muscle at rest. This is itself of diagnostic significance since it will exclude such presynaptic abnormalities as continuous muscle fibre activity. If the muscle is now stimulated by voluntary activity or by moving the electrode, myotonic runs can usually be detected. These are essentially prolonged bursts of repetitive activity of individual potentials with amplitude rapidly increasing to a peak, followed by a prolonged and gradual decline. The visual record is characteristic (Fig. 13–2), but even more so is the auditory effect, often described as a "divebomber" sound. The intensity of myotonia recorded electromyographically is usually comparable to that seen clinically, and is generally greater in myotonia congenita than in most cases of myotonic dystrophy.

Brumlik et al (1970) have attempted to define more accurately the electrical properties of the myotonic discharge, particularly in relation to repetitive electrical discharges of other types. They found a mean discharge frequency of around 70 per second in patients with myotonic dystrophy, with myotonic discharges mostly lasting from 2 to 11 seconds. More prolonged discharges lasting up to 1 minute were seen in polymyositis and some denervating disorders. The myotonic discharge showed a decrescendo more in amplitude than in frequency, the frequency tending to stabilise during the later part of the discharge.

The finding of myotonia alone, whether electromyographic or clinical, does not distinguish myotonic dystrophy from other myotonic disorders. A variety of other changes may be seen, however, which are not found to any extent in the non-dystrophic myotonic disorders. These include reduced size of muscle action potentials, indicating loss of fibres within a motor unit, and polyphasic potentials. Figure 13–3 illustrates some of these abnormalities.

The electromyographic distinction between myotonic dystrophy and other progressive neuromuscular diseases is occasionally a difficult one. Other primary dystrophies show the features of fibre injury and loss already mentioned, but lack myotonia, and neuropathies and anterior horn cell disorders will show changes of denervation. The essentially normal conduction times in myotonic dystrophy are a further distinguishing feature from peripheral neuropathies and the peripheral form of Charcot-Marie-Tooth disease. Repetitive discharges of presynaptic origin may prove confusing, and in some disorders (e.g., the Schwarz-Jampel syndrome) such discharges may coexist with true myotonic discharges (Taylor et al, 1972). In general these "pseudomyotonic discharges" tend to be more prolonged, with less decrescendo of amplitude (Brumlik et al, 1970), and to occur spontaneously as well as in response to stimulation, so that electrical silence at rest may be impossible to obtain. Persistence of stiffness and electrical activity during sleep, and abolition by curare are further distinguishing points. Confusing features may also be noted in some cases of polymyositis, in which a variety of bizarre electromyographic changes may occur, including repetitive changes similar to those

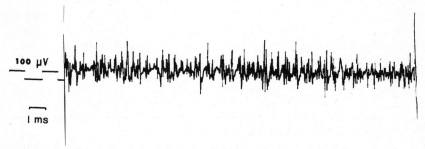

100 μV

1 ms

Figure 13–3. "Dystrophic" features in electromyogram of a patient with myotonic dystrophy, showing variation in size of action potentials, with polyphasic potentials. (Courtesy of Dr. J. Graham.)

seen in true myotonic disorders. Fortunately, such cases are rarely confusing on clinical grounds, for not only is clinical myotonia exceptional, but the other specific features, such as the distribution of muscle involvement, the characteristic lens opacities, and the familial occurrence, are all lacking.

NEUROGENIC ASPECTS

From the practical diagnostic viewpoint the most obvious electromyographic features of myotonic dystrophy, the myotonia itself and the "dystrophic" changes, are those of a primary disorder of muscle. During the past decade, however, there has been extensive argument over whether muscular dystrophies as a group may not be essentially neurogenic disorders, rather than the defect being primarily in muscle, the evidence being partly electrophysiological (McComas et al, 1971) although also from other sources. The conflict over this issue has largely bypassed myotonic dystrophy, since it has always been clearly recognised to be a multisystem disorder, and the existence of neurogenic features in no way diminishes the importance of any primary muscle defect.

The evidence for neurogenic abnormalities in myotonic dystrophy has been discussed in Chapter 7. The electromyographic studies of McComas et al (1971) and of Ballantyne and Hansen (1974, 1975) both agree in showing a reduced number of motor units in recording from the extensor digitorum brevis muscle, even though their findings in Duchenne dystrophy were radically different. In addition McComas et al noted that many motor units were of normal size, rather than reduced as would be expected from a primary myopathy. Ballantyne and Hansen also found an increase in mean amplitude and duration of motor unit potentials, as well as prolonged latency of individual potentials; these authors suggested that abnormal conduction was present in the intramuscular nerve fibres in myotonic dystrophy, correlating with the histological abnormalities already discussed. McComas et al (1971) and Engel (1974) have argued that these neurogenic changes are the primary cause of the other electrophysiological changes seen in myotonic dystrophy, but this view seems to be contradicted by most of the extensive experimental work on the basis of myotonia, which will be outlined.

EXPERIMENTAL STUDIES ON MYOTONIA

Our present understanding of the underlying basis of myotonia rests chiefly on studies utilising the myotonic goat, and owes much to the work of Bryant, who has provided some clear and extensive reviews of the subject (1973, 1976, 1977). The muscle was initially studied in situ, but the later use of isolated intercostal muscle biopsies greatly facilitated the study of single fibres with microelectrodes. The myotonic goat has an intriguing history (White and Plaskett, 1904; Kolb, 1938), albeit somewhat mythical in parts, and has proved much the most fruitful of animal models

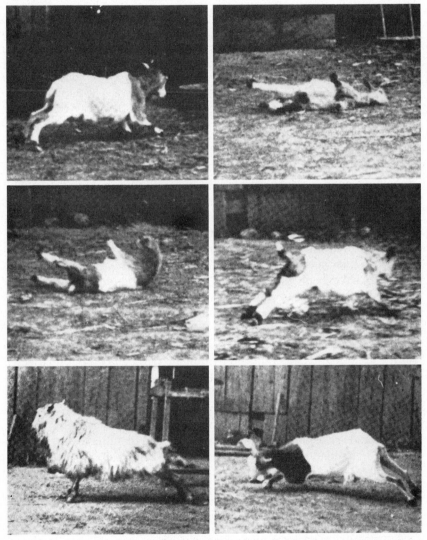

Figure 13-4. Hereditary myotonia in the goat. This disorder is closely comparable to human myotonia congenita, and episodic generalised myotonia resulting in falling is a feature of both diseases. From Kolb, 1938. Congenital myotonia in goats. Bull. Johns Hopkins Hosp. *63*:221–237.

in the study of myotonia. Bryant (1973) describes its origin as follows:

"About 1880, a stranger called Tinsley brought with him 4 to 6 affected, i.e. myotonic, goats and 1 zebu ("sacred cow") to the farm of a Dr Mayberry in Marshall County of central Tennessee. In an interview over 50 years later Dr Mayberry recalled that Tinsley was not native in Tennessee and that he worked on his farm for one season and then left for parts unknown. Tinsley never stated where he obtained the goats or gave any pertinent details of his personal history. One account states that he wore a small hat presumed to be a fez. Before leaving Marshall County he left the goats with Dr Mayberry, and it is commonly assumed that all of the myotonic (nervous) goats in the United States are descendants of these original animals. According to the early accounts, myotonic goats were first found in a few counties of central Tennessee, and from there the breed spread throughout Tennessee, southern Kentucky, northern Alabama and, to a lesser extent, throughout the remainder of the southern states. These areas today still contain the major concentrations of these animals. Farmers sometimes prefer the myotonic goats because they usually do not jump over obstacles higher than 0.5 m. This useful feature plus their curious behaviour appear to be the main reasons why the breed has survived."

Although quiet activity is almost unaffected, muscle stiffness appears on more marked exertion, wearing off after less than half-a-minute. In particular a sudden fright may induce generalised muscle stiffness with falling, comparable to the episodes seen in myotonia congenita. The goats show no progressive dystrophic features and no systemic disturbance, again resembling myotonia congenita rather than myotonic dystrophy. Surprisingly, although the condition is thought to be inherited as an autosomal dominant trait (Burns et al, 1965), few formal breeding studies appear to have been done. Bryant et al (1968) noted two degrees of severity in their inbred colony and suggested that the more severe form might represent the homozygous state for the gene.

The initial electrophysiological studies showed clearly that the defect was a true myotonia, comparable to that seen in the human disorders, and that the abnormality was relieved by quinine (Kolb, 1938) but unaffected by curarisation (Brown and Harvey, 1939). This was confirmed by Denny-Brown and Nevin (1941) although they drew attention to the fact that some part of the clinical syndrome might also have a reflex basis. Bryant (1962) showed that the resting membrane potential was normal, but that the membrane resistance was high, and suggested that this resulted from a decreased conductance to chloride ions. The principal evidence to sup-

---

Figure 13–5. Intracellular potentials recorded from intercostal muscle fibre of the goat.
A, Normal goat in normal Ringer's solution (resting potential – 76mv).
B, Normal goat in sulphate Ringer's solution (resting potential – 87mv).
C, Myotonic goat in normal Ringer's solution (resting potential – 80mv).
In both (B) and (C) repetitive potentials are produced by a stimulus which is without effect in (A). (From Adrian and Bryant, 1974, by permission.)
See illustration on the opposite page.

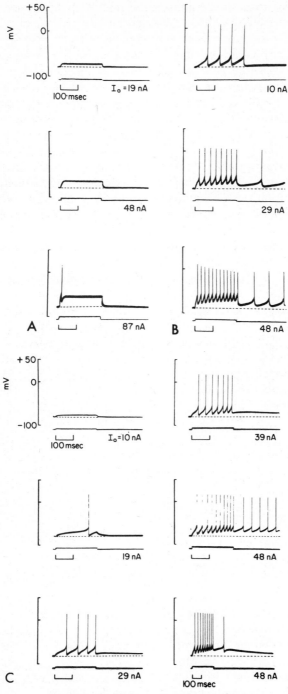

Figure 13-5 *See legend on opposite page*

port this came from the demonstration that, if chloride was replaced by sulphate in the bathing fluid, a normal muscle fibre exhibited the same repetitive activity as one from a myotonic goat (see Fig. 13–5). A variety of other anion substitutions showed the same effect (Bryant and Morales-Aguilera, 1971). More direct evidence came from studies with isotopically labelled chloride (Lipicky and Bryant, 1966) which confirmed reduced permeability to chloride in the myotonic goat from measurement of cable properties (Bryant, 1969), and from the finding that aromatic monocarboxylic acids inducing myotonia also caused a lowered chloride conductance.

Other investigators, notably Bretag (1971), Adrian and Marshall (1976) and Barchi (1975), have developed mathematical models to simulate the situation, and have confirmed that a reduced chloride conductance alone is sufficient to produce the membrane instability necessary for myotonia.

Other naturally-occurring forms of myotonia have been recorded in the horse and dog, as well as in dystrophic animal disorders (see Chapter 14). None have so far received the same detailed investigation as the goat. A parallel source of information, however, has come from study of experimental animals treated with various myotonia-inducing agents, the biochemical aspects of which are also discussed in the next chapter. In the same way as these agents appear to be heterogeneous biochemically, so electrophysiological studies have shown different modes of action in producing myotonia.

The hypocholesterolaemic group of drugs, in particular 20,25-diazacholesterol, depend on the replacement of cholesterol by desmosterol as the major neutral lipid component of the muscle cell membrane, whereas this does not occur in the other main group, the aromatic monocarboxylic acids such as 2,4-dichlorphenoxyl acetic acid (2–4D). Both groups of drugs, however, produce a reduced chloride conductance in the muscle membrane similar to that seen in the myotonic goat (Rudel and Keller, 1975), although it is possible that in the case of the aromatic monocarboxylic acids not only the surface membrane is affected, but also processes in the tubular system such as potassium accumulation (Rudel, 1976).

The rapidity of onset and directness of action of myotonia produced by 2–4D and related agents facilitates its experimental study in isolated muscle. The myotonic potentials can be followed when 2–4D is added to the bathing fluid in the presence of an uncoupling agent of contraction such as dantrolene. A greatly prolonged and increased after-depolarisation is the characteristic feature (Rudel and Senges, 1972; Rudel, 1976). Bryant and Morales-Aguilera (1971) tested a variety of related aromatic monocarboxylic acids and showed all of them to produce a reduced chloride conductance as a common feature.

By contrast, 20,25-diazacholesterol and similar hypocholesterolaemic drugs have no effect on the isolated muscle preparation, but only
induce myotonia when a sufficient dose has been given, either orally or by
injection, to produce a critical level of replacement of cholesterol by
desmosterol in the muscle (Peter et al, 1975).

RESPONSE TO DRUGS IN MYOTONIC DISORDERS

The existence of a number of drugs that may diminish or abolish
myotonia is not only of therapeutic importance (Chapter 15), but affords
opportunities for studying the basis of myotonia similar to those given by
agents producing myotonia. Surprisingly little attention has been given to
this approach since the introduction of microelectrode techniques, and
most of the work has depended on less precise methods of assessment.

Wolff (1936) described the therapeutic application of quinine in relieving myotonia, and Geschwind and Simpson (1955) showed that the
related drug procainamide had similar properties. Electromyographic
documentation of the effects of quinine was shown for the myotonic goat
by Kolb (1938) and by Brown and Harvey (1939), and in human myotonia
congenita by Denny-Brown and Nevin (1941). These workers also demonstrated the lack of effect of curare and the tendency of prostigmine to
aggravate myotonia, in contrast to its effect in myasthenia gravis. Caughey studied the effects of a variety of drugs electromyographically in
patients with myotonic dystrophy (Caughey and Myrianthopoulos, 1963).
He confirmed the effects of quinine and procainamide, and also showed
that adrenal steroids and infusion of glucose and insulin diminished myotonia.

Phenytoin, probably the most satisfactory therapeutic agent in myotonia because of its relative safety and lack of effect on cardiac conduction (Griggs et al, 1976), is of special interest since it has been shown to
reverse the changes in membrane fluidity found in red blood cells from
patients with myotonic dystrophy. So far the electrophysiological mechanism of its effects on myotonia has not been studied thoroughly.

In the myotonic goat there is marked sensitivity to potassium, and
intra-arterial injection of KCl or increase of its concentration in fluid
bathing the muscle results in a marked increase of the myotonia (Brown
and Harvey, 1939). Bryant (1973) showed that potassium lowered the
threshold for excitation, whereas increased calcium concentration had the
reverse effect. Despite these findings and the intimate relationship of
these and other ions to the processes of muscle excitation and contraction, the effects in the intact animal or patient are of less significance, and
there is no evidence of marked improvement or deterioration in either
myotonic dystrophy or myotonia congenita in response to oral potassium

administration, in contrast to the situation in hypokalaemic periodic paralysis. Hypokalaemia produced by chlorothiazide has been reported to improve myotonia (Isaacs, 1959), but again the relationship is much less clear than in periodic paralysis.

A final factor that should be noted is the effect of water deprivation in relieving myotonia. This is well-documented in the myotonic goat (Hegyeli and Szent-Györgi, 1961; Burns et al, 1965). Bryant (1973) found this effect to be associated with increased haematocrit, plasma osmolality and plasma sodium, but without change in concentration of potassium or calcium. There is no clear relationship between either dehydration or excessive dilution in human myotonic dystrophy or myotonia congenita, but it is possible that the increased myotonia sometimes noted in pregnancy may be related to water retention.

STUDIES ON HUMAN MYOTONIC DISORDERS

The studies on naturally-occurring and drug-induced myotonia in animals so far discussed have clearly indicated that a reduced chloride conductance of the muscle membrane is the main factor necessary for the production of myotonia, but until recently it has been uncertain whether the myotonia of human myotonic disorders has a similar basis.

Early electromyographic studies (Denny-Brown and Nevin, 1941; Brown and Harvey, 1939) showed that the electrical properties of human myotonia congenita closely resembled those of the myotonic goat in terms of resistance to curarisation and denervation, and in response to various drugs. Microelectrode studies of single fibres have been carried out in situ by several groups (McComas and Mrozek, 1968), but more detailed information has come from the use of isolated fibres obtained by muscle biopsy, particularly the intercostal muscle studies of Lipicky and colleagues (Lipicky et al, 1971; Lipicky, 1977). A further aid has been the use of the drug dantrolene which, by uncoupling excitation from contraction, prevents the damage to fibres frequently caused by profound myotonic contractions, but leaves electrical activity at the surface membrane intact. These studies have shown that, whereas myotonia congenita indeed shows close similarity to the animal models, myotonic dystrophy does not.

Study of the cable properties of isolated muscle fibres showed that in myotonia congenita there was an increased resistance of the surface membrane, and that chloride conductance was specifically reduced as in the myotonic goat. One difference noted was that potassium conductance was also reduced in myotonia congenita, whereas in the goat it is normal. In myotonic dystrophy little change in total membrane resistance was found, and there was only a minimal reduction in chloride and potassium conductance, with considerable variability between patients.

A further distinction between myotonic dystrophy and myotonia congenita has been the finding by several investigators of a reduced resting membrane potential in myotonic dystrophy (McComas and Mrozek, 1968; Hoffman and DeNardo, 1968; Lipicky and Bryant, 1973), whereas in both myotonia congenita and the myotonic goat this is normal. A value of around 70 mV has been found in most studies of myotonic dystrophy, in comparison with a level of 80 to 85 mV in normal individuals and those with myotonia congenita. How far secondary dystrophic changes in the muscle fibre contribute to this reduction is uncertain at present. Analysis of the ion and water content of muscle has not shown striking changes in either disorder. Lipicky (1977) found slightly increased intracellular potassium concentration in myotonia congenita and in the myotonic goat; in myotonic dystrophy potassium concentration was normal but intracellular sodium concentration was reduced, as was the water content of muscle.

It thus seems clear that the electrophysiological basis of myotonia in myotonic dystrophy is distinct from that seen in other myotonic disorders, whereas myotonia congenita in man and goat and the various forms of drug-induced myotonia show at least one common feature, the reduced chloride conductance. Such heterogeneity comes as no surprise when the clear evidence of clinical and genetic distinction between myotonic dystrophy and myotonia congenita is considered; it is perhaps more surprising that the other myotonic conditions should show so much similarity. It must be noted that the electrophysiological studies of myotonia congenita have rarely made it clear whether the dominant or recessive form is under study; this distinction will be relevant when it becomes possible to identify the precise primary defect underlying the myotonia in each.

Human myotonic disorders other than myotonia congenita and myotonic dystrophy so far have received relatively little detailed electrophysiological study, but may well contribute valuable information. McComas et al (1968) found a reduced resting membrane potential in five patients with normokalaemic periodic paralysis. Burke et al (1974) studied two patients with paramyotonia congenita and showed that electromyographic myotonia was increased by repeated forceful contractions, in keeping with the clinical picture in paramyotonia, and in contrast to the improvement after repeated contraction seen in other myotonic disorders. They also noted that persistent contraction was seen after electrical evidence of myotonia had ceased, and suggested that an abnormality in the contractile system was involved over and above that produced by the myotonia. A somewhat similar situation is observed in the syndrome of myotonia congenita with painful cramps, in which true myotonia is accompanied by electrically silent muscle contractures (Stohr et al, 1975).

The clear demonstration of a reduced chloride conductance as the principal abnormality in myotonia congenita of man and goat and in drug-induced myotonia, although not in myotonic dystrophy, raises the question of what are the normal processes responsible for maintaining chloride conductance in normal muscle. Little is known at present about the enzymes involved in active transport, the carrier molecules or the postulated "chloride channels" in the membrane. Peter and Campion (1977) have discussed the possible sites of a defect affecting chloride conductance, and suggest that whereas myotonia congenita may result from a defective macromolecular component in the conductance system, aromatic monocarboxylic acids act by a reversible attachment to a chloride carrier molecule. This is inevitably speculative in the absence of detailed knowledge of the mechanisms of chloride conductance, and at present it is impossible to explain the electrophysiological changes of myotonia in terms of the disordered membrane biochemistry, for which information is steadily accumulating and which will be discussed in the next chapter.

For myotonic dystrophy itself the situation is even more puzzling; it is now clear that neither human nor caprine myotonia congenita produce myotonia by an identical mechanism, nor do the various forms of drug-induced myotonia have the same electrophysiological basis. It would seem that for myotonic dystrophy, even more than for myotonia congenita, the solution to its basis will be likely to come from the biochemical rather than the electrophysiological approach.

UNEXPLAINED FEATURES

It would be wrong to give the impression that all the electrophysiological findings in myotonia can be explained on the basis of a defect in chloride conductance, and there are a number of puzzling features which suggest that other abnormalities are involved, as well as some features that are entirely unexplained. The relationship of myotonia to direct percussion, the exacerbation by cold, the diminution with repeated activity and the occurrence of sudden generalised attacks of myotonia are all prominent features in myotonia congenita of man and the goat, which have no ready explanation. The original suggestion of Denny-Brown and Nevin (1941) that a reflex process might contribute to myotonia has not been excluded, and the microscopic evidence of muscle spindle involvement provides a possible method, even though no electrophysiological disturbance in the muscle spindle has been detected (Rudel, 1977). Another unexplained feature is the occurrence of a degree of weakness in various non-progressive myotonic disorders. Brown (1974) has demonstrated a fading of the muscle action potential in response to repetitive motor nerve stimulation which appeared to be independent of agents affecting the myotonia. Wiles and Edwards (1977) and Aminoff et al (1977) have discussed the possible causes for such weakness and show that both nerve-mediated and a variety of myogenic influences could produce such effects.

Some pieces of evidence, at present fragmentary, suggest that not just the sarcolemmal membrane but other muscle membrane components, such as the transverse tubular system, may be involved in the production of myotonia. Thus, Adrian and Bryant (1974) found that exposure of myotonic fibres to high osmotic pressure Ringer's solution (Ringer's with 400 mM glycerol), followed by return to normal Ringer's solution, abolished the prolonged after-depolarisation and after-discharge usually seen in these fibres (Fig. 13–6). They suggested that potassium accumulation in

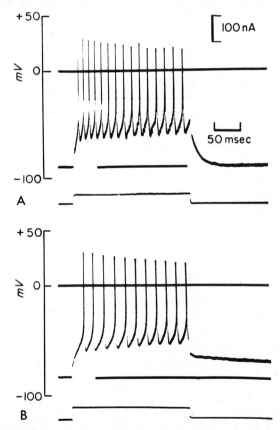

Figure 13–6. Effect of tubular disruption by glycerol on myotonic potentials in the external intercostal muscle fibre of the myotonic goat.

   A, After treatment for one hour in Ringer's plus 400 mM glycerol.

   B, Before glycerol treatment.

   Note absence of after-depolarisation in *A*. (From Adrian and Bryant, 1974, by permission.)

the tubular system might be responsible for this phenomenon. Another finding by Bryant (1976) is that there may be an abnormality of excitation-contraction coupling. When studied by a microelectrode voltage-clamp technique, myotonic fibres showed a higher mechanical threshold than normal fibres, an effect comparable to that of the drug dantrolene, which is known to abolish excitation–contraction coupling. Similar effects were seen when sulphate was substituted for chloride in the bathing fluid, and when normal animals were pre-treated with 20,25-diazacholesterol, but not with monocarboxylic acids. Appel and Roses (1977) have found a reduced calcium-promoted potassium efflux in red cell membranes from myotonic dystrophy patients; they suggest that a comparable process in muscle may be controlled by an enzyme in the transverse tubular system (possibly an ATPase) related to excitation–contraction coupling.

Although the underlying basis of myotonia remains elusive, the work described in this chapter shows that we are not far from a thorough understanding of the process. Already work on the inherited and experimental myotonias has served to define some of the major normal processes in muscle excitation and contraction, the heterogeneity of the phenomenon has been clearly recognised, and the electrophysiological and biochemical approaches are beginning to interact and converge, rather than pursue separate parallel courses. In a similar way it is becoming possible to compare the electrophysiological changes in muscle with changes in comparable processes in other systems. The growing realisation that myotonia in human genetic disorders, especially in myotonic dystrophy, is but one aspect of a generalised process has transformed the experimental approach, and forms the basis of much of the work to be described in the next chapter.

REFERENCES

Adrian R. H. and Bryant S. H. (1974): On the repetitive discharge in myotonic muscle fibres. J. Physiol. *240*:505–515.

Adrian R. H. and Marshall W. M. (1976): Action potentials reconstructed in normal and myotonic muscle fibres. J. Physiol. (Lond.) *258*:125–143.

Aminoff M. J., Layzer R. B., Satya-Murti S. and Faden A. I. (1977): The declining electrical response of muscle to repetitive nerve stimulation in myotonia. Neurology *27*:812–816.

Appel S. H. and Roses A. D. (1977): Membranes and myotonia. *In* Pathogenesis of Human Muscular Dystrophies (Ed.: L. P. Rowland). Excerpta Medica, Amsterdam, pp. 747–758.

Ballantyne J. P. and Hansen S. (1974): New method for the estimation of the number of motor units in a muscle. 2. Duchenne, limb-girdle, facioscapulohumeral and myotonic muscular dystrophies. J. Neurol. Neurosurg. Psychiatry *37*:1195–1201.

Ballantyne J. P. and Hansen S. (1975): Computer method for the analysis of evoked motor unit potentials. 2. Duchenne, limb-girdle, facioscapulohumeral and myotonic muscular dystrophies. J. Neurol. Neurosurg. Psychiatry *38*:417–428.

Barchi R. L. (1975): Myotonia. An evaluation of the chloride hypothesis. Arch. Neurol. *32*:175–180.

Bretag A. H. (1971): Proc. Aust. Physiol. Pharmacol. Soc. 2:22.

Brown G. and Harvey A. M. (1939): Congenital myotonia in the goat. Brain 62:341–363.

Brown J. C. (1974): Muscle weakness after rest in myotonic disorders: an electrophysiological study. J. Neurol. Neurosurg. Psychiatry 37:1336–1342.

Brumlik J., Drechsler B. and Vannin T. M. (1970): The myotonic discharge in various neurological syndromes: a neurophysiological analysis. Electromyography 10:369–383.

Bryant S. H. (1962): Muscle membrane of normal and myotonic goats in normal and low external chloride. Fed. Proc. 21:312.

Bryant S. H. (1969): Cable properties of external intercostal muscle fibres from myotonic and non-myotonic goats. J. Physiol. (Lond.) 204:539–550.

Bryant S. H. (1973): The electrophysiology of myotonia, with a review of congenital myotonia of goat. In New Developments in Electromyography and Clinical Neurophysiology, Vol. 1, (Ed.: J. E. Desmedt). Karger, Basel, pp. 420–450.

Bryant S. H. (1976): Altered membrane properties in myotonia. In Membranes and Disease (Eds.: L. Bolis, J. F. Hoffman and A. Leaf). Raven Press, New York, pp. 197–206.

Bryant S. H. (1977): The physiological basis of myotonia. In Pathogenesis of Human Muscular Dystrophies (Ed.: L. P. Rowland). Excerpta Medica, Amsterdam, pp. 715–728

Bryant S. H., Lipicky R. J. and Herzog W. H. (1968): Variability of myotonic signs in myotonic goats. Am. J. Vet. Res. 29:2371–2381.

Bryant S. H. and Morales-Aguilera A. (1971): Chloride conductance in normal and myotonic muscle fibres and the action of monocarboxylic aromatic acids. J. Physiol. 219:367–383.

Burke D., Skuse N. F. and Lethlean A. K. (1974): An analysis of myotonia in paramyotonia congenita. J. Neurol. Neurosurg. Psychiatry 37:900–906.

Burke D., Skuse N. F. and Lethlean A. K. (1974): Contractile properties of the abductor digiti minimi muscle in paramyotonia congenita. J. Neurol. Neurosurg. Psychiatry 37:894–899.

Burns T. W., Dale H. E. and Langley P. L. (1965): The lipid and electrolyte composition of plasma and the erythrocyte of the myotonic goat. Clin. Res. 13:235.

Caughey J. E. and Myrianthopoulos N. C. (1963): Dystrophia Myotonica and Related Disorders. Charles C Thomas, Springfield, Ill.

Denny-Brown D. and Nevin S. (1941): The phenomenon of myotonia. Brain 64:1–18.

Geschwind N. and Simpson J. A. (1955): Procaine amide in the treatment of myotonia. Brain 78:81–91.

Griggs R. C., Davies R. J., Anderson D. C. and Dove J. T. (1975): Cardiac conduction in myotonic dystrophy. Am. J. Med. 59:37–42.

Hoffman W. W. and DeNardo G. L. (1968): Sodium flux in myotonic muscular dystrophy. Am. J. Physiol. 214:300–336.

Isaacs H. (1959): The treatment of myotonia congenita. S. Afr. Med. J. 33:984.

Kolb L. C. (1938): Congenital myotonia in goats. Bull. Johns Hopkins Hosp. 63:221–237.

Lipicky R. J. (1977): Studies in human myotonic dystrophy. In Pathogenesis of Human Muscular Dystrophies (Ed.: L. P. Rowland). Excerpta Medica, Amsterdam, pp. 729–738.

Lipicky R. J. and Bryant S. H. (1966): Sodium, potassium and chloride fluxes in intercostal muscle from normal goats and goats with hereditary myotonia. J. Gen. Physiol. 50:89–111.

Lipicky R. J. and Bryant S. H. (1973): A biophysical study of the human myotonias. In New Developments in Electromyography and Clinical Neurophysiology, Vol. 1 (Ed.: J. E. Desmedt), Karger, Basel, pp. 451–463.

Lipicky R. J., Bryant S. H. and Salmon J. H. (1971): Cable parameters, sodium, potassium, chloride and water content, and potassium efflux in isolated external intercostal muscle of normal volunteers and patients with myotonia congenita. J. Clin. Invest. 50:2091–2103.

McComas A. J., Campbell M. J. and Sica R. E. P. (1971): Electrophysiological study of dystrophia myotonica. J. Neurol. Neurosurg. Psychiatry 34:132–139.

McComas A. J. and Mrozek K. (1968): The electrical properties of muscle fibre membranes in dystrophia myotonica and myotonia congenita. J. Neurol. Neurosurg. Psychiatry 31:441–447.

McComas A. J., Mrozek K. and Bradley W. G. (1968): The nature of the electrophysiological disorder in adynamia episodica. J. Neurol. Neurosurg. Psychiatry 31:448–452.

Peter J. B. and Campion D. S. (1977): Animal models of myotonia. In Pathogenesis of Human Muscular Dystrophies (Ed.: L. P. Rowland). Excerpta Medica, Amsterdam, pp. 739–746.

Peter J. B., Dromgoole S. H. M., Campion D. S., Stemple K. E., Bowman R. L., Andiman R. M. and Nagatomo T. (1975): Experimental myotonia and hypocholesterolemic agents. Exp. Neurol. 49:115–122.

Peter J. B., Dromgoole S. H., Campion D. S., Stemple K. E., Bowman R. L., Andiman R. M. and Nagatomo T. (1975): The effects of a high cholesterol diet on 20,25-diazacholesterol-induced myotonia. Exp. Neurol. 49:429–438.

Rudel R. (1976): The mechanism of pharmacologically induced myotonia. In Membranes and Disease (Eds.: L. Bolis, J. F. Hoffmann and A. Leaf). Raven Press, New York, pp. 207–213.

Rudel R. and Keller M. (1975): Intracellular recording of myotonic runs in dantrolene-blocked myotonic muscle fibres. In Recent Advances in Myology (Eds.: W. G. Bradley et al). Excerpta Medica, Amsterdam, pp. 441–445.

Rudel R. and Senges J. (1972): Experimental myotonia in mammalian skeletal muscle: changes in membrane properties. Pfluegers Arch. 331:324–334.

Stohr M., Schlote W., Bundschu H. D. and Reichenmiller H. E. (1975): Myopathia myotonica. Fallbericht über eine neuartige hereditare metabolische Myopathie. J. Neurol. 210:41–66.

Taylor R. G., Layzer R. B., Davis H. S. and Fowler W. M. (1972): Continuous muscle fiber activity in the Schwartz-Jampel syndrome. Electroencephalogr. Clin. Neurophysiol. 33:497–509.

White G. R. and Plasket J. (1904): "Nervous", "stiff-legged", or "fainting" goats. Am. Vet. Rev. 28:556–560.

Wiles C. M. and Edwards R. H. T. (1977): Weakness in myotonic syndromes. Lancet 2:598–601.

Wolff A. (1936): Quinine — an effective form of treatment for myotonia. Arch. Neurol. Psychiatry 36:382–383.

CHAPTER FOURTEEN

The Metabolic Basis of Myotonic Dystrophy

The structural abnormalities found in msucle and the studies on the nature of myotonia have so far failed to identify a specific causative factor in myotonic dystrophy, nor has it been possible to find a single common factor that will explain the multiplicity of clinical features so characteristic of this disease. This chapter examines the large body of experimental work that exists and which has given a clear indication of where the primary defect is likely to lie, even though it has not yet isolated it precisely.

There are a number of general features of myotonic dystrophy that provide a framework for hypotheses on the basis of the disorder, and it is important to consider these before examining the detailed experimental data. First, the disease follows mendelian inheritance, despite the presence of some anomalous features such as the maternal transmission of the congenital form. Thus, it can be confidently stated that the primary defect will reside in a specific deoxyribonucleic acid (DNA) sequence, which in turn is reflected in structure of a specific protein. Since there is no evidence for genetic heterogeneity in the sense of more than one locus being involved, a single specific metabolic defect is a logical objective for which to search.

Second, there is the multisystem nature of the disease. Previous chapters have illustrated the involvement of the eye, central nervous system and endocrine glands in addition to smooth, cardiac and voluntary muscle. This strongly suggests that the primary metabolic defect is not confined to muscle but is expressed in a wide variety of cell types. Arising from this is the view, accepted somewhat reluctantly by some neurologists, that it may be easier and more rewarding to study simpler cell types than muscle itself, and that these other cell types, such as red and white

291

blood cells and cultured fibroblasts, may show the primary defect although they are free from many of the secondary changes found in involved muscle. This approach has been amply rewarded in other groups of neurological disorders, notably the lipidoses, and has provided some of the most exciting recent developments in our understanding of myotonic dystrophy and other muscular dystrophies.

The third general property of myotonic dystrophy is its autosomal dominant inheritance. The fact that the disease is expressed in the heterozygote argues against the primary defect lying in an enzyme of intermediary metabolism, for in almost all such disorders the heterozygote is essentially healthy and the disease is confined to the affected homozygote — i.e., recessive inheritance. At present the molecular basis of very few dominantly inherited disorders is understood; in some of these an unstable or otherwise abnormal non-enzymic protein is involved (e.g., certain haemoglobinopathies); in others, such as the porphyrias, enzyme control of a critical pathway is so finely balanced that the heterozygote is involved. Thus, if an enzyme defect is indeed the primary abnormality in myotonic dystrophy, it must be one for which a relatively small reduction in activity has critical effects, or in which the spatial distribution of the molecules is directly related to their function, as in the cell membranes.

MEMBRANE BIOCHEMICAL ABNORMALITIES

The hypothesis that myotonic dystrophy results from an abnormality of structure and function of the cell membranes of muscle, and possibly other tissues, has received powerful indirect support for many years from the evidence on the electrophysiological basis of myotonia, discussed in Chapter 13. Further general support comes from the finding of ionic shifts in some other disorders accompanied by myotonia, such as the periodic paralyses, and from the leakage of creatine kinase and other muscle enzymes into the serum characteristic of Duchenne, and to a lesser extent of other dystrophies. Much of the direct biochemical evidence of a membrane abnormality in myotonic dystrophy, however, has come from study not of muscle but of red blood cell membranes, and has stimulated a new approach to this disease and to muscle dystrophies in general.

In 1973 Roses and Appel reported an abnormality in the phosphorylation of membrane proteins in isolated red blood cell membranes from patients with myotonic dystrophy. They had failed to find any difference in the structural protein or lipid constituents of these membranes, but when exposed to radioactive adenosine triphosphate (ATP) labelled with $^{32}PO_4$ the membranes from myotonic dystrophy patients showed a definite reduction in phosphorylation in comparison with those of normal individuals. This phosphorylation is mediated by a group of enzymes, protein

kinases, located in the cell membrane, and the suggestion was made that
the defect in myotonic dystrophy might lie in one of these.

Initially the changes seen were not large and could be demonstrated
only in frozen stored samples, but further work (Roses and Appel, 1975)
showed that fresh cells did indeed behave similarly and that the decreased
phosphorylation could be located on a particular band of proteins separat-
ed by SDS polyacrilamide gel electrophoresis. Subsequent studies have
concentrated on trying to identify a single component within this band
that shows the abnormality; Wong and Roses (1979) have found a glyco-
protein fraction that accounts for most of the phosphorylation decrease
even though comprising only 0.3 per cent of total membrane protein, but
so far this has not been isolated and characterized sufficiently to be
considered a primary defect.

This exciting work has led to a number of other developments. Roses
and Appel (1974) studied sarcolemmal membranes from muscle biopsies
obtained from six unrelated myotonic dystrophy patients, and showed
reduced phosphorylation to around half the normal level in two elec-
trophoretic bands corresponding to proteins of around 50,000 and 30,000
molecular weight. This suggested that the membrane abnormality in myotonic dystrophy was indeed a generalised one, and that the changes found
in red blood cells were relevant to the disease as a whole and to the
muscular defect in particular. A further and unexpected development was
the discovery that red blood cell membranes from patients and carriers
with Duchenne dystrophy also showed a distinct but quite different abnormality of protein phosphorylation (Roses et al, 1975). Here the phosphorylation is increased, not reduced, and the band involved is band 2,
which contains the major red cell membrane protein spectrin, the structure of which is allied to that of myosin. Roses et al (1977) have suggested
that a mutation in the myosin molecule might be the primary defect in
Duchenne dystrophy, but this remains unconfirmed.

The biochemical studies of cell membranes in myotonic dystrophy
have been considered at some length and before other areas of work,
since they appear to come nearer than any other approach to identifying
the specific molecular basis of this disorder, and possibly of other muscular dystrophies also. It is important, however, to point out some reservations that so far have not been fully resolved. First, no other group as yet
has adequately confirmed the results of Roses, Appel and colleagues on
myotonic dystrophy. Second, the use of the red cell as a source of
membranes is open to question in some respects; although conveniently
obtained in large quantities it is a specialised and incomplete cell, and is
particularly exposed to modification by other circulating factors. On the
other hand, much more is known about its normal properties and constituents than is the case for muscle or the cultured fibroblast. Third, the work
on Duchenne dystrophy conflicts directly with all previous studies in a

number of ways, particularly regarding the findings in carriers. Not only did the known carriers studied by Roses et al (1975) show identical abnormalities to the affected patients, but also the findings on mothers of isolated cases of Duchenne dystrophy suggested that almost all were carriers, whereas at least one-third of such mothers would not have been classed as carriers on the basis of creatine kinase studies or on genetic grounds. Until these doubts on the Duchenne dystrophy findings are resolved there is bound to be hesitation in accepting the results of similar techniques applied to myotonic dystrophy.

Finally, it is becoming apparent that muscular dystrophies are not the only disorders to show abnormalities of protein phosphorylation in the red cell membrane. Both hereditary spherocytosis (Greenquist and Shohet, 1976) and sickle cell anaemia (Hosey and Tao, 1976) have been reported to show reduced protein kinase activity of erythrocytes, suggesting that although such changes may be a valuable indication of involvement of the red cell membrane, they may not necessarily represent the specific primary defect in these or other disorders.

ACTIVITY OF MEMBRANE ADENOSINE TRIPHOSPHATASES (ATPases)

These have been extensively studied in both muscle and red blood cells, although most of the work has been on Duchenne dystrophy and on "dystrophic" animal models. The activity of sodium-potassium ATPase was found to be normal in myotonic dystrophy muscle biopsies by Roses and Appel (1974), and both Peter et al (1973) and Hull and Roses (1976) found normal red cell activity of this enzyme. The latter authors showed abnormal stoichiometry of sodium and potassium transport, with a reduction of sodium extrusion in relation to potassium uptake. They suggested that this might indicate an abnormality in ATPase structure even though activity was unaffected. Studies on ATPases in experimental myotonia have been inconclusive; Peter and Fiehn (1973) showed an increase in sodium-potassium ATPase in red cell and sarcolemmal membranes from rats fed with 20,25-diazacholesterol, and a similar increase was found by Fiehn and Seiler (1975); however, Dromgoole et al (1975), repeating this work with the use of a single dose of diazacholesterol to induce myotonia, were unable to detect any changes in ATPase activity. Fiehn and Seiler also claimed to find an increase in both sodium-potassium and calcium-dependent ATPase in the cardiac sarcolemma of diazacholesterol-fed rats. Appel and Roses (1977) have recently found an abnormality in calcium-dependent potassium efflux in energy-depleted red blood cells, and have suggested that a calcium-dependent ATPase may be involved.

Reddy et al (1977) have studied the activity of the enzyme adenyl cyclase in the sarcolemmal membrane of both patients with myotonic dystrophy and animals with diazacholesterol myotonia. In both groups activity of the enzyme was reduced by 30 to 60 per cent. It will be interesting to see if this observation proves to be consistent and how it can be related to the other evidence for abnormality of membrane enzymes.

CALCIUM TRANSPORT

The possibility that a defect in calcium transport might be responsible for myotonia was raised by Seiler and Kuhn (1970), who studied isolated sarcoplasmic vesicles from the muscle of patients with both myotonic dystrophy and myotonia congenita. They found that both groups showed an increase in the rate of calcium uptake and the total quantity of calcium accumulated by the vesicles, and the rate of calcium efflux from the vesicles was reduced.

Plishker et al (1978) suggested the possibility that this abnormality may reflect a general disturbance of calcium transport across cell membranes, having studied calcium transport in the red blood cells of myotonic dystrophy patients. They found an increased rate of calcium accumulation in the myotonic red cells comparable to that shown in muscle by Seiler et al. However, they noted that the efflux of calcium was also increased, suggesting that a change in membrane permeability rather than a specific transport defect was the cause.

At present these abnormalities have not been satisfactorily related to the changes in membrane protein phosphorylation discussed above, nor to the electrophysiological basis of myotonia. They provide further evidence, however, for a generalised membrane abnormality in myotonic dystrophy. An increased entry of calcium into muscle could also be responsible for some of the dystrophic changes by the activation of proteases.

OTHER EVIDENCE OF MEMBRANE ABNORMALITIES

Physical Properties of Cell Membranes

The technique of electron spin resonance provides a measure of the fluidity of the cell membrane, and Butterfield et al (1974) have shown a significant alteration in membrane fluidity in red cell membranes from patients with myotonic dystrophy. Support for the relevance of this to the disease process comes from the finding that drugs influencing myotonia, such as phenytoin, also normalise the membrane fluidity of the red blood cells as measured by electron spin resonance, although the drug does not affect the membrane fluidity of red cells from normal individuals (Butterfield et al, 1975). It has been suggested that the technique may identify presymptomatic carriers of myotonic dystrophy, but this so far has not been rigorously tested. In an attempt to make this approach more specific, Butterfield et al (1976, 1977) have utilised two different probes measuring different components of membrane fluidity. They found red cells from myotonic dystrophy patients abnormal with both, whereas patients with myotonia congenita showed only abnormal surface fluidity, a specific membrane protein probe giving normal results.

It is not easy for those unfamiliar with this technique to assess it critically, and whether it is as specific as is claimed must remain an unanswered question until other approaches confirm or disprove the findings. It is perhaps unfortunate that its evaluation has not been undertaken in parallel with detailed clinical assessment and the use of other established criteria of investigation. Recent reports that similar abnormalities are found in red cell membranes of patients with such radically different disorders as Huntington's chorea (Butterfield et al, 1977) must also raise serious doubts as to how far electron spin resonance is influenced by the variety of secondary factors to which the red blood cell is inevitably exposed in vivo.

Scanning Electron Microscopy of Red Blood Cells

Initial reports of morphological abnormalities in the red blood cell in a variety of human muscular dystrophies (Matheson and Howland, 1974; Miller et al, 1976) as well as in the "dystrophic" strains of mouse Dy and Dy^{2J} (Morse and Howland, 1974), raised hopes that a visible defect corresponding to the biochemical changes in the cell membrane might exist, and that this might be of use in diagnosis and carrier detection. The abnormal cells showed varying degrees of distortion, with surface projections ("echinocytes"), and abnormalities were more marked after washing in saline. Most of these reports dealt primarily with Duchenne dystrophy, although positive findings were mentioned also for myotonic dystrophy (Roses and Appel, 1974; Miller et al, 1976).

Subsequent studies have either failed to demonstrate consistent morphological red cell abnormalities (Matheson et al, 1976) or have shown only minor changes (Miale et al, 1975); one point of agreement is that morphology of the red cell is very variable, particularly in response to different external conditions. In view of this it seems most unlikely that morphology of red cells will provide a simple diagnostic test in myotonic or other dystrophies, although it is distinctly possible that the abnormal membrane may show a difference in response to specific environmental agents. This work again shows that the red blood cell, although convenient, is not necessarily the ideal subject for study in the muscular dystrophies.

Studies on Cultured Fibroblasts and Lymphocytes

Swift and Finegold (1969) reported an abnormal pattern of cell growth in cultured fibroblasts grown from skin biopsies of patients with myotonic dystrophy. Their findings of increased cell density, with heaping up of cells and loss of the normal pattern of cell orientation, suggested a possible defect in the surface membrane. A subsequent report (Lo Curto et al, 1975) found accumulation of metachromatic material in fibroblasts. Unfortunately the toluidine blue staining used to demonstrate this is non-specific, and no significant abnormalities in fibroblasts could be found by Harper (1972) or Thomas and Harper (1978) in either staining properties, morphology or growth rate in culture.

A recent approach has been to examine the "capping" response of the lymphocyte to labelled immunoglobulin. Abnormalities have been claimed to occur in Duchenne and other dystrophies, but were not found in myotonic dystrophy (Pickard et al, 1978). This is surprising if the technique does indeed indicate a membrane abnormality.

EVIDENCE FROM OTHER "MEMBRANE DISEASES"

In evaluating the possibility that myotonic dystrophy may result from a defect in a specific membrane component, it is relevant to examine the evidence provided by more clearly defined membrane disorders. Festoff (1977) has reviewed the range of these, and their relation to the known properties of normal cell membranes. Two disorders in particular may provide information relevant to myotonic dystrophy, although clinically they are entirely different. Hereditary spherocytosis is the best documented example of an inherited disorder of the red cell membrane (Jacob, 1972). Here both shape and fragility of the cell are affected, and it has been suggested that one of the microfilamentous membrane proteins related to actin may be the primary abnormality. Reduced protein phosphorylation has been found in the red cells (Greenquist and Shohet, 1976) and this has been interpreted as being secondary to the structural deformation of the cells. In this respect it may be questioned why, if such a generalised defect exists in myotonic dystrophy, there is no comparable shortening of red cell lifespan? The second disorder that may be relevant is type II hyperlipoproteinaemia, shown by Brown and Goldstein (1975) to be due to a defective membrane receptor for low density lipoprotein, with a secondary reduction of the regulatory enzyme HMG CoA reductase, and consequent accumulation of cholesterol.

These two disorders, like myotonic dystrophy, show autosomal dominant inheritance, and provide models of the broad type of defect that might also explain at least some of the features of myotonic dystrophy. The complexity of membrane structure, in terms of both the number of molecular components involved and their functional interrelationship, leaves little doubt that before long an entire class of "inborn errors" of membrane structure and function will be delineated.

ABNORMALITIES IN LIPID METABOLISM

A large amount of work has been done on the composition and metabolism of lipids in muscle, serum and red blood cells from patients with Duchenne dystrophy, but myotonic dystrophy has received little attention. The Duchenne studies are fully reviewed by Kunze (1977), and the results have been disappointing. Plasma lipids of all types have shown few changes, and the abnormalities in muscle are difficult to interpret in view of the intense fatty degeneration that is seen particularly in Duchenne dystrophy. Fibroblasts in Duchenne dystrophy have so far shown no lipid abnormality (Kohlschutter et al, 1976; Kunze, 1977). Kunze's studies on red cell lipds included two patients with myotonic dystrophy; only minimal changes were found (Kunze et al, 1973).

Initial studies on plasma lipids and liproproteins in myotonic dystrophy were unremarkable (Kuhn and Weiker, 1957), but the possibility of a significant lipid abnormality was raised by the reports of Wakamatsu et al (1970, 1972) that the serum levels of desmosterol, the immediate precursor of cholesterol, were raised in myotonic dystrophy. This finding was given particular relevance by the work on experimental drug-induced myotonia, discussed below, in which accumulation of desmosterol in the cell membrane appears to be a major factor in the production of myotonia.

A further relevant piece of information in the possible relationship of myotonic dystrophy to a defect in sterol synthesis was the finding that a mouse tumour cell line, the L cell, showed accumulation of desmosterol (Fig. 14–1) and that this was due to the absence of the enzyme, sterol Δ^{24}reductase, responsible for the conversion of desmosterol to cholesterol (Rothblat et al, 1970). This enzyme has been located by cell hybridisation techniques on chomosome 20 in man (Croce et al, 1973). An attractive hypothesis thus existed which explained the myotonia of myotonic dystrophy on the basis of desmosterol accumulation, resulting from a specific enzyme deficiency of sterol Δ^{24}reductase, with the gene concerned located on chromosome 20.

Unfortunately, like many attractive hypotheses, this one has foundered on irreconcilable facts. The desmosterol accumulation claimed by

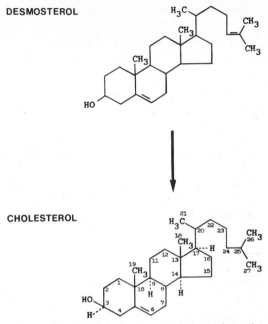

Figure 14-1. The conversion of desmosterol to cholesterol, regulated by the enzyme sterol Δ^{24} reductase, is the point of action of myotonia-inducing agents such as 20,25-diazacholesterol, and is defective in certain tumour cells such as the "L" cell.

Wakamatsu et al has not been found in either myotonic dystrophy or myotonia congenita by other investigators using improved techniques (Peter et al, 1975), and a similar absence of significant accumulation of desmosterol has been noted in both red cell membranes (Peter and Campion, 1977) and cultured fibroblasts (Thomas and Harper, 1978). It seems clear that the biochemical basis of myotonic dystrophy and of experimental myotonia cannot be simply equated, and that myotonic dystrophy is not the result of a block of cholesterol synthesis. Despite this, however, there are sufficient similarities between myotonic dystrophy and the various types of drug-induced myotonia to make worthwhile a careful examination of the biochemical basis of the latter, since the fact that the basis is not identical does not mean that information on the one is irrelevant to the factors underlying the other. The present state of our knowledge on the biochemical basis of drug-induced myotonia is therefore summarised here; the electrophysiological aspects have already been discussed in Chapter 13.

Table 14–1.   DRUG-INDUCED MYOTONIA

Agents blocking conversion of desmosterol to cholesterol
   20,25-diazacholesterol
   Triparanol

Monocarboxylic acids
   2,4-dichlorophenoxyacetic acid (2,4-D)
   Clofibrate

β-adrenergic blocking agents
   Propranolol

EXPERIMENTAL MYOTONIA

The extensive studies on experimental myotonia in the rat, and to a lesser extent in other species, have been well reviewed by Peter and Campion (1977) in relation to human myotonic dystrophy. A variety of agents have been found to be associated with myotonia on occasion (see Table 14–1), but two main groups have been studied in detail. The first group includes a number of hypocholesterolaemic agents blocking the conversion of desmosterol to cholesterol; the second group contains certain aromatic monocarboxylic acids, some of which (e.g., clofibrate) are also hypocholesterolaemic.

The prototype in the first group is the drug 20,25-diazacholesterol, which was originally shown by Winer et al (1966) to produce myotonia in rats and to cause accumulation of desmosterol in the serum (Fig. 14–2A). Desmosterol accumulation in muscle was also found, and a direct relationship between myotonia and degree of desmosterol accumulation was noted by Dromgoole et al (1975) and Peter et al (1975). Using a single large dose of diazacholesterol, these workers found myotonia appearing about five days after peak levels of desmosterol were reached. At this stage desmosterol represented between one-quarter and one-half of all muscle sterols. If the animals were fed on a high cholesterol diet during this time, desmosterol did not accumulate, nor did the animals develop myotonia, confirming the specific relationship between desmosterol and myotonia.

Triparanol (Fig. 14–2B) is a similar drug that produces myotonia by desmosterol accumulation, although a much higher dose is needed. It is of interest that in man the main adverse effect of this drug leading to its withdrawal was cataract, not myotonia (Kirby et al, 1962); this is also seen after diazacholesterol administration, although less commonly (Peter et al, 1973).

In the second group of aromatic monocarboxylic acids, the agent 2,4-dichlorophenoxyacetic acid (2,4-D) has been best studied (Fig. 14–2C). Introduced as a weedkiller, it was initially thought to be harmless,

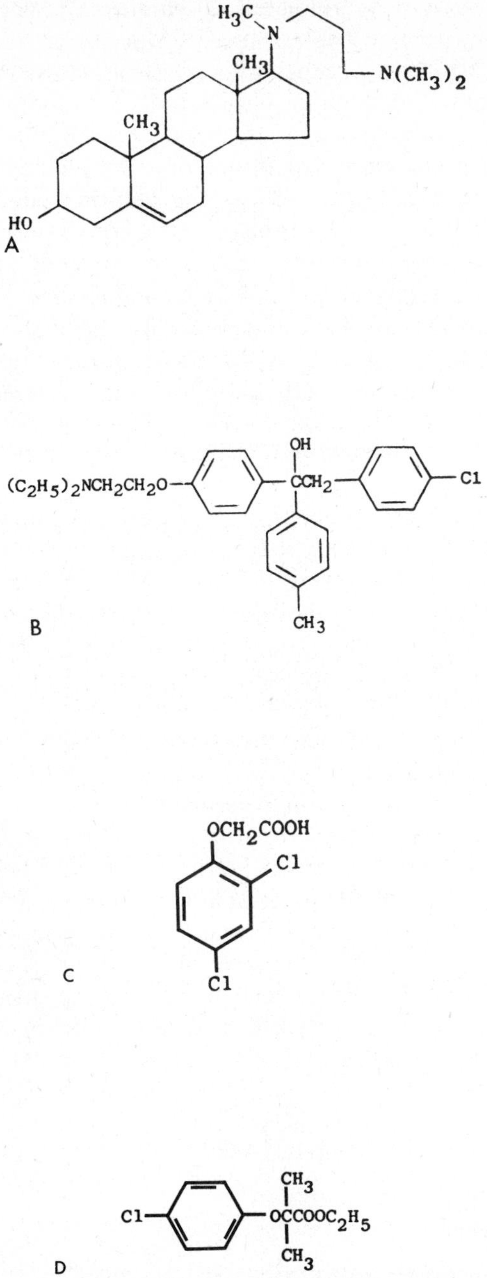

Figure 14–2. The formulae of some major myotonia-inducing drugs.
A, 20,25-diazacholesterol.
B, Triparanol.
C, 2,4-dichlorophenoxyacetic acid (2,4-D).
D, Clofibrate.

but myotonia was noted early in animal studies (Eyzaguirre et al, 1948), and accidental poisoning has produced a variety of neurological problems, notably fibrillary twitches and paralysis (Berwick, 1970) and a syndrome of continuous muscle fibre activity. Brody (1973) studied the mechanism underlying the myotonia and showed that muscle microsomal enzymes were increased in activity. As already discussed, this agent, like diazacholesterol, reduces the chloride conductance of the muscle cell membrane, but 2,4-D has no effect on desmosterol accumulation; the rapidity of its action suggests a direct effect on membrane enzymes to produce the lowered chloride conductance.

Although 2,4-D is not used therapeutically, the hypocholesterolaemic drug clofibrate (Fig. 14–2D) is metabolised to a related substance (chlorophenoxy-isobutyric acid). Despite its use for many years with apparent safety, myotonia has now been found to occur in patients treated with clofibrate, and can also be produced in the rat (Dromgoole et al, 1975).

A third group of drugs that has recently been incriminated in producing myotonia are the β-adrenergic blocking drugs such as propranolol. At present it is not clear whether these actually produce myotonia in a normal individual or whether they merely unmask it in a person with early myotonic dystrophy (Blessing and Walsh, 1977; Satya-Murti et al, 1977). If the latter is the case, this might give the possibility of a provocative test for the carrier state (see Chapter 11); if all individuals are susceptible the wide and increasing use of these drugs makes it likely that more reports will soon be forthcoming.

It is clear from the work on experimental myotonia that not one but several mechanisms exist whereby drugs may induce myotonia, and that the end-point in electrophysiological terms of a reduced chloride conductance in the muscle membrane can result from separate biochemical disturbances. It is equally clear that no model of drug-induced myotonia is an exact counterpart of any of the inherited myotonic disorders of man or other species. This should not lead to their being dismissed as of no relevance, however, since they provide a series of experimental tools by which the factors involved in and necessary for myotonia can be analysed; they form a counterpart to the experiments of nature provided by inherited myotonic disorders, which give a corresponding though less well understood series of models for elucidating the underlying metabolic processes.

THE CONTRACTILE PROTEINS

With such profound disturbance of muscle function and structure seen in the muscular dystrophies, it is natural that the possibility of defects in the molecules actually involved in the contraction process should have been considered. The fact that such proteins are not confined to muscle, and that filamentous and contractile proteins are important constituents of membranes, would make a defect of this type compatible with the current view that myotonic dystrophy and other dystrophies may be due to abnormalities of the muscle cell membranes. The considerable work done on this, mostly in relation to Duchenne dystrophy, has been summarised by Gergely (1977), and it is fair to say that in none of the dystrophies is there significant evidence for a defect of this type.

Samaha and Gergely (1969) studied the composition of actin and myosin in myotonic dystrophy, using material obtained from muscle biopsies in three patients. They found no difference from normal myosin in ATPase activity, nor in the effects of calcium, but did show increased stability of myosin ATPase activity at alkaline pH. No further abnormalities have been reported subsequently.

If any of the myotonic disorders are indeed the result of a defect in contractile proteins, they are more likely to be the non-dystrophic myotonias than myotonic dystrophy. Paramyotonia and the syndrome of myotonia congenita with painful cramps are both characterised by electrically silent contractures in addition to myotonia, and deserve investigation from this angle.

PLATELETS

Platelets are not only a conveniently available source of material rich in membranes, but also contain contractile proteins similar to those occurring in muscle. Any abnormality found in platelets might well be relevant to the primary defect in muscle, although, like the red blood cell, platelets are particularly susceptible to influence by circulating factors.

Bousser et al (1975) found platelets from myotonic dystrophy patients to have an increased sensitivity to epinephrine (adrenaline), increased aggregation in response to epinephrine being seen in all but two of 12 patients. The response to adenosine diphosphate was normal. These authors postulated that this might result from a defect in platelet actomyosin, or might reflect a generalised membrane defect, since phosphorylation of the membrane is considered to be involved in keeping platelets de-aggregated. If this work is confirmed and proves to be as consistent as suggested in the initial report, it could be of diagnostic and predictive value.

HUMORAL FACTORS AND MYOTONIA

The attractive possibility that some abnormal circulating metabolite or other humoral factor could be responsible for the myotonia and perhaps other features of myotonic dystrophy has been considered by a number of workers. However, no such factor has yet materialised, although in myasthenia gravis the identification of such a factor has contributed greatly to our understanding of the aetiology of the disorder. The discovery of drug-induced myotonia showed that a humoral mechanism was indeed possible for myotonia, but subsequent work has failed to show similar changes in myotonic dystrophy. A more direct demonstration of a circulating factor appeared to come from the work of Krull et al (1966), who found a factor in the serum of a patient with a non-dystrophic myotonic disorder (probably adynamia episodica) which would induce myotonia in normal individuals and in experimental animals. Unfortunately this has never been confirmed by other workers, and attempts to show a similar factor in myotonic dystrophy and myotonia congenita have been negative (Peter and Campion, 1977).

A further indication of a humoral factor in myotonic dystrophy comes from the finding of myotonia in a patient with bronchial carcinoma (Humphrey et al, 1976). Most metabolic effects of such tumours result from peptide fragments, but no such peptide was found in this instance, nor could myotonia be induced in animals by the patient's serum.

An indirect piece of evidence arises from the finding of almost exclusive maternal transmission of congenital myotonic dystrophy (Harper and Dyken, 1972). As discussed in Chapter 9, it seems clear that some maternal environmental factor is involved in the production of this form of disease, but what this is is entirely unknown. Although a humoral factor is possible, the combination of a defect in maternal and fetal placental membranes would provide an alternative mechanism. Again, the parallel with congenital myasthenia gravis suggests itself, but the restriction of congenital myotonic dystrophy to those possessing the abnormal gene as well as an affected mother makes it unlikely that a simple immunological basis exists.

For the present, therefore, we have no clear evidence for a humoral factor being directly involved in myotonic dystrophy, but the knowledge that such factors can produce myotonia in other situations is a reminder of the variety of ways by which myotonia may be produced, and of the necessity to consider a wide range of mechanisms in forming hypotheses concerning the basis of myotonic dystrophy.

ANIMAL MODELS

The use of experimental animals, in particular the rat, for the study of drug-induced myotonia has already been discussed, but there also exist several genetically determined abnormalities in animals that may

Table 14–2. ANIMAL MODELS OF MYOTONIC DISEASE

Goat	– Extensively studied electrophysiologically, comparable to myotonia congenita; no dystrophic features
Mouse (Dy and Dy^{2J})	– Dystrophic changes may largely result from denervation; "myotonic" discharges abolished by curare
Dog	– Dystrophy and myotonia reported in Labrador retrievers; non-progressive myotonia reported in chows
Horse	– Non-progressive myotonic disorders reported
Quokka	– Myotonia recorded in association with hereditary myopathy

provide some clues regarding the nature of the abnormality in human myotonic dystrophy (Table 14–2). It must be stressed from the outset that animal models rarely form counterparts of the human situation, a fact all too often ignored by those using them as convenient experimental material. The X-linked genetic disorders are an exception to this, for the X-chromosome has remained remarkably conservative during mammalian evolution; thus, an X-linked animal model would have much greater significance for Duchenne dystrophy than a model for myotonic dystrophy can hope to have.

The Mouse (Dy and Dy^{2J})

The original strain of dystrophic mouse (Dy) discovered at the Jackson Laboratory, Bar Harbor, in 1951 has provided the basis for a large volume of histological and biochemical work, as well as for studies on muscle development and muscle in tissue culture (Meier, 1969).

Most of these studies have used the dystrophic mouse as a model for Duchenne dystrophy, an assumption of doubtful validity in view of the different mode of inheritance (autosomal recessive) as well as other clear differences in muscle pathology. The discovery of another dystrophic allele, Dy^{2J}, at the same locus (Meier and Southard, 1970) shifted the emphasis of the animal model from Duchenne to myotonic dystrophy, since it was found that the Dy^{2J} mouse showed myotonia as a prominent feature in addition to progressive dystrophic changes in muscle (Gilbert et al, 1973). Re-examination of the original Dy strain indicated that electrical myotonia may occur in this too, although masked by the greater severity of the dystrophy and the limited lifespan of this form.

The question now needs to be assessed: how closely do the changes in the Dy^{2J} mouse resemble those in human myotonic dystrophy? Already there is a tendency for the Dy^{2J} strain to be referred to as "the myotonic mouse", and a critical attitude needs to be maintained if the same unjustified assumptions made in relation to Duchenne dystrophy are to be avoided. It has recently been shown that the myotonia of the Dy^{2J} mouse is in fact abolished by curare (Eberstein et al, 1975), a finding which if confirmed would clearly distinguish the abnormality of true myotonia, and would suggest a presynaptic origin of the discharges. This would also correlate with some of the histological and developmental studies, which have also suggested a neurogenic rather than a primary myopathic origin for the changes in the muscle. Thus, Pachter et al (1975) showed not only changes in the muscle fibres (see Chapter 12) but abnormal morphology and increased numbers of axonal terminals, suggesting that the defect was not confined to muscle.

In our present state of knowledge neither the Dy^{2J} nor the original Dy strain of dystrophic mouse seem to be adequate models for myotonic dystrophy.

The Goat

The hereditary non-dystrophic form of myotonia found in the goat has already been described in relation to the electrophysiological studies for which it has been the principal subject. Biochemical investigation has been limited, but no accumulation of desmosterol has been found in the muscle (Peter et al, 1975), showing that in this respect the disorder is closer to the human hereditary myotonic disorders than to diazacholesterol-induced myotonia. Studies on protein phosphorylation in muscle and red blood cell membranes have not yet been reported, possibly because their ready application to human material makes the use of the goat model unnecessary. It will be important however, to know whether the biochemical changes in the goat are indeed the same as in human myotonia congenita, since so much of the fundamental electrophysiological work has been done on the former.

The Horse

Congenital myotonia in the horse is restricted to a single example, fortunately well-documented. Steinberg and Botelho (1962) studied a "thoroughbred" filly in which muscle stiffness was noted from 3 weeks of age. Myotonic potentials were found at 7 months and persisted despite total curarisation. No progressive dystrophic features were noted, and the condition seems to be analogous to congenital myotonia in the goat, and to human myotonia congenita rather than to myotonic dystrophy.

The Dog

Few well-documented reports exist, and there certainly seems to be no common canine counterpart to the myotonic goat — presumably the immobilising effects of such a disorder would not be regarded as desirable by dog-breeders in the way that they were for the goat! Griffiths and Duncan (1973) give electromyographic details of several isolated cases, but no breeding experiments or other investigations were performed. The same authors (1978) have recently found a strain of chow with non-progressive myotonia.

An interesting, although so far only briefly reported, myotonic disorder has been described in a strain of Labrador retrievers (Chatburn and Meyers, 1977). In these animals clinical and electromyographic myotonia was accompanied by progressive muscle wasting and by electrocardiographic abnormalities. The myotonic discharges were uninfluenced by curare, but there were also some changes in peripheral nerve conduction. It is to be hoped that a colony of these dogs will be established so that a thorough study of the disorder and its possible relationship to myotonic dystrophy can be carried out.

In summary, none of the animal models, apart possibly from the retrievers described above, are adequate, let alone satisfactory for myotonic dystrophy, although the myotonic goat seems to be close to human myotonia congenita. The lack of a good model is unfortunate in some ways, but is less so than would have been the case a few years ago; the improvement of ultrastructural and histochemical techniques of studying muscle, the development of tissue culture, and the increasing use of other cell types such as blood cells have all made it increasingly feasible to use human material and to avoid the necessity of studying what will almost certainly prove to be defects with a very different molecular basis.

OTHER METABOLIC CLUES

The work discussed so far has mostly centred on the possible factors underlying the myotonia and the progressive dystrophic changes which are the hallmarks of myotonic dystrophy, and have had the central hypothesis of a molecular defect in the cell membrane of muscle and probably other organs. There are various other pieces of evidence regarding biochemical abnormalities in myotonic dystrophy which cannot at present be fitted into the overall picture that is gradually being built up, and which give no immediate prospect of a satisfactory alternative hypothesis. They are mentioned here because it is possible that their further investigation might throw light on the underlying primary defect, and because they themselves may become better understood when we have a clearer idea of what that primary defect may be.

Endocrine Abnormalities

The various endocrine defects discussed in Chapter 6 cannot at present be explained in terms of a common molecular abnormality. Any hypothesis of abnormal membrane function is entirely speculative at the moment, and the only observation that relates to a possible specific defect is the finding of Hamilton (1974) that enzymes of testosterone synthesis, in particular 17,20-desmolase and 17-reductase, were reduced in the prepubertal testis of patients with an infantile onset of the disease. This is intriguing in view of the production of myotonia by drugs inhibiting sterol synthesis.

The possible explanations for the abnormality in carbohydrate metabolism have already been discussed, and an abnormality of insulin binding either in peripheral tissues or to specific receptor sites on the pancreatic β cell deserves further investigation. The discovery that cultured fibroblasts show specific insulin binding sites should make this approach testable, although insulin receptor sites on monocytes have been shown to be normal (Kobayashi et al, 1977).

Cataract

The paucity of biochemical studies on the lens in myotonic dystrophy has already been noted, and although the development of cataract would be compatible with a defective membrane of the cells of the lens, there is no evidence that this is the case; similarly, there is no clear evidence that the lipid composition of the lens is in any way abnormal, although lipid droplets in the lens have been demonstrated by electron microscopy (Dark and Streeten, 1977). It cannot be entirely irrelevant that the drugs affecting cholesterol synthesis, in particular diazacholesterol and triparanol, cause both myotonia and cataract, whereas quinine and its derivatives not only relieve myotonia but can produce a pigmentary retinopathy closely resembling that occurring in myotonic dystrophy itself.

Immunoglobulin Metabolism

A reduction in the γ globulin fraction of the serum of myotonic dystrophy patients was an early metabolic finding (Lowenthal and van Sande, 1956; Kuhn and Weiker, 1957), and a defect in breakdown rather than synthesis was indicated from the outset by the finding of Zinneman and Rotstein (1956) that labelled γ globulin showed a reduced half-life. A more precise defect was noted by Wochner et al (1966) who found levels of IgG alone to be reduced, and that it was this immunoglobulin fraction that showed an increased rate of catabolism. Although Wochner et al claimed that myotonic dystrophy represented a specific inborn error of immunoglobulin metabolism, the true significance of the increased IgG catabolism has never been resolved. Other authors have confirmed its existence but relevant questions remain unanswered; in particular, no experiments using labelled immunoglobulin fragments have been carried out, nor has the binding of immunoglobulin to cell membranes in myotonic dystrophy been examined. It seems more likely that the abnormality reflects impaired binding rather than an abnormality in the immunoglobulin molecule itself, and further investigation along these lines might help to throw light on the nature of any membrane defect in the disorder.

Attempts have been made to utilise the reduction of IgG in the identification of the presymptomatic gene carrier, as discussed in Chapter 10. Bundey et al (1970) found it too variable to be useful, and indeed some authors have failed to find significant IgG reduction in their patients (Grove et al, 1973). For this reason the attempt of Roberts and Bradley (1977) to use immunoglobulin levels in genetic counselling seems unwise.

Grove et al (1973) have suggested that there may be a more widespread disturbance of humoral immunity in myotonic dystrophy. In particular they found failure to respond to tetanus toxoid in more than half the patients studied. Clinically, however, myotonic dystrophy shows no features resembling an immune deficiency state; there is no particular susceptibility to bacterial or viral infections except in advanced disease, there is no increase in "autoimmune" disorders of any type, and there is no association with malignancy.

Seay et al (1978) have reported defective function of neutrophil leucocytes in a series of ten patients, with reduced chemotaxis. Phagocytosis and killing power of the cells were normal. The authors suggest that the abnormalities result from a primary defect of the white cell membrane, and it will be important to see if these changes are observed consistently in early cases.

Creatine and Amino Acid Metabolism

Increased excretion of creatine is commonly seen in wasting disorders of muscle, and early observations of lack of increased creatine excretion in myotonic dystrophy (Zierler et al, 1949) raised the possibility of a defect in creatine synthesis. More variable rates of creatine and creatinine excretion were found by Caughey and Myrianthopoulos (1963). Harvey (1969) studied creatine synthesis in both myotonic dystrophy and myotonic goats and claimed that a reduction existed in both conditions in the renal enzyme arginine-glycine transamidase, as well as in the urinary excretion of guanidinoacetic acid; however, Bolton and Emery (1972) could find no abnormality in blood or urine levels of guanidinoacetic acid, and a metabolic defect of this type seems improbable.

Blood levels and urinary excretion of a variety of amino acids were studied in 12 patients by Emery and Burt (1972); results were mostly normal, although excretion of threonine and some other amino acids was somewhat increased. There was no indication of a specific metabolic abnormality of amino acid metabolism.

CONCLUSION

In conclusion, the primary biochemical defect in myotonic dystrophy remains unknown and it is not yet possible to provide a unifying explanation for the variety of clinical features that exist, nor for the equal variety of metabolic abnormalities that have been detected. The weight of evidence strongly favours a defect of a specific constituent of the cell membrane, and it is most unlikely that it will be confined to muscle. It is too early to say at present whether the currently debated abnormalities in membrane biochemistry will prove to be related to the primary defect, but it is likely that the final answer will have to await a better understanding of the molecular structure of normal mammalian cell membranes. The identification of the primary defect will be of crucial importance for preclinical diagnosis and prenatal detection, and quite possibly may open the way to more satisfactory approaches to therapy.

REFERENCES

Appel S. H. and Roses A. D. (1977): Membranes and myotonia. *In* Pathogenesis of Human Muscular Dystrophies (Ed.: L. P. Rowland). Excerpta Medica, Amsterdam, pp. 747–758.

Berwick D. (1970): 2,4-Dichlorophenoxyacetic acid poisoning in man. Some interesting clinical and laboratory findings. J.A.M.A. *214*:114–117.

Blessing W. and Walsh J. C. (1977): Myotonia precipitated by propranolol therapy. Lancet *1*:73–74.

Bolton C. E. and Emery A. E. H. (1972): Myotonic dystrophy: investigation of the proposed defect in guanidoacetic acid synthesis. J. Neurol. Neurosurg. Psychiatry *35*:801–803.

Brown M. S. and Goldstein J. L. (1974): Familial hypercholesterolemia: defective binding of lipoproteins to cultured fibroblasts associated with impaired regulation of 3-hydroxy-3-methylglutaryl coenzyme A reductase activity. Proc. Natl. Acad. Sci. USA *71*:788.

Bousser M. G., Conard J., Lecrubier C. and Samama M. (1975): Increased sensitivity of platelets to adrenaline in human myotonic dystrophy. Lancet *2*:307–309.

Brody I. A. (1973): Myotonia induced by monocarboxylic aromatic acids. A possible mechanism. Arch. Neurol. *28*:243–246.

Bundey S., Carter C. O. and Soothill J. F. (1970): Early recognition of heterozygotes for the gene of dystrophia myotonica. J. Neurol. Neurosurg. Psychiatry *33*:279–293.

Butterfield D. A. (1977): Electron spin resonance investigations of membrane proteins in erythrocytes in muscle diseases. Duchenne and myotonic muscular dystrophy and congenital myotonia. Biochim. Biophys. Acta 470:1–7.

Butterfield D. A., Chesnut D. B., Appel S. H. and Roses A. D. (1976): Spin label study of erythrocyte membrane fluidity in myotonic and Duchenne dystrophy and congenital myotonia. Nature 263:159–161.

Butterfield D. A., Oeswein J. Q. and Markesbery W. R. (1977): Electron spin resonance study of membrane protein alteration in erythrocytes in Huntington's disease. Nature 267:453–455.

Butterfield D. A., Roses A. D. and Cooper M. L. (1974): A comparative electron spin resonance study of the erythrocyte membrane in myotonic muscular dystrophy. Biochemistry 13:5078–5082.

Caughey J. E. and Myrianthopoulos N. C. (1963): Dystrophia Myotonica and Related Disorders. Charles C Thomas, Springfield, Ill.

Chatburn C. C. and Meyers K. M. (1977): Electromyographic abnormalities of Labrador retriever dogs with familial myotonic dystrophy. Fed. Proc. 36:556.

Croce C. M., Keiba I., Korrowski H., Molino M. and Rothblat G. M. (1973): Restoration of the conversion of desmosterol to cholesterol in L-cells after hybridization with human fibroblasts. Proc. Natl. Acad. Sci. USA 71:110–113.

Dark A. J. and Streeten B. W. (1977): Ultrastructural study of cataract in myotonia dystrophica. Am. J. Ophthalmol. 84:666–674.

Dromgoole S. H., Campion D. S. and Peter J. B. (1975): Myotonia induced by clofibrate and sodium chlorophenoxy isobutyrate. Biochem. Med. 14:238–240.

Dromgoole S. H., Campion D. S. and Peter J. B. (1975): Myotonia induced by single doses of 20,25-diazacholesterol: increased muscle and desmosterol levels, unaltered (Na + K+) ATPase activity of erythrocyte ghosts. Biochem. Med. 13:307–311.

Eberstein A., Goodgold J. and Pachter B. R. (1975): Effect of curare on electromyographic and contractile response in the myotonic mouse. Exp. Neurol. 49:612–616.

Emery A. E. H. and Burt D. (1972): Amino acid, creatine and creatinine studies in myotonic dystrophy. Clin. Chim. Acta 39:361–365.

Eyzaguirre C., Folk B., Zierler K. L., and Lilienthal J. L., Jr. (1948): Experimental myotonia and repetitive phenomena: the veratrine effects of 2,4-dichlorophenoxyacetate (2,4-D) in the rat. Am. J. Physiol. 155:69–77.

Festoff B. W. (1977): Genetic alterations in surface membranes. In Pathogenesis of Human Muscular Dystrophies (Ed.: L. P. Rowland). Excerpta Medica, Amsterdam, pp. 521–545.

Fiehn W. and Seiler D. (1975): Alteration of erythrocyte–ATPase by replacement of cholesterol by desmosterol in the membrane. Experientia 31:773–775.

Gergely J. (1977): Contractile proteins. In Pathogenesis of Human Muscular Dystrophies (Ed.: L. P. Rowland). Excerpta Medica, Amsterdam.

Gilbert J. J., Steinberg M. C. and Banker B. Q. (1973): Ultrastructural alterations of the motor end plate in myotonic dystrophy of the mouse. J. Neuropathol. Exp. Neurol. 32:345.

Greenquist A. C. and Shohet S. B. (1976): Phosphorylation in erythrocyte membranes from abnormally shaped cells. Blood 48:877–886.

Griffiths I. R. and Duncan I. D. (1973): Myotonia in the dog: a report of four cases. Vet. Rec. 93:184–188.

Griffiths I. R. and Duncan I. D. (1978): Neuromuscular disease in dogs. 4th International Congress of Neuromuscular Diseases, Montreal (abstr.).

Grove D. I., O'Callaghan S. J., Burston T. O. and Forbes I. J. (1973): Immunological function in dystrophia myotonica. Br. Med. J. 3:81–83.

Hamilton W. (1974): Testicular function in myotonic dystrophy of childhood. Clin. Endocrinol. 3:215–222.

Harper P. S. (1972): Genetic studies in myotonic dystrophy. (Thesis.) Oxford University.

Harper P. S. and Dyken P. R. (1972): Early onset dystrophia myotonia — evidence supporting a maternal environmental factor. Lancet 2:53–55.

Harvey J. C. (1969): Reduced renal arginine-glycine transamidinase activity in myotonic goats and in patients with myotonic muscular dystrophy. Johns Hopkins Med. J. 125:270–275.

Hosey M. M. and Tao M. (1976): Altered erythrocyte membrane phosphorylation in sickle cell disease. Nature 263:424–425.

Hull K. L. Jr. and Roses A. D. (1976): Stoichiometry of sodium and potassium transport in erythrocytes from patients with myotonic muscular dystrophy. J. Physiol. 254:169–181.

Humphrey J. G. et al (1976): Myotonia associated with small cell carcinoma of the lung. Arch. Neurol. 33:375–376.

Jacob H. S. (1972): The abnormal red-cell membranes in hereditary spherocytosis: evidence for the causal role of mutant microfilaments. Br. J. Haematol. 23 (Suppl.):35–44.

Kirby J. J., Achor R. W. R., Perry H. O. and Winkelmann R. K. (1962): Cataract formation after triparanol therapy. Arch. Ophthalmol. 68:486–489.

Kobayashi M., Meek J. C. and Streib E. (1977): The insulin receptor in myotonic dystrophy. J. Clin. Endocrinol. Metab. 45:821–825.

Kohlschutter A., Wiesmann U. N. and Herschkowitz N. N. (1976): Phospholipid composition of cultivated skin fibroblasts in Duchenne's muscular dystrophy. Clin. Chim. Acta 70:463–465.

Krull G. H., Leijnse B., DeVlieger M., Vietor W. P. J., Ter Bank J. W. G. and Gerbrandy J. (1966): Myotonia produced by an unknown humoral substance. Lancet 2:668–672.

Kuhn E. and Weiker H. (1957): Serumproteine und Lipide bei myotonischer Dystrophie. Schweiz. Med. Wochenschr. 87:460–462.

Kunze D. (1977): Lipids: composition and metabolism in human dystrophy. In Pathogenesis of Human Muscular Dystrophies (Ed.: L. P. Rowland). Excerpta Medica, Amsterdam, pp. 404–414.

Kunze D., Reichmann G., Egger E., Leuschner G. and Eckhard J. H. (1973): Erythrozytenlipide bei progressiver Muskeldystrophie. Clin. Chim. Acta 43:333–341.

Lo Curto F., Castello A., Magrini U. and Nappi G. (1975): Cytochemistry of cultured fibroblasts in myotonic dystrophy. J. Genet. Hum. (Suppl.) 23:173–178.

Lowenthal A. and van Sande M. (1956): Nouvelles déterminations des fractions protéiniques dans le sérum de patients atteints d'affections musculaires. Rev. Fr. Etud. Clin. Biol. 1:765–771.

Matheson D. W., Engel W. K. and Derrer E. C. (1976): Erythrocyte shape in Duchenne muscular dystrophy. Neurology 26:1182–1183.

Matheson D. W. and Howland J. L. (1974): Erythrocyte deformation in human muscular dystrophy. Science 184:165–166.

Meier H. (1969): Muscular dystrophy, a hereditary disorder in mice. Proc. 2nd Int. Cong. Neuro-genet. Neuro-ophthal., Vol 1, pp. 72–78.

Meier H. and Southard J. L. (1970): Muscular dystrophy in the mouse caused by an allele at the Dy-locus. Life Sci. 9:137–144.

Miale T. D., Frias J. L. and Lawson D. L. (1975): Erythrocytes in human muscular dystrophy. Science 187:453–454.

Miller S. E., Roses A. D. and Appel S. H. (1976): Scanning electron microscopy studies in muscular dystrophy. Arch Neurol. 33:172–174.

Morse P. F. and Howland J. L. (1974): Erythrocytes from animals with genetic muscular dystrophy. Nature 245:156–157.

Pachter B. R., Davidowitz, J. and Breinin G. M. (1975): Muscle fiber and motor end plate involvement in the extraocular muscles of the myotonic mouse. Invest. Ophthalmol. 14:481–427.

Peter J. B., Andiman R. M., Bowman R. L. and Nagatomo T. (1973): Myotonia induced by diazacholesterol: increased ($Na^+ + K^+$) ATPase activity of erythrocyte ghosts and development of cataracts. Exp. Neurol. 41:738–744.

Peter J. B. and Campion D. S. (1977): Animal models of mytonia. In Pathogenesis of Human Muscular Dystrophies (Ed.: L. P. Rowland). Excerpta Medica, Amsterdam, pp. 739–746.

Peter J. B., Dromgoole S. H., Campion D. S., Stempel K. E., Bowman R. L., Andiman R. M. and Nagatomo T. (1975): Experimental myotonia and hypocholesterolemic agents. Exp. Neurol. 49:115–122.

Peter J. B. and Fiehn W. F. (1973): Diazacholesterol myotonia: accumulation of desmosterol and increased adenosine triphosphatase activity of sarcolemma. Science 179: 910–912.

Peter J. B., Stempel K. E., Dromgoole S. H., Campion D. S., Bowman R. L., Nagatomo T. and Andiman R. M. (1975): The effect of a high cholesterol diet on 20,25-diazacholesterol-induced myotonia. Exp. Neurol. 49:429–438.

Pickard N. A., Gruemer H. D., Verrill H. L., Isaacs E. R., Robinow M., Nance W. E., Myers E. C. and Goldsmith B. (1978): Systemic membrane defect in the proximal muscular dystrophies. N. Engl. J. Med. 299:841–846.

Plishker G. A., Gitelman H. J. and Appel S. H. (1978): Myotonic muscular dystrophy: altered calcium transport in erythrocytes. Science 200:323–325.

Reddy N. M., Oliver K. L. and Engel W. K. (1977): Alterations in the sarcolemmal adenylate cyclase activity (AC-0) in myotonia. Neurology 8:378–379.

Roberts D. F. and Bradley W. G. (1977): Immunoglobulin levels in dystrophia myotonica. J. Med. Genet. 14:16–19.

Roses A. D. and Appel S. H. (1973): Protein kinase activity in erythrocyte ghosts of patients with myotonic muscular dystrophy. Proc. Natl. Acad. Sci. USA 70:1855–1859.

Roses A. D. and Appel S. H. (1974): Muscle membrane protein kinase in myotonic muscular dystrophy. Nature 250:245–247.

Roses A. D. and Appel S. H. (1975): Phosphorylation of component "a" of the human erythrocyte membrane in myotonic muscular dystrophy. J. Membr. Biol. 20:51–58.

Roses A. D. Butterfield D. A., Appel S. H. and Chesnut D. B. (1975): Phenytoin and membrane fluidity in myotonic dystrophy. Arch. Neurol. 32:535–538.

Roses M. S., Nicholson M. T., Kircher C. S. and Roses A. D. (1977): Evaluation and detection of Duchenne's and Becker's muscular dystrophy carriers by manual muscle testing. Neurology (Minneap.) 27 (1):20–25.

Rothblat G. H., Burns C. H., Conner R. L. and Landrey J. R. (1970): Desmosterol as the major sterol in L-cell mouse fibroblasts grown in sterol-free culture medium. Science 169:880–882.

Samaha F. J. and Gergely J. B. (1969): Biochemistry of normal and myotonic dystrophic myosin. Arch. Neurol. 21:200–207.

Satya-Murti S., Heiman T. and Martinez L. B. (1977): Possible propranolol–myotonin association. N. Engl. J. Med. 297:233–224.

Seay A. R., Ziter F. A. and Hill H. R. (1978): Defective neutrophil function in myotonic dystrophy. J. Neurol. Sci. 35:25–30.

Seiler D. and Kuhn E. (1970): Kalzium Transport der isolierten Vesikel des Sarkoplasmatischen Retikulums von Patienten mit Myotonia congenita und Myotonia dystrophica. Schweiz Med. Wochenschr. 100:1374–1376.

Steinberg S. and Botelho S. (1962): Myotonia in a horse. Science 137:979–980.

Swift M. R. and Finegold M. J. (1969): Myotonic muscular dystrophy: abnormalities in fibroblast culture. Science 165:294–295.

Thomas N. S. T. and Harper P. S. (1978): Myotonic dystrophy: studies on the lipid composition and metabolism of erythrocytes and skin fibroblasts. Clin. Chim. Acta 83:12–23.

Wakamatsu H., Nakamura H. and Ito K. (1972): Concentration and fatty acid composition of serum lipids in myotonia dystrophica with special reference to pathogenesis. Horm. Metab. Res. 4:458–462.

Wakamatsu H. Nakamura H. and Ito K. (1970): Serum desmosterol and other lipids in myotonic dystrophy. A possible pathogenesis of myotonic dystrophy. Keio J. Med. 19:145–149.

Winer N., Klachko D. M., Baer R. D., Langley P. L. and Burns T. W. (1966): Myotonic response induced by inhibition of cholesterol biosynthesis. Science 153:312–313.

Wochner R. D., Drews G., Strober W. and Waldmann T. A. (1966): Accelerated breakdown of IgG in myotonic dystrophy. J. Clin. Invest. 45:321–329.

Wong P. and Roses A. D. (1977): Altered component "a" phosphorylation in erythrocyte membrane in myotonic muscular dystrophy. In press.

Zierler K. L., Folk B. P., Magladery J. W. and Lilienthal J. L. (1949): On creatinuria in man. The roles of the renal tubule and of muscle mass. Bull. Johns Hopkins Hosp. 85:370–395.

Zinneman H. H. and Rotstein J. (1956): A study of gamma globulins in dystrophia myotonica. J. Lab. Clin. Med. 47:907–916.

CHAPTER FIFTEEN

Problems of Management and Therapy

There is at present no treatment that will significantly alter the natural history of the progressive dystrophic changes seen in myotonic dystrophy, nor can the onset of the disease be modified in any way. This situation is not likely to alter until we have a much fuller understanding of the biochemical basis of the disease than we have now, and it therefore may be felt that a chapter on therapy is irrelevant. This is far from being the case: there are numerous aspects of the disease in which medical intervention has the potential for either improving the patient's condition or, equally important, making it worse. The approach taken in this chapter will be to consider the overall management, taking preventive measures along with active therapy, and dealing with the disorder in a chronological sequence since the problems encountered vary so greatly with the age of the patient.

MANAGEMENT BEFORE BIRTH

It may reasonably be argued that the most effective measure in myotonic dystrophy is to ensure that an individual destined to be affected is not conceived, and the importance of genetic counselling and the various ancillary measures to increase its effectiveness have been discussed in Chapter 11. Once a pregnancy at high risk of ending in an affected infant is under way, the question of whether it should be terminated again arises, and the possibility has been mentioned of using the secretor linkage in some cases to increase the precision of the risk estimate. For a pregnancy that is to continue, the next measures depend on whether the affected parent is male or female. If male, there are unlikely

314

to be any problems relating to the disorder in the perinatal period or in infancy. If the mother is affected, the possibility exists that a child with the congenital form may be born, with the severe hazards described fully in Chapter 9.

Hydramnios and poverty of fetal movement may give further warning of a congenitally affected child, but even if the pregnancy is progressing normally it is wise for delivery to be in a hospital with full supportive measures, for maternal complications may occur even if the infant proves to be normal. The risk of overestimating the stage of gestation because of hydramnios should make the obstetrician cautious about artificial induction of labour; other problems (see Chapter 6) include post partum haemorrhage and abnormal sensitivity to sedative and anaesthetic drugs used in labour.

NEONATAL PROBLEMS

It must be clearly stated at the outset that absence of neonatal complications is no guarantee that the individual will not develop the disease in later life, even if born to an affected mother. The existence of severe neonatal problems from the time of birth, however, may give an urgency to the situation which is still not appreciated by neurologists who see myotonic dystrophy as an "adult" disease and are unaware of the congenital form.

The overriding immediate problem in the most severely affected infants is the respiratory distress and failure that result from a combination of pulmonary immaturity and hypoplasia of the respiratory muscles. In some cases the respiratory distress improves spontaneously, in others artificial ventilation is required, and in some infants there is a fatal outcome before, or in spite of, these measures. Throughout this period of ventilatory inadequacy there is the ever-present danger of hypoxaemia, with the possibility of resulting brain damage. It is arguable how closely the mental retardation so commonly seen in affected children is related to perinatal anoxia; the data discussed in Chapter 9 suggest that it is largely independent, but it is clearly essential that no added cerebral damage from anoxia is imposed on an affected child.

Many infants with congenital myotonic dystrophy are not diagnosed in the neonatal period, or at least not until after the initial respiratory difficulties are over. A serious ethical problem has to be considered, however, in the case of the increasing number of infants diagnosed immediately after birth, as to whether active measures should be undertaken in the first place. Clearly, once resuscitative procedures are under way, they should be performed as well as possible, but in the infant showing grossly inadequate ventilation and likely to die, with no other remediable cause for the problem, it seems reasonable not to embark on artificial ventilation. This is particularly relevant in view of the relatively good prognosis for life once the neonatal period has been passed, together with the high incidence of mental retardation and of eventual severe and progressive physical handicap. It is important that these factors, as well as the question of immediate survival, are taken into account when these initial decisions are being made, and that the parents as well as the medical personnel involved are aware of them in making what can and should be a very difficult decision.

INFANCY AND LATER CHILDHOOD

Once the hazards of the initial weeks are passed, it is essential to recognise that an affected child will not only survive but will tend to improve over a prolonged period, often throughout the first decade of life. Only two in the author's series of 70 congenitally affected patients had died after the age of 1 month (Harper, 1975), and none of the survivors was so disabled as to be confined to a wheelchair. In most the physical disability was much less of a problem than that resulting from mental retardation. Many parents and their doctors were of the opinion that their children would rapidly deteriorate and die, or in the case of those with severe neonatal complications would never be able to walk or function independently in other ways. Many families were pleasantly surprised by this unexpected progress; others were confused and unprepared for it.

It is clear that the static or improving course of the disorder during childhood demands an active approach to any disabilities that may be present. These may be surgically correctible, such as talipes, strabismus, undescended testis or hernia. There were no postoperative deaths in the author's series, which included repair of atrial septal defect among other major surgery. This may seem surprising in view of the high mortality in relation to surgery seen in adults, but it is probably related to the fact that these children were all recognised as having a serious neuromuscular problem, with great care consequently taken by surgeon and anaesthetist alike.

It is particularly important that active orthopaedic measures are taken to help the child with myotonic dystrophy since, unlike such conditions as Duchenne dystrophy or the spinal atrophies, most affected children will have a prolonged period of potentially active life ahead of them. Scoliosis is not a common problem, and satisfactory correction of talipes is probably the single most important measure. Most cases of hip dislocation do not appear to require surgery.

The high incidence of mental retardation in childhood myotonic dystrophy has already been discussed in Chapter 9, and the distribution in the author's series is given in Figure 9–11. From the viewpoint of management it is important that the degree of retardation, if any, should be assessed early to allow optimal school placement, and that it should not be overestimated as a result of facial immobility, dysarthria, or other physical problems, some of which may respond to speech therapy. It is important to note its essentially static nature, too, in contrast to the progressive deterioration sometimes seen in adults.

Mental retardation is not confined to those children with physical complications at birth, and it may be the presenting feature in older children in whom there are few physical abnormalities. Some of these children give an impression of having behavioural and school problems greater than would be expected from their IQ level.

Progressive muscle weakness is rarely encountered in the child with myotonic dystrophy, and myotonia usually is not severe enough to require drug treatment, even in later childhood when it generally can be detected clinically. The presence of severe myotonia in a child should suggest that the diagnosis is incorrect and that he has myotonia congenita or an allied condition. Other physical problems are not common; probably the most severe and frequent is a tendency to constipation, sometimes leading to faecal soiling and to megacolon, which may be extreme (Chapter 4). Regular laxative treatment can help if applied early, but enemas may be needed to prevent recurrence in severe cases. Liquid paraffin should be avoided in view of the dangers of bronchial aspiration. A further symptom present in several of the author's patients is recurrent colicky abdominal pain, of "spastic colon" type. This may occur without constipation, and in one patient was accompanied by normal barium appearance and motility of the colon.

Dental problems may be considerable in children with congenital myotonic dystrophy: dental crowding, a narrow palate and the sagging lower jaw may all need orthodontic measures; one patient studied by the author benefited from surgery to the mandibular muscles.

PROBLEMS OF ADULT LIFE

Drug Treatment of Myotonia

Although often effective in pharmacological terms, drug treatment is disappointing clinically when judged by the degree to which it helps the patient. Successive authors have noted how a high proportion of patients do not persevere with treatment (Thomasen, 1948; Klein, 1958; Caughey and Myrianthopoulos, 1963). The author's experience has been no different in this respect. Even in patients who are obviously hampered by severe myotonia it is surprising how frequently their myotonia is ignored, explained away or frankly denied. One woman, with myotonia of 20 years' duration before she was diagnosed, thought it was something everyone experienced. Even in patients admitting its existence few consider it a symptom worthy of treatment, and most come to terms with it over the years.

In myotonia congenita, myotonia may be extremely disabling, and drug therapy may enable the patient to live a near-normal life. Particular indications for treatment are the characteristic episodes of generalised sudden myotonia that may result in falling; blepharospasm, especially after sneezing, which may be dangerous when driving; and involvement of tongue and jaw muscles, which may impede speech.

The beneficial effects of warmth and of alcohol on myotonia have long been recognised, but the first specific treatment to prove effective was quinine. Wolff (1936) and Kennedy and Wolff (1937, 1938) thoroughly investigated the effects of quinine given at first intravenously, but later orally, and found it effective in both myotonic dystrophy and myotonia congenita. A single dose relieved myotonia for 15 to 20 hours, and there was no significant loss of effect with repeated doses. Numerous workers subsequently have confirmed these effects (Kolb, 1938; Thomasen, 1948), although a variability in response between patients is seen, more in myotonic dystrophy than in myotonia congenita. Thomasen found definite loss of effect after about one week of treatment. A daily dose of 1 to 1.5 g is usually sufficient, given as oral quinine sulphate.

The effect of quinine was shown to be largely peripheral by Kennedy and Wolff (1938) who found it effective after spinal anaesthesia; studies on the myotonic goat (Kolb, 1938; Brown and Harvey, 1939) demonstrated both that it was effective in relieving myotonia and that this effect was independent of curarisation. These workers also showed that the clinical effects were paralleled by a reduction in electromyographic myotonia. The mechanism of its action, still poorly understood, has been discussed in Chapter 13.

No serious cardiac or other effects were found to result from quinine therapy, and although the retinal degeneration seen in some patients was initially attributed to this it was soon shown that most affected patients had not received quinine (Mansoelf et al, 1972). Tinnitus was a frequent side-effect, and quinine became less used when it was found that procainamide was equally effective in most patients, and was free from this and other side-effects. Leyburn and Walton (1959) conducted a trial to compare the two agents and found procainamide the more effective. A dose of 0.5 to 1 g four times a day is generally sufficient.

Both quinine and procainamide are open to the objection that they have depressant effects on myocardial function and ventricular conduction. Since in any case these are problems in some myotonic dystrophy patients, it seems unwise to use such drugs in those with clinical or electrocardiographic evidence of a conduction defect, even though no fatalities seem to have been directly related to these drugs. For this reason the discovery that phenytoin (diphenylhydantoin) has a powerful effect in reducing myotonia has led to its use in preference to other agents, certainly in patients with cardiac involvement, and probably as first choice in others. Griggs et al (1975) investigated the effect of phenytoin, procainamide and quinine on cardiac conduction as recorded by the His bundle electrogram, and showed phenytoin to be free from any effect on conduction, whereas both the others depressed it significantly. All three drugs were equally effective in relieving myotonia at the dose used. Most patients respond to 100 mg three times daily, a dose at which the undesirable effects of hirsutism, gum hyperplasia and ataxia are rarely seen. Caution should be taken in using the drug in women in the reproductive age group in view of the existence of teratogenic effects (Hanson and Smith, 1975), although these are probably rare in relation to the risk of congenital myotonic dystrophy in the offspring. The action of phenytoin appears to be one of increasing fluidity in the cell membrane (Roses et al., 1975).

A variety of other agents have been claimed to benefit myotonia. Leyburn and Walton (1959) found prednisone (10 mg twice daily) as effective as procainamide, and its efficacy was confirmed electromyographically by Caughey and Myrianthopoulos (1963). Although its other effects clearly rule it out for long-term use, it might be considered as a temporary measure in myotonia congenita if severe myotonia were likely to pose problems after anaesthesia or surgery. Drugs affecting the dopamine-GABA pathways have also been shown to improve myotonia, including levodopa (Pendefunda et al, 1974) and baclofen (Karli and Bergström, 1974), but their central effects make them undesirable and they have no clear advantage over more established drugs. Griggs (1977) has found acetazolamide useful in treating myotonia in myotonia congenita, in addition to its more established use in treating the weakness of hypokalaemic and hyperkalaemic periodic paralysis. He found it of little help in myotonic dystrophy, principally because few of the patients were willing to persist with any form of therapy for their myotonia.

In summary, phenytoin is a suitable first choice of drug for treating myotonia in both myotonic dystrophy and myotonia congenita, provided there is no risk of pregnancy during therapy. Procainamide provides a second choice, and quinine can still be tried if the others are unsatisfactory, but it is wise to check for clinical and electrocardiographic evidence of conduction defects before either procainamide or quinine is used. None of these drugs need be employed if the myotonia is not troubling the patient greatly. However gratifying it may be for the physician to see the myotonia disappear, this is irrelevant if it was not bothering the patient in the first place. It may be preferable to reserve drug treatment for short courses in those patients whose myotonia varies in severity. It must also be remembered that, although all the major drugs used for treating myotonia are relatively safe, even a small risk becomes significant when the symptom is relatively benign and the underlying condition a lifelong one.

Dystrophic Changes

The progressive muscle weakness rather than myotonia is the most disabling symptom for most patients, and is the symptom for which least can be done. Weakness of specific muscle groups may give problems long before generalised weakness becomes disabling; thus, sternomastoid weakness may prevent a patient raising his head in bed, and foot drop may contribute to frequent falls. Extraocular muscle weakness may contribute significantly to visual deterioration. It is rare that surgical treatment of such specific disabilities is helpful, although tendo Achillis lengthening may be needed in those few patients (usually with childhood onset) who develop severe contractures. Ocular muscle surgery is likewise helpful, mostly in children with strabismus.

Physiotherapy has two main roles to play. The development of regular breathing exercises may help to combat the tendency to hypoventilation found in many patients, and also reduce the accumulation of secretions that occurs in severely disabled individuals. Postural drainage may help reduce the effects of bronchial aspiration of food and secretions, and is particularly important if bronchiectasis is already established. The role of physiotherapy in maintaining general muscle power and mobility is more limited, and few patients persevere with this approach. Fortunately, the tendency to contractures is less than in many neuromuscular disorders, and indeed few patients are confined to a wheelchair even when in an advanced stage of the disease. The limited mobility that most maintain is sufficient to avert the severe contractures seen in such conditions as Duchenne or other limb-girdle dystrophies, in which selective involvement of proximal muscles confines the patient to a wheelchair relatively early in the course of the disease.

Some patients with particular weakness of lower limb muscle groups may be helped by below-knee calipers and toesprings or by plastic moulded splints to control foot drop.

Cardiorespiratory Problems

Neither angina pectoris nor cardiac failure are major complications in myotonic dystrophy, and both generally respond to standard therapy; a combination of a diuretic with a small dose of digoxin for heart failure, and glyceryl trinitrate with a β-adrenergic blocking drug for angina, have proved suitable in the author's patients. Myotonic dystrophy patients rarely are physically active, even when relatively mildly affected by muscle weakness, a factor which may contribute to lessening these symptoms. Arrhythmias are the main cardiac problem to be encountered, and as discussed in Chapter 5 may be the presenting symptom. Most are episodic and arise spontaneously, although in a few instances anaesthesia or investigative procedures appear to be precipitating factors. It seems wise to avoid drug therapy that may provoke arrhythmias, such as epinephrine (adrenaline) and related bronchodilator agents. There is no evidence to suggest that arrhythmias in myotonic dystrophy, most commonly atrial flutter, respond differently to the various forms of treatment from those with other underlying causes. Quinidine now is less often used, as is DC cardioversion, and β-adrenergic blockers and verapamil have not been noted as giving untoward effects.

In view of the risk of sudden death in myotonic dystrophy, presumably due to ventricular fibrillation, the question arises of long-term antiarrhythmic therapy as a preventive measure. It would be extremely difficult to validate the efficacy of such measures, and if β-blocking agents such as propranolol were chosen the possible aggravation of myotonia (Blessing and Walsh, 1977) would have to be considered.

On the respiratory side the main problem, as already noted, is the tendency to bronchial aspiration as a result of a defective swallowing mechanism and oesophageal reflux associated with low pressure at the cardiac sphincter. Although prompt antibiotic treatment of the consequent chest infections is important, it is still more important to recognise their cause and to reduce the risk of aspiration by such measures as thickening the consistency of liquid foods, avoiding large meals particularly at night, and by sleeping well-propped. Drug treatment of the other main respiratory problem, hypoventilation, has been attempted with use of respiratory stimulants, but with little success as a long-term measure.

Other General Aspects

Endocrine defects do not generally require treatment. Although most patients show a degree of carbohydrate intolerance, overt diabetes is not common (Chapter 6) and insulin is rarely required. The gonadal failure in males is not usually accompanied by loss of libido or potency; fertility is only moderately reduced, and measures to restore this in either sex seem doubtful wisdom from a genetic viewpoint. The risks of pregnancy have been mentioned both in this chapter and in Chapter 6. Thyroid and adrenal insufficiency are exceptional, and there is a greater danger of treatment being given unnecessarily than of these being overlooked. The early balding prominent in many males and in few females does not seem to be related to, or to respond to, any endocrine factors.

Cataract

Most patients have a good result from cataract surgery, and probably the majority will require this by late middle age. Ophthalmic opinion varies as to the optimum stage for surgery, but there seem to be no special characteristics of the myotonic cataract in this respect. Many patients in whom early lens opacities are found on slit-lamp examination at the time of diagnosis are alarmed by the findings, and cannot easily be convinced that such early opacities do not interfere with vision and may not cause trouble for many years. Clear explanation and firm reassurance are needed if symptoms are not to be created.

Surgery for cataract can usually be undertaken even in patients with severe muscle disease or cardiac involvement, provided that the existence of these aspects is recognised and taken into account in planning the procedure and the anaesthetic. Before it is performed a careful search for evidence of retinal dysfunction is wise, and the involvement of extraocular muscles must also be checked before visual symptoms are attributed to cataract alone.

Surgery and Investigative Procedures*

The high risk of abdominal surgery, notably cholecystectomy, has already been noted; Kaufman's survey showed four deaths and five cases of severe postoperative respiratory problems in a total of 25 unselected operations, and numerous case reports bear further witness to the hazards. It is clear from most of these that difficulties have mainly arisen either because the diagnosis of myotonic dystrophy had not been made at the time, or because the hazards of respiratory insufficiency were not recognised. There seems no reason to consider myotonic dystrophy an absolute contraindication to necessary surgery, but every reason for surgery and anaesthesia to be avoided when not necessary, and to be undertaken in the full knowledge of the possible problems that may arise. This caution applies to the mildly affected person even more than to the severe case in which it is obvious that special care must be taken.

---

*See Chapters 4 and 5.

In conclusion, it is important to stress that general management and specific therapeutic measures in myotonic dystrophy have to be seen against the background of a disease the natural history of which is usually a very slow deterioration, and which in many patients is relatively benign. The hospital physician sees only the more severe cases, and family studies show that many patients go through much of their life without troubling or being troubled by the medical profession. In such mildly affected patients an over-zealous approach to therapy is rarely helpful, and the best service the physician can provide is to be alert for the variety of problems that may arise, to consider the possible role of the disease in any apparently unrelated illnesses that the patient may develop, and to alert the patient and all involved in his care to the factors that might aggravate the condition.

For the smaller number of patients severely disabled by progressive muscle weakness and wasting, the therapeutic situation remains sadly unsatisfactory, and hope must be pinned on the rapid advance in our understanding of the biochemical basis of this and other dystrophies to provide a specific therapeutic agent. Until then, preventive genetic measures offer the best hope of controlling this disorder; it is salutary to remember that almost all patients with myotonic dystrophy are born to an affected parent. If genetic counselling and related aspects of prevention were always undertaken with the same vigour as diagnostic investigations, it is possible that myotonic dystrophy could be greatly reduced in incidence. At present this is far from the case, and the variability in onset and severity of the disorder, as well as the frequent reluctance of patients to heed genetic advice, makes it likely that myotonic dystrophy will not decline greatly in frequency in the immediate future. The author hopes that this book, with its emphasis on prevention, will contribute in the longer term to a reduction in the prevalence of this disease and a better outlook for those who suffer from it.

REFERENCES

Blessing W. and Walsh J. C. (1977): Myotonia precipated by propranolol therapy. Lancet *1*:73–74.

Brown G. L. and Harvey A. M. (1939): Congenital myotonia in the goat. Brain 62:341–363.

Caughey J. E. and Myrianthopoulos N. C. (1963): Dystrophia Myotonica and Related Disorders. Charles C Thomas, Springfield, Ill.

Griggs R. C. (1977): The myotonic disorders and the periodic paralyses. *In* Advances in Neurology, Vol. 17 (Eds.: R. C. Griggs and R. T. Maxley). Raven Press, New York, pp. 143–159.

Griggs R. C., Davies R. J., Anderson D. C. and Dove J. T. (1975): Cardiac conduction in myotonic dystrophy. Am. J. Med. *59*:37–42.

Hanson J. W. and Smith D. W. (1975): The fetal hydantoin syndrome. J. Pediatr. *87*:285.

Harper P. S. (1975): Congenital myotonic dystrophy in Britain. 1. Clinical aspects. Arch. Dis. Child. *50*:505–513.

Harper P. S. (1975): Congenital myotonic dystrophy in Britain. 2. Genetic Basis. Arch. Dis. Child. *50*:514–521.

Karli P. and Bergström L. (1974): Effect of baclofen on myotonia. Lancet *1*:1285–1286.

Kennedy F. and Wolff A. (1937): Experiments with quinine and Prostigmin in treatment of myotonia and myasthenia. Arch. Neurol. Psychiatry *37*:68.

Kennedy F. and Wolff A. (1938): Quinine in myotonia and Prostigmin in myasthenia. J.A.M.A. *110*:198.

Klein D. (1958): La dystrophie myotonique (Steinert) et la myotonie congénitale (Thomsen) en Suisse. J. Genet. Hum. (Suppl.) *7*:1–328.

Kolb L. C. (1938): Congenital myotonia in goats. Bull. Johns Hopkins Hosp. *63*:221–237.

Leyburn P. and Walton J. N. (1959): The treatment of myotonia. A controlled clinical trial. Brain *82*:81–91.

Mansoelf F. A., Burns C. A. and Burian H. M. (1972): Morphologic and functional retinal changes in myotonic dystrophy unrelated to quinine therapy. Am. J. Ophthalmol. *74*: 1141–1143.

Pendefunda G., Stefanache F. and Cozma V. (1974): The treatment of myotonia with L-dopa. 1. Clinical and electromyographic study. Rev. Med. Chir. Soc. Med. Nat. Iasi *78*:591–602.

Roses A. D., Butterfield D. A., Appel S. H. and Chesnut D. B. (1975): Phenytoin and membrane fluidity in myotonic dystrophy. Arch. Neurol. *32*:535–538.

Thomasen E. (1948): Myotonia. Universitetsforlaget Aarhus.

Wolff A. (1936): Quinine—an effective form of treatment for myotonia. Arch. Neurol. Psychiatry *36*:382–383.

Index

Page numbers in *italics* refer to illustrations.